W9-BYU-722

CONTEMPORARY CARDIOLOGY™

CHRISTOPHER P. CANNON, MD
SERIES EDITOR

ANNEMARIE M. ARMANI, MD
EXECUTIVE EDITOR

Atrial Fibrillation: From Bench to Bedside, edited by *A. Natale, MD, and J. Jalife, MD, 2008*

Cardiovascular MRI: 150 Multiple-Choice Questions and Answers, by *Peter G. Danias, MD, 2008*

Pulmonary Hypertension, edited by *Nicholas S. Hill, MD, and Harrison W. Farber, MD, 2008*

Nuclear Cardiology: The Basics: How to Set Up and Maintain a Laboratory, Second Edition, by *Frans Wackers, MD, PhD, Barry L. Zaret, MD, PhD, and Wendy Bruni, CNMT, 2008*

Rapid ECG Interpretation, Third Edition, by *M. Gabriel Khan, MD, FRCP, 2008*

Cardiovascular Magnetic Resonance Imaging, edited by *Raymond Y. Kwong, MD, 2008*

Therapeutic Lipidology, edited by *Michael H. Davidson, MD, Kevin C. Maki, PhD, and Peter P. Toth, MD, PhD, 2007*

Essentials of Restenosis: For the Interventional Cardiologist, edited by *Henricus J. Duckers, PhD, MD, Patrick W. Serruys, MD, and Elizabeth G. Nabel, MD, 2007*

Cardiac Drug Therapy, Seventh Edition, by *M. Gabriel Khan, MD, FRCP, 2007*

Essential Echocardiography: A Practical Handbook With DVD, edited by *Scott D. Solomon, MD, 2007*

Cardiac Rehabilitation, edited by *William Kraus, MD, and Steven Keteyian, MD*

Management of Acute Pulmonary Embolism, edited by *Stavros Konstantinides, MD, 2007*

Stem Cells and Myocardial Regeneration, edited by *Marc S. Penn, MD, PhD, 2007*

Handbook of Complex Percutaneous Carotid Intervention, edited by *Jacqueline Saw, MD, Jose Exaire, MD, David S. Lee, MD, Sanjay Yadav, MD, 2007*

Current Concepts in Cardiology: Cardiac Rehabilitation, edited by *William E. Kraus, MD, FACC, FACSM, and Staven J. Keteyian, PhD, 2007*

Preventive Cardiology: Insights Into the Prevention and Treatment of Cardiovascular Disease, Second Edition, edited by *JoAnne Micale Foody, MD, 2006*

The Art and Science of Cardiac Physical Examination: With Heart Sounds and Pulse Wave Forms on CD, by *Narasimhan Ranganathan, MD, Vahe Sivaciyan, MD, and Franklin B. Saksena, MD, 2006*

Cardiovascular Biomarkers: Pathophysiology and Disease Management, edited by *David A. Morrow, MD, 2006*

Cardiovascular Disease in the Elderly, edited by *Gary Gerstenblith, MD, 2005*

Platelet Function: Assessment, Diagnosis, and Treatment, edited by *Martin Quinn, MB BCh BAO, PhD, and Desmond Fitzgerald, MD, FRCPI, FESC, APP, 2005*

Diabetes and Cardiovascular Disease, Second Edition, edited by *Michael T. Johnstone, MD, CM, FRCP(C), and Aristidis Veves, MD, DSc, 2005*

PULMONARY HYPERTENSION

by

NICHOLAS S. HILL, MD
*Division of Pulmonary, Critical Care
and Sleep Medicine
Tufts Medical Center
Boston, MA*

HARRISON W. FARBER, MD
*Pulmonary Center
Boston University, Boston, MA*

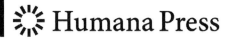 Humana Press

Editors
Nicholas S. Hill
Division of Pulmonary, Critical Care
  and Sleep Medicine
Tufts Medical Center
Boston, MA

Harrison W. Farber
Pulmonary Center
Boston University
Boston, MA

Series Editor
Christopher P. Cannon
Senior Investigator
TIMI Study Group Cardiovascular Division
Brigham and Women's Hospital
Associate Professor of Medicine
Harvard Medical School
Boston, MA

Executive Editor
Annemarie Armani

ISBN: 978-1-58829-661-0   e-ISBN: 978-1-60327-075-5

Library of Congress Control Number: 2007940760

Cover illustration: Image provided courtesy of Wendolyn Hill. Modified with permission.

Printed on acid-free paper

9 8 7 6 5 4 3 2 1

springer.com

To the many patients with pulmonary hypertension whom we have been privileged to care for and who have inspired us to learn as much as possible about the disease, help educate others and work on the ultimate shared goal of finding a cure.

Preface

Enormous gains have been made in the pathophysiologic understanding and therapy of pulmonary hypertension, particularly over the past decade. *Pulmonary Hypertension* aims to provide a current, comprehensive, and clinically relevant perspective on these gains, with contributions from accomplished experts. As background, Alfred P. Fishman, MD, a leader in the field for more than four decades, offers his unique perspective on developments in the field over the past century, including the development of right heart catheterization techniques by individuals with whom he subsequently worked, the first descriptions of "primary" pulmonary hypertension, the formation of the NIH registry, and earlier attempts to classify the disease.

The subsequent text provides an overview of the current state of the art. Descriptions of the present iteration of the classification system (as refined by the World Health Organization [WHO] consensus conference in 2003) and diagnostic approach occupy the next two chapters, followed by insights into pathophysiology, genetics, and the role of the right ventricle. These provide the foundation for Chapters 6–10, which discuss specific conditions associated with pulmonary hypertension, including those from WHO Groups 1, 2, 4, and 5. Chapter 10 is authored by experts from the center (University of California, San Diego) with the greatest experience in surgical management of the disease.

Chapters 11–16 deal with currently available therapies, starting with a general discussion of the therapeutic approach and traditional therapies for pulmonary hypertension. The three classes of drugs currently approved in the United States for therapy of pulmonary hypertension—prostacyclins, endothelin receptor antagonists, and phosphodiesterase-5 inhibitors—are examined in separate chapters. Results of clinical trials that have evaluated these therapies are analyzed and critiqued, and newer potential therapies, such as statins, are discussed. The last chapter in this grouping addresses the issues of transitioning from one therapy to another and combining different therapies. These are promising therapeutic avenues that are currently of great interest to the pulmonary hypertension community and are undergoing intense investigation in a number of recently completed and ongoing clinical trials.

Surgical and interventional approaches to the management of pulmonary hypertension, including lung transplantation and atrial septostomy, are considered in the penultimate chapter. The final chapter casts a forward glance, as Christopher M. Carlin and Andrew J. Peacock attempt to prognostigate on the future directions the field is likely to follow.

The editors hope that interested readers including cardiologists, pulmonologists, rheumatologists, medical trainees, and nurses with an interest in the field will find the scope of the topics and the depth of coverage useful and informative in their everyday clinical practice and that researchers will gain perspective on developments in the field that will be helpful in charting future directions. We are deeply indebted to all of our contributors and express our profound thanks to them for the hard work that went into each of their outstanding contributions.

Nicholas S. Hill
Harrison W. Farber

Contents

Preface   vii

Contributors   xi

List of Color Plates   xv

1 Historical Perspective: *A Century of Primary (Idiopathic)*
    Pulmonary Hypertension   1
    Alfred P. Fishman

2 Classification of Pulmonary Hypertension   15
    C. William Hargett and Victor F. Tapson

3 Diagnostic Approach to Pulmonary Arterial Hypertension   33
    Ronald J. Oudiz

4 Pathophysiology of Pulmonary Arterial Hypertension   51
    Harrison W. Farber

5 Pulmonary Hypertension Genes   73
    Elisabeth Donlevy Willers and Ivan M. Robbins

6 The Right Ventricle in Pulmonary Hypertension   93
    Andrew C. Stone and James R. Klinger

7 Congenital Heart Disease Associated with Pulmonary
    Arterial Hypertension   127
    Michael J. Landzberg

8 Connective Tissue Disease Associated Pulmonary
    Hypertension   145
    **Kimberly A. Fisher, Nicholas S. Hill,
    and Harrison W. Farber**

9 Pulmonary Hypertension Associated with HIV, Liver Disease,
    Sarcoidosis, and Sickle Cell Disease   173
    Kimberly A. Fisher and Elizabeth S. Klings

10 Chronic Thromboembolic Pulmonary Hypertension 199
Victor J. Test, William R. Auger, and Peter F. Fedullo

11 General Therapeutic Approach and Traditional Therapies 231
Nicholas S. Hill and Elizabeth S. Klings

12 Prostacyclin Therapy for Pulmonary Arterial Hypertension . . . 255
Nicholas S. Hill, Todd F. Vardas, and Vallerie McLaughlin

13 Endothelin and Its Blockade in Pulmonary Arterial
Hypertension 283
David Langleben

14 PDE5 Inhibitors and the cGMP Pathway in Pulmonary
Arterial Hypertension 305
Ioana R. Preston

15 Statins for Treatment of Pulmonary Hypertension 321
*John L. Faul, Peter N. Kao, Toshihiko Nishimura,
Arthur Sung, Hong Hu, and Ronald G. Pearl*

16 Transitions and Combination Therapy for Pulmonary Arterial
Hypertension 337
Todd Hirschtritt, M. Kathryn Steiner, and Nicholas S. Hill

17 Acute Right Ventricular Dysfunction: *Focus on Acute Cor
Pulmonale* 363
Antoine Vieillard-Baron and François Jardin

18 Lung Transplantation and Atrial Septostomy for Pulmonary
Arterial Hypertension 383
E. P. Trulock

19 New Directions in Pulmonary Hypertension Therapy 405
Christopher M. Carlin and Andrew J. Peacock

Index 431

Contributors

WILLIAM R. AUGER, MD • *University of California San Diego, La Jolla, CA*

CHRISTOPHER M. CARLIN, BSc (HONS), MB, CHB (HONS), MRCP • *Scottish Pulmonary Vascular Unit, Western Infirmary, Glasgow, Scotland*

HARRISON W. FARBER, MD • *Pulmonary Center, Boston University, Boston, MA*

JOHN L. FAUL, MD • *Stanford University Medical Center, Palo Alto, CA*

PETER F. FEDULLO, MD • *University of California San Diego, La Jolla, CA*

KIMBERLY A. FISHER, MD • *Division of Pulmonary, Allergy, and Critical Care Medicine, University of Massachusetts Medical Center, North Worcester, MA*

ALFRED P. FISHMAN, MD • *University of Pennsylvania School of Medicine, Philadelphia, PA*

C. WILLIAM HARGETT, MD • *Division of Pulmonary, Allergy, and Critical Care Medicine, Duke University Medical Center, Durham, NC*

NICHOLAS S. HILL, MD • *Division of Pulmonary, Critical Care and Sleep Medicine, Tufts Medical Center, Boston, MA*

TODD HIRSCHTRITT, MD • *Division of Pulmonary and Critical Care Medicine, Loyola University Medical Center, Chicago, IL*

HONG HU, MD • *Stanford University Medical Center, Palo Alto, CA*

FRANÇOIS JARDIN, MD • *Service de Réanimation Médicale Hôpital Ambroise Paré, Boulogne Cedex, France*

PETER N. KAO, MD • *Pulmonary and Critical Care, Stanford University School of Medicine, Stanford, CA*

JAMES R. KLINGER, MD • *Division of Pulmonary, Sleep and Critical Care Medicine, Rhode Island Hospital, Providence, RI*

ELIZABETH S. KLINGS, MD • *The Pulmonary Center, Boston University School of Medicine, Boston, MA*

MICHAEL J. LANDZBERG, MD • *Boston Adult Congenital Heart (BACH) and Pulmonary Hypertension Group Children's Hospital, Brigham and Women's Hospital, and Beth Israel Deaconess Medical Center, Boston, MA*

DAVID LANGLEBEN, MD • *McGill University Jewish General Hospital, Montreal, Quebec, Canada*

VALLERIE MCLAUGHLIN, MD • *Division of Cardiology, University of Michigan Medical Center, University of Michigan School of Medicine, Ann Arbor, MI*

TOSHIHIKO NISHIMURA, MD • *Stanford University Medical Center, Palo Alto, CA*

RONALD J. OUDIZ, MD, FACP, FACC • *David Geffen School of Medicine, Liu Center for Pulmonary Hypertension, Harbor-UCLA Medical Center, Torrance, CA*

ANDREW J. PEACOCK, MD, FRCP • *Scottish Pulmonary Vascular Unit, Western Infirmary, Glasgow, Scotland*

RONALD G. PEARL, MD, PHD • *Department of Anesthesia, Stanford University School of Medicine, Stanford, CA*

IOANA R. PRESTON, MD • *Division of Pulmonary, Critical Care and Sleep Medicine, Tufts Medical Center, Boston, MA*

IVAN M. ROBBINS, MD • *Division of Allergy, Pulmonary and Critical Care Medicine, Department of Medicine, Vanderbilt University School of Medicine, Vanderbilt Medical Center, North Nashville, TN*

M. KATHRYN STEINER, MD • *Pulmonary Unit, Massachusetts General Hospital, Boston, MA*

ANDREW C. STONE, MD • *Division of Pulmonary, Sleep and Critical Care Medicine, Rhode Island Hospital, Providence, RI*

ARTHUR SUNG, MD • *Stanford University Medical Center, Palo Alto, CA*

VICTOR F. TAPSON, MD • *Division of Pulmonary, Allergy, and Critical Care Medicine, Duke University Medical Center, Durham, NC*

VICTOR J. TEST, MD, FCCP • *Division of Pulmonary Medicine and Critical Care, University of California, San Diego, CA*

E. P. TRULOCK, MD • *Division of Pulmonary and Critical Care Medicine, Washington University School of Medicine, St Louis, MO*

TODD F. VARDAS, MD • *Division of Cardiology, University of Michigan Medical Center, University of Michigan School of Medicine, Ann Arbor, MI*

ANTOINE VIEILLARD-BARON, MD • *Service de Réanimation Médicale, Hôpital Ambroise Paré, Boulogne Cedex, France*
ELISABETH DONLEVY WILLERS, MD • *Division of Allergy, Pulmonary and Critical Care Medicine, Department of Medicine, Vanderbilt University School of Medicine, Vanderbilt Medical Center, North Nashville, TN*

List of Color Plates

Color plates follow page 144.

Color Plate 1   The process leading to the discovery of mutations in bone morphogenetic protein receptor type-2 (*BMPR2*) as the cause of familial pulmonary arterial hypertension is depicted. (Fig. 2, Chapter 5; *See* complete caption on p. 77.)

Color Plate 2   Consequences of bone morphogenetic protein type-2 receptor (*BMPR2*) mutations on signaling. (Fig. 3, Chapter 5; *See* complete caption on p. 80.)

Color Plate 3   Serotonin receptors and transporter in pulmonary artery smooth muscle cells. (Fig. 4, Chapter 5; *See* complete caption on p. 83.)

Color Plate 4   Adaptive and maladaptive cardiac hypertrophic intracellular signaling pathways. (Fig. 3, Chapter 6; *See* complete caption on p. 101.)

Color Plate 5   Increase in six-minute walk distance (m) in BREATHE-1, the major outcome variable in the pivotal trial testing the clinical efficacy of bosentan in PAH. (Fig. 1, Chapter 13; *See* complete caption on p. 288.)

Color Plate 6   Increase in six-minute walk distance, the major outcome variable in the STRIDE-2 study. (Fig. 2, Chapter 13; *See* complete caption on p. 293.)

Color Plate 7   Kaplan–Meier curves for rate of discontinuation for liver enzyme elevations (larger than fivefold elevation over normal) in the STRIDE-2X study. (Fig. 3, Chapter 13; *See* complete caption on p. 294.)

Color Plate 8   The three main therapeutic pathways currently targeted in the treatment of PAH are schematized. (Fig. 1, Chapter 16; *See* complete caption on p. 346.)

1

Historical Perspective: A Century of Primary (Idiopathic) Pulmonary Hypertension

Alfred P. Fishman

CONTENTS

INTRODUCTION
THE STUDY OF PULMONARY HEMODYNAMICS
CONTROL OF THE PULMONARY CIRCULATION
PULMONARY HEMODYNAMICS IN PRIMARY
   (IDIOPATHIC) PULMONARY HYPERTENSION
THE AMINOREX EPIDEMIC
THE FIRST WORLD HEALTH ORGANIZATION
   MEETING, GENEVA, 1973
THE NATIONAL REGISTRY, 1981
THE SECOND PULMONARY HYPERTENSION
   EPIDEMIC
THE SECOND WORLD HEALTH ORGANIZATION
   MEETING, EVIAN, 1998
FAMILIAL IDIOPATHIC PULMONARY ARTERIAL
   HYPERTENSION
CONCLUSION
REFERENCES

From: *Contemporary Cardiology: Pulmonary Hypertension*
Edited by: N. S. Hill and H. W. Farber © Humana Press, Totowa, NJ

Abstract

   During the past century, great progress has been made in the understanding
of pulmonary hemodynamics and in the control of the normal and hypertensive
pulmonary circulations. In large measure, the door to new knowledge was
opened by the introduction and standardization of right heart catheterization in
normal individuals and subsequently in patients with pulmonary hypertension.
A byproduct of this remarkable progress has been the development of a classification schema for pulmonary hypertensive diseases based more on pathophysiology. Unfortunate experiments of nature giving rise to pulmonary hypertension
epidemics related to appetite suppressant ingestion have nonetheless provided
insights into its pathogenesis. The progress over the past century has laid the
foundation for the gains in management that we have witnessed in recent
years. In the near future, newer and less invasive technologies for detection
and assessment, such as echocardiagraphic and magnetic resonance imaging,
and novel, more effective medications are raising hopes for steadily improving
outcomes.

   Key Words: pulmonary hypertension; appetite suppressants; Aminorex;
NIH Registry; pulmonary hemodynamics.

1. INTRODUCTION

   For more than a century before pulmonary arterial pressures could
be measured directly in humans, pulmonary arteriosclerosis was widely
accepted as morphological evidence of chronic pulmonary arterial
hypertension *(1,2)*. In 1891, Ernst von Romberg, a German physician
and pathologist, puzzled by his inability to discover at autopsy the
etiological basis for pulmonary vascular lesions now recognized to
be the hallmark of primary hypertension, categorized the disease
simply as "pulmonary vascular sclerosis." Features of the disease
began to be elucidated in 1901 by Dr. Abel Ayerza, professor
of medicine at the University of Buenos Aires, Argentina. Ayerza
did not publish his findings but described the clinical features of
the disease in his lectures. He recognized that the clinical constellation of chronic cyanosis, dyspnea, and polycythemia was associated
with sclerosis of the pulmonary arteries at autopsy. Arrillaga, one
of his students, subsequently designated the syndrome as "Ayerza's
disease."

   The first reports of the disease described as "primary pulmonary
hypertension" were clinical-pathological correlations accompanied by
speculations about etiology *(1–7)*. These began in 1913 with Arrillaga,
who attributed the disease to syphilitic pulmonary endarteritis and
spurred a controversy about the etiological role of the spirochete that
lasted for two decades. Oscar Brenner, a physician from Birmingham,

England, finally laid to rest the belief that the disease had a syphilitic etiology in 1935, while serving as a Rockefeller Traveling Fellow at Massachusetts General Hospital (MGH) *(8)*. After reviewing 100 case reports of pulmonary hypertension in the MGH autopsy files, 25 of which were considered to have "Ayerza's disease," Brenner concluded that the disease was neither a clinical nor a pathological entity and that syphilis was not the cause. In a major contribution to the growth of understanding of the disease, he pinpointed the small muscular arteries and arterioles as the source of the pulmonary hypertension and described their histopathological features. However, Brenner was a histopathologist and not a physiologist, so he failed to recognize the functional role vasoconstriction plays in the pathogenesis of pulmonary hypertension. Nor did he appreciate the causal relationship between the pulmonary vascular lesions and the enlargement of the right side of the heart, considering these as separate consequences of a shared insult. The recognition of the connection between the two awaited the insights of pulmonary physiologists later during the 20th century.

2. THE STUDY OF PULMONARY HEMODYNAMICS

At the start of the 20th century, studies of pulmonary hemodynamics were largely confined to measurements of pulmonary arterial pressures in anesthetized, open-chest animals undergoing artificial respiration *(9,10)*. By then, pressure recording was fairly well standardized, and pressures recorded in animals by different manometric systems were similar in form and generally accurate. In large measure, credit for standardizing pressure recording goes to Otto Frank (1865–1944), a distinguished German physiologist and physician, whose name is well known to circulatory physiologists as one of the discoverers of the Frank–Starling law of the heart *(11)*. These standards played a key role in shaping the design and application of cardiac catheters for recording pulmonary arterial pressures in humans. However, the concept of measuring pulmonary artery outflow pressure, needed for the calculation of pulmonary vascular resistance and estimation of pulmonary venous pressure, did not become available until mid-century *(12–14)*.

Ernest Henry Starling (1866–1927) sorted out the individual mechanisms involved in the regulation of the pulmonary circulation. For this purpose, Starling developed heart-lung preparations that enabled him to focus on individual physiological factors and to analyze them in mechanical and physiological terms. From such preparations were derived the Frank–Starling law of the heart and the forces that govern the trans-capillary exchange of water. However, Starling's observations, made under such artificially controlled conditions, paid the price of obscuring automatic adjustments that occur under more physiological conditions.

The modern era of the understanding of pulmonary hemodynamics began in 1912 with August Krogh and Johannes Lindhard, who used nitrous oxide to measure blood flow and popularized the use of gas uptake methods in humans *(15,16)*. However, these indirect methods for measuring pulmonary blood flow were handicapped by two major problems: (1) early recirculation that artificially decreased the value for cardiac output by diminishing the uptake of gas from the alveoli, and (2) reliance on alveolar gas samples to provide a measure of the content of the respiratory gases in mixed venous blood.

In 1870 Adolph Fick suggested a direct approach for measuring cardiac output. In a short commentary to his local medical society in Würzburg, Germany *(19)*, Fick pointed out that the cardiac output could be measured by dividing the oxygen uptake, measured at the mouth, by the corresponding arteriovenous difference in oxygen content. Carbon dioxide, as well as oxygen, could serve as the test gas. However, his concept was not immediately applied; not until two decades later did physiologists begin to apply the Fick principle in animals *(10)*.

Application of the Fick principle in humans was handicapped from the start by the difficulty in obtaining samples of mixed venous blood. Sporadic attempts were made to obtain mixed venous blood by invasive procedures such as the transthoracic needling of the right ventricle or the passage of a tube into the right atrium via a large neck vein. However, these procedures were too formidable for popular use.

While a surgeon-in-training in Sauerbruch's prestigious surgical department in Berlin in 1929, Werner Forssmann demonstrated a novel and safe way to obtain mixed venous blood *(21)*. Forssmann was interested in injecting medications directly into the heart for cardiac resuscitation without resorting to transthoracic puncture or the passage of a tube into the right ventricle via a neck vein. By repeated experiments on himself, he showed that the right side of the heart could be safely catheterized, occasionally walking about and even climbing stairs with a catheter in place to demonstrate the safety of the procedure. His experiment became well known in his institution. However, instead of plaudits and a promotion, Forssmann was subjected to criticism and ridicule.

Forssmann's demonstration of the safety of cardiac catheterization attracted more attention in Europe and in South America than in Germany. In the United States, the Cardiopulmonary Laboratory at

Bellevue Hospital in New York City *(22,23)*, headed by André Cournand, took the lead. Cournand was the director of the Laboratory, which was jointly sponsored by the Chest Service, headed by J. Burns Amberson, and the Medical Division of Columbia University, headed by Dickinson Richards, Jr. I rotated through the laboratory in 1951 as part of my program as an Established Investigator of the American Heart Association. A few years later, after completing the prescribed series of rotations at other universities and hospitals, I was invited back to the Cardiopulmonary Laboratory as a member of both the research team and the faculty of the College of Physicians and Surgeons of Columbia University *(22)*.

Spurred in large measure by reports from the Bellevue laboratory, the use of cardiac catheterization for diagnostic purposes spread quickly throughout medical centers in the United States and abroad. Ureteral catheters were modified for cardiac catheterization, recording equipment was greatly improved, and the diagnostic procedures were standardized. In 1956, Cournand and Richards shared the Nobel Prize with Forssmann for their respective roles in introducing and standardizing cardiac catheterization.

Gradually, modifications in equipment and technique made it possible to move cardiac catheterization from the fluoroscopy room to the bedside using hemodynamic monitoring instead of visualization by X-ray to localize the tip of the catheter. In 1953, Michael Lategola and Hermann Rahn showed in dogs how to obtain a measure of outflow pressures for the determination of pulmonary vascular resistance *(12)*. They used a flow-directed catheter with an inflatable balloon at its tip to measure pulmonary arterial pressure. In 1950, Hellems, Haynes, and Dexter modified the technique to measure pulmonary "capillary" pressure in humans *(13)*. The final step in moving the technique from the fluoroscopy suite to the bedside was taken by William Ganz and Harold J. C. Swan in 1970. They developed a multi-lumen, balloon-tipped catheter that could be advanced and the tip positioned under hemodynamic monitoring, thereby enabling simultaneous recording of pressures in the pulmonary artery and left atrium *(14)*.

3. CONTROL OF THE PULMONARY CIRCULATION

Control of the pulmonary circulation was first studied in open-chest, anesthetized animals *(15)*. Although these studies showed that stimulation of nerves to the lungs could affect pulmonary hemodynamics, by the 1940s there was a consensus that the pulmonary nerves played little, if any, role in regulating the normal pulmonary circulation. In 1946, attention shifted from nerves to local self-regulatory mechanisms, prompted by the demonstration by von Euler and Liljestrand, in anesthetized cats, that acute hypoxia elicits pulmonary vasoconstriction *(16,18)*. Shortly thereafter in the Cournand–Richards Laboratory, Motley et al. *(20)* repeated the experiments with acute hypoxia in normal, awake humans. They exposed five human subjects to 10% O_2 in N_2 for 10 minutes and observed an increase in pulmonary arterial pressure and pulmonary vascular resistance, indicating that acute hypoxia elicited pulmonary vasoconstriction *(20)*. These observations on hypoxic pulmonary vasoconstriction suggested the possibility that the lungs contained a self-regulatory mechanism that would automatically direct mixed venous blood to well-aerated alveoli, thereby optimizing gas exchange.

Included in the results of Motley's experiments was the puzzling observation that the increase in pulmonary arterial pressure induced by acute hypoxia was accompanied by a decrease in cardiac output. Subsequent investigation showed that this unanticipated outcome was an artifact due to the failure to allow sufficient time during hypoxia for a new steady state of the respiration and circulation to be established *(22)*. Clarification of this issue played a key role in establishing guidelines for the valid application of the Fick principle.

While Cournand and Richards were exploring the pulmonary circulation in adult humans, Geoffrey Dawes was doing the same for the pulmonary circulation of the fetal lamb *(23,24)*. Dawes had been trained in physiology and pharmacology at several of the foremost laboratories in the United States but spent the remainder of his research career as director of the Nuffield Institute for Medical Research in Oxford, England. Using the pregnant ewe as the experimental model, he pursued this line of research in the footsteps of Sir Joseph Barcroft of Cambridge, England, whose research had been interrupted by the outbreak of the First World War. Although his research was done in animals, it was directly applicable to humans *(24)*.

4. PULMONARY HEMODYNAMICS IN PRIMARY (IDIOPATHIC) PULMONARY HYPERTENSION

Clinical studies on control of the pulmonary circulation followed soon after the experimental studies on animals *(16,17)*. In 1951, Dresdale, Michtom, and Schultz demonstrated that acute administration of tolazoline (priscoline), a pulmonary vasodilator, alleviated pulmonary hypertension in adult humans *(26)*. However, since tolazoline is not only a pulmonary vasodilator but also a systemic vasodilator, the possibility remained that the effect on the pulmonary circulation was secondary to systemic vasodilation. To eliminate this uncertainty, Harris et al. resorted to the intravenous injection of acetylcholine, which is destroyed during a single passage through the lungs *(27)*. The acetylcholine elicited pulmonary vasodilation in normal subjects with pulmonary hypertension induced by inhalation of a hypoxic gas mixture (10% O_2 in N_2) *(27,28)*. Soon thereafter, Wood et al. obtained similar responses in patients with pulmonary hypertension secondary to mitral stenosis, demonstrating that pulmonary vasoconstriction contributes to their pulmonary hypertension *(25,29)*.

5. THE AMINOREX EPIDEMIC

Against this physiological backdrop, an epidemic of aminorex-induced pulmonary hypertension broke out in the late 1960's *(30)*. A catechol derivative, Aminorex fumarate (2-amino-5-phenyl-2-oxazoline) was sold over-the-counter as an appetite suppressant to promote weight loss. Its actions include release of norepinephrine at nerve endings and an increase in levels of serotonin in the circulation. The drug was introduced to the Swiss, German, and Austrian markets in November 1965 and withdrawn in October 1968 because it was held responsible for the epidemic. Patients with aminorex-induced pulmonary hypertension who came to autopsy had pulmonary vascular lesions that were identical with those of primary pulmonary hypertension. The aminorex outbreak raised two major questions about the pathogenesis of primary pulmonary hypertension: First, stemming from the fact that relatively few who took the drug developed pulmonary hypertension, was there a genetic predisposition that played a role in the pathogenesis of the disease; and second, what are the initiating and pathogenetic mechanisms of the disease? Both questions continue to be the foci of intense inquiry.

6. THE FIRST WORLD HEALTH ORGANIZATION MEETING, GENEVA, 1973

Prompted by the outbreak of aminorex-induced pulmonary hypertension, the World Health Organization convened a group of experts in 1973 to take stock of the state of knowledge about primary (idiopathic) pulmonary hypertension (PPH) and to standardize clinical and pathological nomenclature *(31)*. In addition, the 1973 meeting called for an international registry that would accumulate standardized data about the rare disease.

7. THE NATIONAL REGISTRY, 1981

The international registry did not materialize but, in 1981, the National Heart, Lung and Blood Institute of the National Institutes of Health in the United States created a National Registry of Patients with primary pulmonary hypertension *(32)*. The Registry consisted of three components: a statistical-epidemiological core, a pathology core, and 32 clinical centers. By the time of Registry closure in 1987, clinical, physiological, and therapeutic data had been collected according to a preset protocol on more than 200 patients with primary pulmonary hypertension. Moreover, the participants, gratified by the success of this collaborative effort, subsequently embarked upon other clinical trials and collaborative efforts.

The National Registry, sponsored by the National Institutes of Health, had several favorable outcomes, including (1) sharpening of clinical and pathological diagnostic criteria *(33,34)*, (2) provision of a standardized format for data collection, (3) encouraging the exploration and systematic evaluation of pulmonary vasodilators, (4) promotion of subsequent cooperative studies among the investigators at various centers, and (5) increased public awareness of the disease *(30)*.

8. THE SECOND PULMONARY HYPERTENSION EPIDEMIC

In a tragic demonstration of the maxim that those who fail to learn from history are doomed to repeat it, a second epidemic of pulmonary hypertension occurred during the late 1990s in Europe and the United States. Against the staunch opposition of several prominent members of the pulmonary hypertension community, in April 1996 the Food and Drug Administration approved dexfenfloramine and phentermine/fenfloramine (phen/fen) for the treatment of obesity. Sales of the drugs soared, as did reports of pulmonary hypertension and valvular heart disease associated with drug ingestion. The epidemiological association of these drugs and PAH was established by the International Primary Pulmonary Hypertension Study Group, which reported a 23-fold increase in the incidence of PAH among patients ingesting the drugs for more than 3 months compared to age- and gender-matched controls *(35)*. Well-publicized lethal cases of pulmonary hypertension arising after drug ingestion occurred subsequently in the United States, but concerns about an increase in the incidence of cardiac valvular disease as detected echocardiographically eventually led the FDA to remove the drugs from the market in

September 1997. Cases of PAH continued to appear for several years after the removal of the drugs from the market. Although litigation on some of the cases has continued through the present, clinical cases are now rarely seen. The etiology of this form of pulmonary hypertension has never been defined, partly because no adequate animal model could be developed, but it is thought to involve effects on serotonin uptake as well as a genetic predisposition.

9. THE SECOND WORLD HEALTH ORGANIZATION MEETING, EVIAN, 1998

Held on the 25th anniversary of the original meeting in Geneva, the second WHO meeting was more ambitious than the first, undertaking to revise the classification of all pulmonary hypertensive diseases. This classification has since been modified by the Third WHO Pulmonary Hypertension Symposium, held in Venice in 2003 (see Chapter 2 for details). This meeting was prompted by the remarkable surge in the understanding of the mechanisms involved in the pathogenesis of pulmonary hypertension that occurred during the few years after the 1998 meeting. These advances cover a wide span, ranging from molecular biology, developmental biology, and genetics on the one hand to clinical trials, natural history, and epidemiology on the other.

At this meeting, 14 experts from the United States and abroad were asked to critically review the Evian diagnostic classification with respect to its value for clinical, research, and epidemiological purposes. Virtually all agreed that the classification was primarily useful for clinical and epidemiological purposes and less so for research. This lukewarm endorsement was not unexpected, since research has become increasingly devoted to the molecular and developmental aspects of the disease, whereas the classification was focused on diagnosis and treatment. Although no major changes in the classification arose from the Venice meeting (except for the replacement of the term "primary pulmonary hypertension" with "idiopathic pulmonary arterial hypertension"), future revisions of the nosology are likely to incorporate insights from advances in the research on genetic and molecular mechanisms.

10. FAMILIAL IDIOPATHIC PULMONARY ARTERIAL HYPERTENSION

In recent years, it has become increasingly clear that genetic factors influence both the susceptibility and the heritability of idiopathic pulmonary arterial hypertension. The relatively small number of individuals who actually developed pulmonary hypertension in the face of the large number who took aminorex as an appetite suppressant underlines the role of susceptibility in the development of PAH. The heritability of pulmonary hypertension has been established beyond doubt by the occasional occurrence of familial idopathic pulmonary arterial hypertension (roughly 7% of all patients with IPAH). The pattern of inheritance seems to be autosomal dominant with incomplete penetrance. Consequently, the disease becomes manifest in only up to 20% of individuals at risk *(30)*.

Familial IPAH has provided a unique opportunity to explore the molecular bases of the disease *(36)*. Mutations have been found in two TGF-ß receptor genes [Bone morphogenetic protein receptor gene (*BMPR2*) and Activin-receptor-like-kinase 1 (*ALK1*)]. A mutation in *BMPR2* may lead to a loss of the inhibitory action of *BMPR2* on the growth of smooth muscle cells in the pulmonary vessels *(37,38)*. Mutations in *BMPR2* have been identified in more than 50% of families with multiple members affected by PPH. In some instances, these germ-line mutations are inherited. But in others, the mutation seems to arise *de novo*.

However, more than one-third of families with IPAH do not have identified mutations in *BMPR2* or *ALK1*. The genetic bases for familial IPAH in these instances have yet to be discovered. Incomplete penetrance of PPH and the finding that only about 25% of patients with PPH have a mutation in *BMPR2* suggest that nonheritable factors influence expression of the genes or that there are other, as yet undisclosed, genetic determinants.

In a number of families, primary pulmonary hypertension is associated with hereditary hemorrhagic telangiectasia (Osler-Weber-Rendu syndrome) in which vascular dilations, presumably endothelial in nature, are a predominant feature *(39)*. In this combined disorder, mutations have been found in the gene for *ALK1*, a gene abundant in endothelial cells.

11. CONCLUSION

The past century has seen great progress in the understanding of pulmonary hemodynamics and in the control of the normal and hypertensive pulmonary circulations. The introduction and standardization of right heart catheterization around mid-century was a key step in opening the door to new knowledge about human pulmonary circulatory physiology and pathophysiology. A by-product of this remarkable progress has been the development of a classification schema for pulmonary hypertensive diseases based more on pathophysiology. However, the end is not yet in sight. Newer and less invasive technologies such as cardiac imaging, and novel medications, such as endothelin-receptor blocking agents and many even newer agents, hold great promise for fresh insights into the cellular and molecular mechanisms involved in the control of the pulmonary circulation.

REFERENCES

1. Romberg E. Ueber Sklerose der Lungen arterie. Dsch Archiv Klin Med 1891; 48:197–206.
2. Larrabee WF., Parker RL., Edwards JE. Pathology of intrapulmonary arteries and arterioles in mitral stenosis. Proc Mayo Clin 1949; 24: 316–326.
3. Mönckeberg JG. Ueber die genuine Arteriosklerose der Lungenarterie. D Med Wchnschr 1907; 33:1243–1246.
4. Arrillaga FC. Sclérose de l' artére pulmonaire (cardiagues noirs). Bull Mem Soc Méd Hop Paris 1924; 48:292–303.
5. Brachetto-Brian D. Concepto anatomo-pathologico de los cardiacos engross de Ayerza. Rev Soc Med Int Soc Tisiol 1925; 1:821–931.
6. Posselt, A. Zur Pathologie und Klinik der primären Atherosklerosis pulmonalis. Wien Arch £ Inn Med 1925; 11–357.
7. Brill IC., Krygier CK. Primary pulmonary vascular sclerosis. Arch Intern Med 1941; 68:560–577.
8. Brenner O. Pathology of the vessels of the pulmonary circulation. Arch Intern Med 1935; 56:211–237, 457–497, 724–752, 976–1014, 1190–1241.
9. Wiggers CJ. The Pressure Pulses in the Cardiovascular System. New York. Longmans. 1928.
10. Zuntz N., Hagemann O. Untersuchungen über den Stoffwechsel des Pferdes bei Ruhe und Arbeit. *Landw. jahrb.* XXVII Band, Ergänzungsband III, Paul Parey publisher, Berlin, 1898, pp. 1–438.
11. Frank O. Der Puls in den Arterien. Ztsch Biol 1905; 46:441–543.
12. Lategola M., Rahn H. A self-guiding catheter for cardiac and pulmonary arterial catheterization and occlusion. Proc Soc Exp Biol Med 1953; 84:667–668.
13. Hellems HK., Haynes FW., Dexter L. Pulmonary "Capillary" Pressure in Man. J Appl Physiol 1949–1950; 2:24–29.
14. Swan HJ., Ganz W., Forrester J., Marcus H., Diamond G., Chonette D. Catheterization of the heart in man with use of a flow-directed balloon-tipped catheter. N Engl J Med 1970; 283(9):447–451.
15. Krogh A., Lindhard J. Measurement of the blood flow through the lungs of man. Skand Arch Physiol 1912; 27:100–125.
16. Euler USV., Liljestrand G. Observations on the pulmonary arterial blood pressure in the cat. Acta Physiol Scand 1946; 12:301–320.

17. Cerretelli P., Cruz JC., Fahri LE., Rahn H. Determination of mixed venous O_2 and CO_2 tensions and cardiac output by a rebreathing method. Respir Physiol 1966; 1:258–264.
18. Liljestrand G. Regulation of pulmonary arterial blood pressure. Acta Physiol Scand 1947; 14:162–172.
19. Fick A. Uber die Messung des Blutquantums in den Herzventrikeln. Sitx der Physik-Med ges Wurzburg 1870; 16.
20. Motley HL., Cournand A., Werko L., Himmelstein A., Dresdale D. The influence of short periods of induced acute anoxia upon pulmonary arterial pressures in man. Am J Physiol 1947–1948; 150:315–320.
21. Forssmann W. Die Sondierung des rechten Herzens, Klin Wochnschr 1929; 8:2085–2087.
22. Fishman AP. Respiratory gases in the regulation of the pulmonary circulation. Physiol Rev 1961; 41:214–279.
23. Cournand A. Control of the Pulmonary Circulation in Normal Man. Proc. of the Harvey Tercentenery Congress. Oxford. Blackwell Scientific Publications. 1958; 219–237.
24. Dawes GS. Foetal and Neonatal Physiology: A Comparative Study of the Changes at Birth. Chicago, Yearbook Medical Publishers, 1968.
25. Wood P. Diseases of the Heart and Circulation. Philadelphia, J. B. Lippincott, 1952.
26. Dresdale DT., Michtom RF., Schultz M. Recent studies in primary pulmonary hypertension including pharmacodynamic observations on pulmonary vascular resistance. Bull NY Acad Med 1954; 30:195–207.
27. Harris P. Influence of acetylcholine on the pulmonary arterial pressure. Br Heart J 1957; 19(2):272–278.
28. Fritts HW., Harris P. Jr., Clauss RH., Odell JE., Cournand A. The effect of acetylcholine on the human pulmonary circulation under normal and hypoxic conditions. J Clin Invest 1958; 37:99–108.
29. Wood P., Besterman EM. Towers MK., McIlroy, MB. The effect of acetyleholine on pulmonary vascular resistance and left atrial pressure in mitral stenosis. Br Heart J 1957; 19(2):279–286.
30. Gurtner HP. Aminorex pulmonary hypertension. In: Fishman AP., ed. The Pulmonary Circulation: Normal and Abnormal. Mechanisms, Management and the National Registry. Philadelphia. University of Pennsylvania Press. 1990; 397–411.
31. Hatano S., Strasser R. eds. Primary pulmonary hypertension. World Heath Organization, Geneva, 1975.
32. Fishman, AP. Introduction to the national registry on primary pulmonary hypertension. In: Fishman, AP., ed. The Pulmonary Circulation: Normal and Abnormal. Philadelphia. University of Pennsylvania Press. 1990; 437–439.
33. Pietra, GG. The histopathology of primary pulmonary hypertension. In: Fishman, AP., ed. The Pulmonary Circulation: Normal and Abnormal. Philadelphia. University of Pennslvania Press. 1990; 459–472.

34. Wagenvoort, CA. Pathology of Pulmonary Hypertension. New York. John Wiley and Sons. 1977; 217–231.
35. Abenhaim L., Moride Y., Brenot F et al. Appetite-Suppressant drugs and the risk of primary pulmonary hypertension. N Engl J Med 1996; 335:609–616.
36. Loyd JE., Newman J. Familial primary pulmonary hypertension: clinical patterns. Am Rev Resp Dis 1984; 129:194–197.
37. Newman JH., Lane KB. Hypertensive pulmonary vascular disease: dawn of the age of prevention? Am J Respir Crit Care Med 2000; 162(6): 2020–2021.
38. Newman JH., Trembath RC., Morse JA., Grunig E., Loyd JE., Adnot S., Coccolo F., Ventura C., Phillips JA 3rd, Knowles JA., Janssen B., Eickelberg O., Eddahibi S., Herve P., Nichols WC., Elliott G. Genetic basis of pulmonary arterial hypertension: current understanding and future directions. J Am Coll Cardiol 2004; 43(12 Suppl S):33S–39S.
39. Trembath RC., Thomson JR., Machado RD., Morgan NV., Atkinson C., Winship I., Simonneau G., Galie N., Loyd JE., Humbert M., Nichols WC., Morrell NW., Berg J., Manes A., McGaughran J., Pauciulo M., Wheeler L. Clinical and molecular genetic features of pulmonary hypertension in patients with hereditary hemorrhagic telangiectasia. N Engl J Med 2001; 345(5):325–334.

2 Classification of Pulmonary Hypertension

C. William Hargett
and Victor F. Tapson

CONTENTS

INTRODUCTION
PULMONARY ARTERIAL HYPERTENSION
PULMONARY VENOUS HYPERTENSION
PULMONARY HYPERTENSION ASSOCIATED
    WITH HYPOXIA
PULMONARY HYPERTENSION DUE TO CHRONIC
    THROMBOTIC AND/OR EMBOLIC DISEASE
PULMONARY HYPERTENSION
    DUE TO MISCELLANEOUS CAUSES
FUNCTIONAL CLASSIFICATION OF PULMONARY
    HYPERTENSION
CONTROVERSIES
CONCLUSION
REFERENCES

Abstract

Pulmonary hypertension refers to a variety of conditions characterized by elevations in pulmonary arterial pressure. Major advances in the understanding of PH have led to the current classification in which PH diseases are grouped into five categories according to cause and therapeutic strategy, with each category subdivided to reflect diverse underlying etiologies and sites of injury. The five major categories of the Venice classification include PAH, pulmonary venous hypertension associated with left heart disease, PH associated

From: *Contemporary Cardiology: Pulmonary Hypertension*
Edited by: N. S. Hill and H. W. Farber © Humana Press, Totowa, NJ

with hypoxemia, PH due to chronic thrombotic and/or embolic disease, and PH due to miscellaneous causes. One notable change in the current nomenclature is that the term "idiopathic pulmonary arterial hypertension" (IPAH) has replaced "primary pulmonary hypertension." The WHO functional classification standardizes the comparison of clinical severity among patients with PH. Experts have embraced both the clinical and functional classification systems. Future attempts at refining the classification of this constellation of diseases are likely to embrace new insights into the molecular mechanisms and genetics of PH.

Key Words: pulmonary hypertension classification; idiopathic pulmonary hypertension; connective tissue disease-associated pulmonary hypertension; chronic thromboembolic pulmonary hypertension; pulmonary circulation; pulmonary vascular pathology.

1. INTRODUCTION

The term "pulmonary hypertension" (PH) denotes various conditions in which pulmonary arterial pressure is elevated above normal. The original classification of PH, established at a World Health Organization (WHO) Symposium in 1973, categorized the disorder as "secondary" when an identifiable factor was deemed causal and "primary" when no underlying etiology or risk factor could be identified *(1)*. However, these terms were problematic because the actual "cause" of secondary pulmonary hypertension was often no clearer than with the "primary" group, and the two types were often very similar in presentation, histopathology, and response to therapy. These concerns and the extraordinary advances in the understanding of PH led to a revision of the classification at the Second World Symposium on Pulmonary Hypertension held in Evian, France, in 1998. The Evian group defined PH as a pulmonary artery pressure ≥ 25 mm Hg at rest or ≥ 30 mm Hg with exercise and categorized different types of PH based on clinical similarities, focusing on the biological expression of the disease as well as etiological factors. The Evian classification has subsequently been widely accepted, proving particularly useful in clinical practice and for drug evaluation and registration *(2)*.

More recently, PH was again reclassified by a group of experts at the Third World Symposium on Pulmonary Arterial Hypertension held in Venice, Italy, in 2003 (Table 1). The Venice classification preserved the philosophy and architecture of the Evian classification but included important revisions, most notably the abandonment of the term "primary" pulmonary hypertension. In the current classification,

Table 1
Revised (Venice 2003) Clinical Classification of Pulmonary Hypertension

1. Pulmonary Arterial Hypertension
   1.1. Idiopathic (IPAH)*
   1.2. Familial (FPAH)
   1.3. Associated with (APAH)
      1.3.1. Collagen vascular disease
      1.3.2. Congenital systemic to pulmonary shunts
      1.3.3. Portal hypertension
      1.3.4. HIV infection
      1.3.5. Drugs and toxins
      1.3.6. Other* (thyroid disorders, glycogen storage disease, Gaucher's disease, hereditary hemorrhagic telangiectasia, hemoglobinopathies, myeloproliferative disorders, splenectomy)
   1.4. Associated with significant venous or capillary involvement*
      1.4.1. Pulmonary veno-occlusive disease (PVOD)
      1.4.2. Pulmonary capillary hemangiomatosis (PCH)
   1.5. Persistent pulmonary hypertension of the newborn
2. Pulmonary venous hypertension (associated with left heart disease)
   2.1. Left-sided atrial or ventricular heart disease
   2.2. Left-sided valvular heart disease
3. Pulmonary hypertension associated with hypoxemia
   3.1. Chronic obstructive pulmonary disease
   3.2. Interstitial lung disease
   3.3. Sleep-disordered breathing
   3.4. Alveolar hypoventilation disorders
   3.5. Chronic exposure to high altitude
   3.6. Developmental abnormalities
4. Pulmonary hypertension due to chronic thrombotic and/or embolic disease
   4.1. Thromboembolic obstruction of proximal pulmonary arteries
   4.2. Thromboembolic obstruction of distal pulmonary arteries
   4.3. Non-thrombotic pulmonary embolism (tumor, parasites, foreign material)
5. Miscellaneous*
   5.1. Sarcoidosis, histiocytosis X, lymphangiomatosis, compression of pulmonary vessels (adenopathy, tumor, fibrosing mediastinitis)

* Modifications of the Evian 1998 classification.
** Simonneau G, et al. *(2)*; reproduced with permission.

PH diseases are grouped into five categories according to cause and therapeutic strategy, with each category subdivided to reflect diverse underlying etiologies and sites of injury. This chapter outlines the Venice classification and emphasizes important changes and their rationale.

2. PULMONARY ARTERIAL HYPERTENSION

Pulmonary arterial hypertension (PAH), the first major category in the Venice clinical classification of PH, comprises conditions that share localization of lesions in precapillary segments of the pulmonary vasculature. As such, pulmonary capillary and venous pressures are normal (≤15 mm Hg). Patients may present with varying levels of PH, but the course of the disease is generally progressive and the prognosis poor without therapy. Histopathology may include plexogenic arteriopathy, thrombotic lesions, and medial hypertrophy with intimal fibrosis. This grouping includes multiple risk factors for PH, some potentially avoidable, and underlying conditions that may predispose to development of the disease.

2.1. Idiopathic Pulmonary Arterial Hypertension

Unexplained PAH has been designated "idiopathic PAH" (IPAH), which replaces the term "primary" pulmonary hypertension. For the purposes of this chapter, we will henceforth use this term, even in a historical context. This change in nomenclature reflects the increased understanding of PH, the acknowledgment that the cause of primary pulmonary hypertension is unknown, and the frequent lack of clinical distinction between primary and secondary forms of the disease. The true incidence of IPAH is unknown but has been estimated at one to two cases per million people per year (3). With increases in awareness and improvements in detection capabilities, however, it is likely that the disease will be recognized more often than originally estimated.

IPAH is the most studied form of PAH. The prospective National Institutes of Health (NIH) Registry, the largest natural history study of IPAH, recruited 187 patients from 32 centers and followed them from 1981 through 1987 (4). This cohort provided a wealth of information on IPAH and is often used as a benchmark, providing survival data in untreated patients for comparison with long-term follow-up studies of currently available therapies. Average survival overall was 2.8 years from the time of diagnosis, with New York Heart Association (NYHA) functional class predicting survival in subgroups (6, 3, and 1.8 years, and 6 months for classes I–IV, respectively). Poor survival has also been associated with the severity of elevated mean pulmonary arterial pressure, and even more strongly with right ventricular dysfunction (specifically, elevated mean right atrial pressure and decreased cardiac index) *(5)*.

Patients with IPAH most frequently present in their third and fourth decades and are mostly female (female/male ratio approximately 1.7/1). Enrollment in clinical trials over the past decade, however, would suggest that this ratio is at least twice as high. Dyspnea on exertion is the main presenting symptom in at least 60% of patients, with fatigue, chest pain, near syncope or even syncope, leg edema, and palpitations being other common presenting complaints. IPAH is diagnosed clinically by the absence of any identifiable associated or etiological factors in a patient with PAH and is characterized pathologically by the plexiform lesion. These lesions may be seen in other forms of severe PH and are not pathognomonic of IPAH. They consist of whorls of endothelial cells that some investigators have identified as monoclonal, leading to speculation that they are "quasi-oncogenic" *(6)*.

2.2. Familial Pulmonary Arterial Hypertension (FPAH)

Within a few years of his original description and coining of the term "primary pulmonary hypertension" in 1951, Dresdale reported on a family with several members affected by the disease, initiating speculation about a hereditary cause for PAH *(6,7)*. Since then, IPAH has been described in two or more first-degree relatives in almost 100 American families *(8)*. Familial pulmonary arterial hypertension (FPAH) is clinically indistinguishable from nonfamilial PAH, and the exact incidence is unknown. The NIH Registry Study reported 12 cases (6%) of FPAH *(4)*, but more recent evidence suggests that the familial association with IPAH patients is underrecognized. The actual incidence may be as high as 13.6%, with one study finding FPAH-like mutations in 26% of cases of IPAH *(8–10)*.

FPAH segregates in an autosomal dominant fashion with incomplete penetrance, with about 10–20% of carriers affected *(11)*. The disease has been known to skip entire generations within families, suggesting that other factors (environmental and/or genetic) are required for pathogenesis. FPAH demonstrates a female preponderance and may undergo genetic anticipation *(12)*.

Linkage analysis has localized a responsible gene (*PPH1*) to chromosome 2q33, mutations of which may result in defective function of the bone morphogenetic protein receptor type II (BMPRII) *(13,14)*. The *BMPRII* gene encodes for a receptor member of the transforming growth factor (TGF)-beta superfamily. It is hypothesized that interruption of the BMP-mediated signaling pathway resulting from the mutations predisposes cells within small pulmonary arteries toward growth and proliferation in response to injury. A recently described but less common form of hereditary PAH may be due to a mutation of the activin-like kinase type-1 receptor (*ALK1*) gene in patients with hereditary hemorrhagic telangiectasia *(15)*. A more detailed discussion of the genetic abnormalities associated with PAH may be found in Chapter 3.

2.3. Conditions Associated with Pulmonary Arterial Hypertension (APAH)

PAH occurring in the presence of a known cause or risk factor is termed "associated PAH" (APAH). This is the predominant category within the PAH grouping and includes PH associated with conditions such as connective tissue disease, drugs, HIV, and portal hypertension. Since the likelihood of developing PAH in the company of these known risk factors is relatively low, individual susceptibility and/or genetics must be important factors in the development of APAH.

2.3.1. PAH ASSOCIATED WITH CONNECTIVE TISSUE DISEASE

PAH has been associated with every known type of connective tissue disease (CTD) *(16)*. Most commonly, it complicates the scleroderma spectrum of diseases, systemic lupus erythematosus, and mixed connective tissue disease, but it can also rarely be seen in rheumatoid arthritis, dermatomyositis/polymyositis, and primary Sjogren's syndrome. PAH associated with connective tissue disease may occur as isolated pulmonary vascular disease or in association with parenchymal lung disease. While the term "collagen vascular disease" has been utilized, "connective tissue disease" (CTD) is most commonly used to describe this category of patients.

The pulmonary vascular disease associated with CTD is often indistinguishable from IPAH *(16)*. Both conditions share presenting symptomatology, a female predominance, the presence of Raynaud's phenomenon, and abnormal serologies (elevated antinuclear antibody titers and rheumatoid factor). The histopathologies of APAH due to CTD and IPAH also overlap. Although they often show similar acute hemodynamic and exercise improvements with medical therapy, patients with PAH associated with CTD tend to have a worse prognosis when compared to IPAH, whether treated or not *(17,18)*.

2.3.2. PAH ASSOCIATED WITH CONGENITAL SYSTEMIC-TO-PULMONARY SHUNTS

Pulmonary hypertension is a common manifestation of congenital heart disease (CHD). The Venice classification for congenital systemic-to-pulmonary shunts is outlined in Table 2. The initial association

Table 2
Guidelines for Classification of Congenital Systemic-to-Pulmonary Shunts*

1. Type
     Simple
          Atrial septal defect (ASD)
          Ventricular septal defect (VSD)
          Patent ductus arteriosus
          Total or partial unobstructed anomalous pulmonary venous return
     Combined
          Describe combination and define prevalent defect, if any
     Complex
          Truncus arteriosus
          Single ventricle with unobstructed pulmonary blood flow
          Atrioventricular septal defects
2. Dimensions
     Small (ASD $\leq$ 2.0 cm and VSD $\leq$ 1.0 cm)
     Large (ASD > 2.0 cm and VSD > 1.0 cm)
3. Associated extracardiac abnormalities
4. Correction status
     Noncorrected
     Partially corrected (age)
     Corrected: spontaneously or surgically (age)

* Simonneau G, et al (2); reproduced with permission.

was reported by Eisenmenger in 1897, when he described a 32-year-old man with cyanosis and exercise intolerance who died of massive hemoptysis and in whom a ventricular septal defect and severe pulmonary vascular disease were discovered postmortem (19). This case characterizes the physiology and symptoms now referred to as "Eisenmenger syndrome," which includes all systemic to pulmonary arterial connections leading to PH and a right-to-left or bidirectional shunt. This abnormality begins as a left-to-right shunt that chronically increases blood flow through the pulmonary vascular bed. For reasons not entirely understood, this increased blood flow leads to morphological and histological changes similar to those found in IPAH (20).

The clinical manifestations of PAH associated with CHD, however, have some important differences when compared to IPAH. Cyanosis and exercise oxygen desaturation are common and usually more severe than those of IPAH consistent with the right-to-left shunting. Hemoptysis occurs more frequently in these patients, and stroke is more common due to paradoxical embolization. The vascular disease of PAH associated with CHD progresses more slowly to right ventricular failure, which accounts at least partly for the better survival compared to IPAH *(18,21)*.

The risk of developing Eisenmenger syndrome depends in large part on the size and location of the anatomical defect. Of the simple cardiac anomalies, ventricular septal defects most frequently lead to PH, especially in patients with large defects (>1.5 cm in diameter) *(20,22)*. Early detection of the CHD defect is key, as surgical repair prior to the development of severe pulmonary hypertension halts the progression of pulmonary vascular disease. When the disease is advanced, patients with CHD and severe PH may not benefit or even worsen with surgical correction, and so medical therapy is preferred. At such a severe stage, the differentiation between CHD and IPAPH becomes moot, because differentiating between a small atrial septal defect and a patent foramen ovale (PFO) may be impossible short of autopsy, and therapy will be the same for both.

2.3.3. PAH ASSOCIATED WITH PORTAL HYPERTENSION

Portopulmonary hypertension (PPHTN) is diagnosed when PAH occurs in association with portal hypertension without other risk factors. PPHTN seems to be related to the elevated portal pressure itself and can occur in the presence or absence of underlying liver parenchymal disease. The diagnosis is often indirect, based on the signs and symptoms of portal disease, as the direct measurement and definition of portal hypertension are unclear in the context of an elevated right atrial pressure.

A large autopsy series suggests that PH occurs in patients with cirrhosis at greater than five times the expected frequency and, even after excluding known cases of PPHTN, PH was found to complicate portal hypertension in 2% of over 500 patients studied *(23,24)*. Whether the severity of portal hypertension influences the development of PAH is controversial, but the prevalence of PPHTN appears to be highest in patients with end-stage liver disease undergoing evaluation for liver transplantation *(25)*. It is also possible that PAH is simply more often sought and identified in this group.

PPHTN is histologically and clinically similar to IPAH with a few important differences *(24,26,27)*. PPHTN has no gender predilection and patients tend to be older. Hemodynamically, patients tend to have higher cardiac outputs than patients with other causes of PAH. The prognosis of untreated PPHTN is poor, but patients may respond to intravenous epoprostenol, and liver transplantation may reverse the pulmonary vascular disease *(28,29)*.

2.3.4. PAH Associated with HIV Infection

When present, PH increases the mortality of HIV-infected patients, in whom the incidence of HIV-associated PH may be between 0.1% and 0.5% *(30,31)*. PAH probably develops through the activation of cytokine or growth factor pathways, but the exact mechanism is unknown. IPAH and HIV-associated PAH appear clinically and histologically alike, and survival is also similar with comparable therapy *(30,31)*. Improved survival has been associated with a higher CD4 count and combination highly active anti-retroviral therapy (HAART) *(32,33)*.

2.3.5. PAH Associated with Drugs and Toxins

Although several drugs and toxins have been associated with the development of PAH, the strongest causal association has been with anorectic agents such as aminorex and the fenfluramines *(34,35)*. The adjusted odds ratio for fenfluramine use longer than six months and an associated diagnosis of IPAH was 7.5, and the high prevalence of anorectic use in patients with secondary forms of PH raises the possibility that the drugs precipitate PH in patients with underlying conditions *(36)*. Anecdotally, PAH associated with fenfluramines is more aggressive than IPAH and may carry a worse prognosis, although spontaneous regression may occur as well.

2.3.6. PAH Associated with Other Diseases

Other miscellaneous diseases have been associated with PAH, such as the rare condition Type Ia glycogen storage disease. PH commonly complicates sickle cell disease, although this condition is sometimes related to diastolic dysfunction rather than PAH. Patients with hereditary hemorrhagic telangiectasia may also develop classic PAH or have PH secondary to right-to-left shunting through pulmonary arteriovenous malformations.

2.4. PAH Associated with Significant Pulmonary Venular or Capillary Involvement

Pulmonary veno-occlusive disease (PVOD) and pulmonary capillary hemangiomatosis (PCH) are rare conditions that share with IPAH an overlapping clinical presentation and histopathology. PVOD produces patchy pulmonary venous obstruction, which may confound the diagnosis as pulmonary capillary wedge pressure may be normal or elevated depending on the lung segment that is measured *(37)*. Proliferating capillaries that invade and occlude the pulmonary vasculature characterize PCH. The diagnosis of both diseases may be aided by findings on chest computed tomography (CT), PVOD manifesting septal lines, but lung biopsy may be necessary for confirmation *(38)*. Both PVOD and PCH are unique in the PAH category in that vasodilator therapy (especially epoprostenol) must be used cautiously, if at all, due to the risk of precipitating potentially fatal pulmonary edema *(39,40)*.

2.5. Persistent Pulmonary Hypertension of the Newborn

Persistent pulmonary hypertension of the newborn (PPHN) is characterized by elevated right heart pressures that persist after birth, resulting in right-to-left shunting of blood through fetal circulatory pathways and severe hypoxemia. PPHN is likely an effect of chronic fetal distress, which leads to persistent vasoconstriction and pulmonary hypertension. The prevalence of PPHN is estimated at 1.9 per 1000 live births *(41)*. Therapy is directed toward cardiopulmonary support, with inhaled nitric oxide having been shown to improve oxygenation and outcome *(42)*.

3. PULMONARY VENOUS HYPERTENSION

PH associated with left-sided heart disease, termed "pulmonary venous hypertension," is the second major category in the Venice classification and is the most common cause of PH in clinical practice, although certainly not the most common cause of severe PH (mean pulmonary artery pressure > 50). Any chronic elevation of filling pressures on the left side of the heart passively increases pulmonary artery pressure. Many cardiac abnormalities lead to pulmonary venous hypertension, but the most common include left ventricular systolic failure, diastolic dysfunction, and mitral valve disease.

Corresponding to the difference in pathophysiology, patients with pulmonary venous hypertension often present differently than patients with PAH. Signs and symptoms of left-sided heart disease (e.g., pulmonary edema, orthopnea, paroxysmal nocturnal dyspnea) generally precede evidence of right-sided heart failure. On the other hand, some patients, particularly those with left ventricular diastolic dysfunction, may present with clinical features that are indistinguishable from those of PAH. Also, the picture can be confusing in the presence of advanced disease, and the presentation may be mixed (i.e., with left ventricular failure and PAH seemingly coexisting). An elevated pulmonary capillary wedge pressure, taken as a reflection of left ventricular filling pressure, is usually adequate to diagnose pulmonary venous hypertension, but left ventricular end-diastolic pressure measured via left heart catheterization may sometimes be helpful in confusing situations.

Treatment of the underlying cardiac disorder is essential in managing pulmonary venous hypertension. Typical therapies for PAH have so far been ineffective or even detrimental for patients with severe congestive heart failure and are generally avoided in isolated pulmonary venous hypertension *(43,44)*.

4. PULMONARY HYPERTENSION ASSOCIATED WITH HYPOXIA

Chronic alveolar hypoxia leading to hypoxic pulmonary vasoconstriction and pulmonary vascular remodeling is the hallmark of disorders in the third major category of the Venice classification. Intrinsic lung disease, impaired control of breathing, and residence at high altitude are examples of conditions associated with alveolar hypoxia leading to PH. Patients with chronic hypoxic pulmonary hypertension often have only mild to moderate PH accompanied by cor pulmonale, and treatment is generally aimed at the underlying disease. Supplemental oxygen and/or ventilatory assistance to correct the hypoventilation often provide significant clinical improvement. Pharmacological treatment of PH, when warranted, should be done with care, as some therapies for PH may worsen ventilation perfusion matching and increase the hypoxemia.

5. PULMONARY HYPERTENSION DUE TO CHRONIC THROMBOTIC AND/OR EMBOLIC DISEASE

PH due to chronic pulmonary embolism, the fourth major category of the Venice classification, is often clinically indistinguishable from PAH. Obstruction may be caused by distal or proximal disease and may be due to clot, metastatic tumor, parasites, or foreign material. Premortem diagnosis of the latter few requires clinical suspicion and, often, lung biopsy. Tumor embolism should be considered when patients have relatively rapid progression and are unresponsive to therapy. Chronic thromboembolic pulmonary hypertension may be clinically silent for months or years, is potentially curable by thromboendarterectomy, and must be excluded in every case of PAH.

6. PULMONARY HYPERTENSION DUE TO MISCELLANEOUS CAUSES

Rare causes of pulmonary hypertension are categorized as "miscellaneous" and comprise the fifth Venice category (Table 1). In Western countries, sarcoidosis is probably the most common of these diverse etiologies. In sarcoidosis, PH may result from fibrocystic parenchymal destruction and hypoxemia, but a subset of patients may suffer from sarcoid involvement of the pulmonary circulation. PH due to histiocytosis X may be related to intrinsic pulmonary vascular disease and is independent of the degree of airway and lung parenchymal injury *(45)*. Another miscellaneous cause of PH is extrinsic mechanical compression of the pulmonary vasculature, such as occurs with fibrosing mediastinitis, which may be discovered by radiographic imaging of the chest.

7. FUNCTIONAL CLASSIFICATION OF PULMONARY HYPERTENSION

The 1998 Evian meeting also produced the WHO Functional Classification of Pulmonary Hypertension, which was created to standardize the comparison of clinical severity among patients (Table 3). This was modeled after the New York Heart Association (NYHA) Functional Classification for heart disease but also includes consideration of syncope. As with the clinical classification, use of the functional classification has been widely accepted.

The major limitation of the functional classification of PH is that class III patients are an extraordinarily heterogeneous group, demonstrating varying degrees of disability. This may be particularly important when considering the applicability of clinical trial data and choosing a therapeutic intervention. Some investigators have proposed that class III patients be subcategorized as either IIIa or IIIb depending on symptom severity/progression, but this has not yet been officially embraced by the PH community.

Table 3
A Comparison of the New York Heart Association and World Health Organization Functional Classifications

A. New York Heart Association functional classification
  Class 1: No symptoms with ordinary physical activity.
  Class 2: Symptoms with ordinary activity. Slight limitation of activity.
  Class 3: Symptoms with less than ordinary activity. Marked limitation
  of activity.
  Class 4: Symptoms with any activity or even at rest.

B. World Health Organization functional assessment classification

Class I: Patients with PH but without resulting limitation of physical
activity. Ordinary physical activity does not cause undue dyspnea or
fatigue, chest pain, or near syncope.

Class II: Patients with PH resulting in slight limitation of physical
activity. They are comfortable at rest. Ordinary physical activity causes
undue dyspnea or fatigue, chest pain, or near syncope.

Class III: Patients with PH resulting in marked limitation of physical
activity. They are comfortable at rest. Less than ordinary activity causes
undue dyspnea or fatigue, chest pain, or near syncope.

Class IV: Patients with PH with inability to carry out any physical
activity without symptoms. These patients manifest signs of right heart
failure. Dyspnea and/or fatigue may even be present at rest. Discomfort
is increased by any physical activity.

8. CONTROVERSIES

Despite the remarkable advances in our understanding of pulmonary
hypertension, the present classification of the disease remains
imperfect. While a classification based on clinical principles seems
most useful at this time, new insights may change this, just as they did
when the initial WHO classification that was centered on morphology
shifted to the clinical focus of the Evian and Venice classification
schemes. This may be especially relevant when considering a genetic
classification for PH. Mutations in two receptors of the TGF-beta
family of receptors are present in the majority of FPAH cases, and
BMPR2 mutations have been found in many nonfamilial cases of PAH
as well (2,46). At this time, however, the pathway for the development
of pulmonary hypertension via genetic susceptibility (either through

gene-gene interactions or environmental factors) has yet to be fully elucidated.

PVOD and PCH have been incorporated into the PAH category because of the similarities in risk factors, clinical presentation, familial occurrence, genetic mutations, and arterial histopathology (2,47–50). These disorders are thought to represent a spectrum of a single disease. The current classification of PVOD and PCH is somewhat problematic in that it cannot guide therapy. As noted above, the presence of significant disease distal to the precapillary arterioles makes vasodilator therapy potentially dangerous, and lung transplantation may be the most appropriate therapy for advanced cases (39,40).

9. CONCLUSION

Pulmonary hypertension describes a variety of conditions in which pulmonary arterial pressure is elevated above normal. Major advances in the understanding of PH have led to the current classification in which PH diseases are grouped into five categories according to cause and therapeutic strategy, with each category subdivided to reflect diverse underlying etiologies and sites of injury. The five major categories of the Venice classification include PAH, pulmonary venous hypertension associated with left heart disease, PH associated with hypoxemia, PH due to chronic thrombotic and/or embolic disease, and PH due to miscellaneous causes. One notable change in the current nomenclature is that the term "IPAH" has replaced "primary pulmonary hypertension." The WHO functional classification standardizes the comparison of clinical severity among patients with PH. Experts have embraced both the clinical and functional classification systems. Future attempts at refining the classification of this constellation of diseases are likely to embrace new insights into the molecular mechanisms and genetics of PH.

REFERENCES

1. Hatano S, Strasser T, eds. Primary pulmonary hypertension. Report on a WHO meeting. Geneva: World Health Organization; 1975.
2. Simonneau G, Galie N, Rubin LJ, et al. Clinical classification of pulmonary hypertension. J Am Coll Cardiol 2004;43(12 Suppl S):5S–12S.
3. The International Primary Pulmonary Hypertension Study (IPPHS). Chest 1994;105(2 Suppl):37S–41S.
4. Rich S, Dantzker DR, Ayres SM, et al. Primary pulmonary hypertension. A national prospective study. Ann Intern Med 1987;107(2):216–23.

5. D'Alonzo GE, Barst RJ, Ayres SM, et al. Survival in patients with primary pulmonary hypertension. Results from a national prospective registry. Ann Intern Med 1991;115(5):343–9.

6. Lee SD, Shroyer KR, Markham NE, Cool CD, Voelkel NF, Tuder RM. Monoclonal endothelial cell proliferation is present in primary but not secondary pulmonary hypertension. J Clin Invest. 1998;101:927–34.

7. Dresdale DT, Schultz M, Michtom RJ. Primary pulmonary hypertension. I. Clinical and hemodynamic study. Am J Med 1951;11(6):686–705.

8. Newman JH, Wheeler L, Lane KB, et al. Mutation in the gene for bone morphogenetic protein receptor II as a cause of primary pulmonary hypertension in a large kindred. N Engl J Med 2001;345(5):319–24.

9. McLaughlin VV, Shillington A, Rich S. Survival in primary pulmonary hypertension: the impact of epoprostenol therapy. Circulation 2002; 106(12):1477–82.

10. Thomson JR, Machado RD, Pauciulo MW, et al. Sporadic primary pulmonary hypertension is associated with germline mutations of the gene encoding BMPR-II, a receptor member of the TGF-beta family. J Med Genet 2000;37(10):741–5.

11. Loyd JE, Primm RK, Newman JH. Familial primary pulmonary hypertension: clinical patterns. Am Rev Respir Dis 1984;129(1):194–7.

12. Loyd JE, Butler MG, Foroud TM, Conneally PM, Phillips JA, 3rd, Newman JH. Genetic anticipation and abnormal gender ratio at birth in familial primary pulmonary hypertension. Am J Respir Crit Care Med 1995;152(1):93–7.

13. Lane KB, Machado RD, Pauciulo MW, et al. Heterozygous germline mutations in BMPR2, encoding a TGF-beta receptor, cause familial primary pulmonary hypertension. The International PPH Consortium. Nat Genet 2000;26(1):81–4.

14. Deng Z, Morse JH, Slager SL, et al. Familial primary pulmonary hypertension (gene PPH1) is caused by mutations in the bone morphogenetic protein receptor-II gene. Am J Hum Genet 2000;67(3):737–44.

15. Trembath RC, Thomson JR, Machado RD, et al. Clinical and molecular genetic features of pulmonary hypertension in patients with hereditary hemorrhagic telangiectasia. N Engl J Med 2001;345(5):325–34.

16. Hoeper MM. Pulmonary hypertension in collagen vascular disease. Eur Respir J 2002;19(3):571–6.

17. Badesch DB, Tapson VF, McGoon MD, et al. Continuous intravenous epoprostenol for pulmonary hypertension due to the scleroderma spectrum of disease. A randomized, controlled trial. Ann Intern Med 2000;132(6):425–34.

18. Kuhn KP, Byrne DW, Arbogast PG, Doyle TP, Loyd JE, Robbins IM. Outcome in 91 consecutive patients with pulmonary arterial hypertension receiving epoprostenol. Am J Respir Crit Care Med 2003;167(4):580–6.

19. Eisenmenger V. Die angeboren defects des kammerscheidewand des herzen. Z Klin Med 1897;32:1–28.

20. Kidd L, Driscoll DJ, Gersony WM, et al. Second natural history study of congenital heart defects. Results of treatment of patients with ventricular septal defects. Circulation 1993;87(2 Suppl):I38–51.
21. Hopkins WE, Ochoa LL, Richardson GW, Trulock EP. Comparison of the hemodynamics and survival of adults with severe primary pulmonary hypertension or Eisenmenger syndrome. J Heart Lung Transplant 1996;15(1 Pt 1):100–5.
22. Daliento L, Somerville J, Presbitero P, et al. Eisenmenger syndrome. Factors relating to deterioration and death. Eur Heart J 1998;19(12):1845–55.
23. McDonnell PJ, Toye PA, Hutchins GM. Primary pulmonary hypertension and cirrhosis: are they related? Am Rev Respir Dis 1983;127(4):437–41.
24. Hadengue A, Benhayoun MK, Lebrec D, Benhamou JP. Pulmonary hypertension complicating portal hypertension: prevalence and relation to splanchnic hemodynamics. Gastroenterology 1991;100(2):520–8.
25. Ramsay MA, Simpson BR, Nguyen AT, Ramsay KJ, East C, Klintmalm GB. Severe pulmonary hypertension in liver transplant candidates. Liver Transpl Surg 1997;3(5):494–500.
26. Edwards BS, Weir EK, Edwards WD, Ludwig J, Dykoski RK, Edwards JE. Coexistent pulmonary and portal hypertension: morphologic and clinical features. J Am Coll Cardiol 1987;10(6):1233–8.
27. Herve P, Lebrec D, Brenot F, et al. Pulmonary vascular disorders in portal hypertension. Eur Respir J 1998;11(5):1153–66.
28. Krowka MJ, Frantz RP, McGoon MD, Severson C, Plevak DJ, Wiesner RH. Improvement in pulmonary hemodynamics during intravenous epoprostenol (prostacyclin): A study of 15 patients with moderate to severe portopulmonary hypertension. Hepatology 1999;30(3):641–8.
29. Krowka MJ, Mandell MS, Ramsay MA, et al. Hepatopulmonary syndrome and portopulmonary hypertension: a report of the multicenter liver transplant database. Liver Transpl 2004;10(2):174–82.
30. Opravil M, Pechere M, Speich R, et al. HIV-associated primary pulmonary hypertension. A case control study. Swiss HIV Cohort Study. Am J Respir Crit Care Med 1997;155(3):990–5.
31. Speich R, Jenni R, Opravil M, Pfab M, Russi EW. Primary pulmonary hypertension in HIV infection. Chest 1991;100(5):1268–71.
32. Nunes H, Humbert M, Sitbon O, et al. Prognostic factors for survival in human immunodeficiency virus-associated pulmonary arterial hypertension. Am J Respir Crit Care Med 2003;167(10):1433–9.
33. Zuber JP, Calmy A, Evison JM, et al. Pulmonary arterial hypertension related to HIV infection: improved hemodynamics and survival associated with antiretroviral therapy. Clin Infect Dis 2004;38(8):1178–85.
34. Gurtner HP. Aminorex and pulmonary hypertension. A review. Cor Vasa 1985;27(2–3):160–71.
35. Abenhaim L, Moride Y, Brenot F, et al. Appetite-suppressant drugs and the risk of primary pulmonary hypertension. International Primary Pulmonary Hypertension Study Group. N Engl J Med 1996;335(9): 609–16.

36. Rich S, Rubin L, Walker AM, Schneeweiss S, Abenhaim L. Anorexigens and pulmonary hypertension in the United States: results from the surveillance of North American pulmonary hypertension. Chest 2000;117(3):870–4.
37. Holcomb BW, Jr., Loyd JE, Ely EW, Johnson J, Robbins IM. Pulmonary veno-occlusive disease: a case series and new observations. Chest 2000;118(6):1671–9.
38. Dufour B, Maitre S, Humbert M, Capron F, Simonneau G, Musset D. High-resolution CT of the chest in four patients with pulmonary capillary hemangiomatosis or pulmonary venoocclusive disease. AJR Am J Roentgenol 1998;171(5):1321–4.
39. Palmer SM, Robinson LJ, Wang A, Gossage JR, Bashore T, Tapson VF. Massive pulmonary edema and death after prostacyclin infusion in a patient with pulmonary veno-occlusive disease. Chest 1998;113(1):237–40.
40. Humbert M, Maitre S, Capron F, Rain B, Musset D, Simonneau G. Pulmonary edema complicating continuous intravenous prostacyclin in pulmonary capillary hemangiomatosis. Am J Respir Crit Care Med 1998;157(5 Pt 1):1681–5.
41. Walsh-Sukys MC, Tyson JE, Wright LL, et al. Persistent pulmonary hypertension of the newborn in the era before nitric oxide: practice variation and outcomes. Pediatrics 2000;105(1 Pt 1):14–20.
42. Roberts JD, Jr., Fineman JR, Morin FC, 3rd, et al. Inhaled nitric oxide and persistent pulmonary hypertension of the newborn. The Inhaled Nitric Oxide Study Group. N Engl J Med 1997;336(9):605–10.
43. Califf RM, Adams KF, McKenna WJ, et al. A randomized controlled trial of epoprostenol therapy for severe congestive heart failure: The Flolan International Randomized Survival Trial (FIRST). Am Heart J 1997;134(1):44–54.
44. Rich S, McLaughlin VV. Endothelin receptor blockers in cardiovascular disease. Circulation 2003;108(18):2184–90.
45. Fartoukh M, Humbert M, Capron F, et al. Severe pulmonary hypertension in histiocytosis X. Am J Respir Crit Care Med 2000;161(1):216–23.
46. Newman JH, Trembath RC, Morse JA, et al. Genetic basis of pulmonary arterial hypertension: current understanding and future directions. J Am Coll Cardiol 2004;43(12 Suppl S):33S–9S.
47. Pietra GG, Capron F, Stewart S, et al. Pathologic assessment of vasculopathies in pulmonary hypertension. J Am Coll Cardiol 2004;43(12 Suppl S):25S–32S.
48. Voordes CG, Kuipers JR, Elema JD. Familial pulmonary veno-occlusive disease: a case report. Thorax 1977;32(6):763–6.
49. Langleben D, Heneghan JM, Batten AP, et al. Familial pulmonary capillary hemangiomatosis resulting in primary pulmonary hypertension. Ann Intern Med 1988;109(2):106–9.
50. Runo JR, Vnencak-Jones CL, Prince M, et al. Pulmonary veno-occlusive disease caused by an inherited mutation in bone morphogenetic protein receptor II. Am J Respir Crit Care Med 2003;167(6):889–94.

3 Diagnostic Approach to Pulmonary Arterial Hypertension

Ronald J. Oudiz

CONTENTS

INTRODUCTION
SUSPICION/HISTORY
PHYSICAL EXAMINATION
NONINVASIVE TESTING
INVASIVE TESTING
LABORATORY TESTING
SUMMARY
REFERENCES

Abstract

Detecting pulmonary arterial hypertension (PAH) requires an index of suspicion that is raised by the combination of exertional symptoms and suggestive physical findings such as increased intensity of P2. Cardiac echocardiography is the most useful noninvasive screening test. Diagnosing PAH requires a carefully directed workup that is focused on excluding other causes of pulmonary hypertension. Initially, noninvasive tests are used to confirm the suspicion for pulmonary hypertension and evaluate for secondary contributing factors, and cardiac catheterization is then performed to confirm suspected PAH. Functional testing such as the six-minute walk test and certain blood tests are proving useful in assessing responses to therapy. Additional testing can aid the clinician in determining prognosis and characterizing PAH severity, helping the decision-making process to optimize the choice and timing of treatment.

From: *Contemporary Cardiology: Pulmonary Hypertension*
Edited by: N. S. Hill and H. W. Farber © Humana Press, Totowa, NJ

Key Words: pulmonary   hypertension   diagnosis;   echocardiography; exercise testing; pulmonary function; six-minute walk test.

1. INTRODUCTION

Diagnosing pulmonary hypertension (PH) and, as much as possible, delineating the underlying pathophysiology are important, because differing pathophysiologies necessitate different treatment approaches. For example, PH associated with left ventricular diastolic dysfunction requires different therapy than idiopathic pulmonary arterial hypertension (IPAH). Thus, correctly detecting and diagnosing PH is absolutely essential in order to formulate a sound treatment plan. Since PAH is mainly a diagnosis made after excluding other, usually more common, diagnoses, the diagnostic workup of PAH requires the utilization of many diagnostic modalities. These include clinical history, physical examination, and noninvasive and invasive testing. The following information represents a synthesis of published data, consensus recommendations *(1,2)*, and clinical expertise used to provide a practical approach to diagnosing PAH.

2. SUSPICION/HISTORY

Although PH may be found incidentally, a critical element in the evaluation of PH is the clinical suspicion the diagnostician must have that PH exists, since the symptoms are often nonspecific. This suspicion may be triggered by the patient's history or physical findings, or it may emerge from one or more abnormal laboratory test results.

Dyspnea on exertion is the most common symptom of PH *(3)*, but is, of course, nonspecific. Also, other nonspecific symptoms may predominate, such as fatigue, lack of energy, and/or syncope, and patients may not readily volunteer that they are dyspneic, leading to delays in detection. In one study *(3)*, the average time from symptom onset to diagnosis was approximately two years. This likely reflects not only the reluctance on the part of patients to attribute significance to their symptoms, but also the clinician's unwillingness to associate common symptoms with a rare disease such as PAH. Another impediment to the early diagnosis of PAH lies in the fact that PAH symptoms do not typically manifest themselves until pulmonary vascular resistance (PVR) becomes significantly elevated, perhaps years after the onset of pulmonary vascular disease *(4)*.

A focused history facilitates the consideration of important differential diagnoses in the workup of PAH. Dyspnea and/or fatigue along with symptoms or signs of connective tissue diseases (CTDs), namely, the CREST variant of scleroderma (calcinosis cutis, Raynaud's phenomenon, esophageal motility disorder, sclerodactyly, and telangiectasia), systemic lupus erythematosus, or mixed CTD suggests PAH associated with CTDs. PAH associated with CTDs in fact makes up a large proportion of the total PAH population in the United States. Estimates of the prevalence of PAH in patients with CTDs range from 4.9% to 38%, depending on the diagnostic modality used to detect PH. Interestingly, many patients with IPAH experience symptoms of Raynaud's phenomenon in the absence of other signs of CTDs (5).

Although less frequently encountered now since the FDA mandated the removal of fenfluramine derivatives from the market, a history of anorexigen exposure strongly suggests drug-induced PAH, while a history of high-risk behavior for HIV disease suggests HIV-associated PAH (6,7). In patients exposed to fenfluramine anorexigens, the risk of developing PAH was increased 23-fold (8). Because the prevalence of PAH is so much higher in these individuals, screening is of particular importance.

A family history of PAH (or unexplained cardiovascular death) helps to identify patients with the familial form of PAH, which may account for up to 25% of IPAH cases (9). The offspring of patients with familial PAH have an overall 10% risk of developing overt PAH, with the onset of disease occurring earlier in succeeding generations, and in whom outcome may be worse (10). Thus, taking a detailed

A. Drugs and Toxins
1. Definite
• Aminorex
• Fenfluramine
• Dexfenfluramine
• Toxic rapeseed oil
2. Very likely
• Amphetamines
• L-tryptophan
3. Possible
• Meta-amphetamines
• Cocaine
• Chemotherapeutic agents
4. Unlikely
• Antidepressants
• Oral contraceptives
• Estrogen therapy
• Cigarette smoking

B. Demographic and Medical Conditions
1. Definite
• Gender
2. Possible
• Pregnancy
• Systemic hypertension
3. Unlikely
• Obesity
C. Diseases
1. Definite
• HIV infection
2. Very likely
• Portal hypertension/liver disease
• Collagen vascular diseases
• Congenital systemic-pulmonary-cardiac shunts
3. Possible
• Thyroid disorders

Fig. 1. Risk factors and associated conditions for PAH classified according to the strength of evidence; reproduced with permission from Ref. *11*.

family history in a patient with suspected PH may also facilitate a more focused approach to the diagnostic workup, possibly allowing for earlier intervention.

Figure 1 shows noteworthy risk factors associated with PAH that might increase the clinician's suspicion of the presence of PAH.

3. PHYSICAL EXAMINATION

The physical findings of patients with PAH vary widely, and are often nonspecific. Probably the earliest and single most common physical finding is that of an accentuated pulmonic component of the second heart sound, also referred to as the 'P2'. The loud P2 in patients with PH results from the more forceful closure of the pulmonic valve in response to an elevated diastolic pulmonary artery pressure (PAP). In patients with PH, the P2 is increased in intensity compared to the aortic valve closure sound (3). Occasionally, the second heart sound may also be palpable.

Additional physical findings associated with PH reflect the effects of PH on the heart and other organs. Most patients develop some degree of tricuspid regurgitation due to the pressure overload of the right ventricle. Some patients may not have an audible tricuspid regurgitation murmur, and may not even have detectable tricuspid regurgitation by echocardiogram. The murmur of pulmonic regurgitation (Graham Steell murmur) may be present; however, it is unclear whether its presence or absence correlates with clinical status. A right ventricular lift (heave) may be noted. Jugular venous pulsations may be elevated in the presence of volume overload and/or overt right ventricular failure, and large V-waves may be evident in the presence of significant tricuspid regurgitation.

Hepatomegaly may be present, occasionally with palpable pulsations of the liver edge, related to the underlying tricuspid regurgitation. Ascites may also be the prominent feature of right ventricular failure in these patients, even in the absence of other manifestations of peripheral fluid retention.

The lung examination in most PAH patients is normal, and is thus of limited value in confirming PAH. However, it may be useful in excluding other causes of PH, such as significant airway disease, or pulmonary edema.

The extremities may show pitting edema with or without venous stasis changes. In patients with the scleroderma spectrum of disease, thickened skin, sclerodactyly, telangiectasias, and/or digital ulcers related to Raynaud's phenomenon may be observed.

4. NONINVASIVE TESTING

Once there is a clinical suspicion of PAH, either by history and physical examination or from incidental findings, the ensuing workup should include confirmatory testing and testing to exclude other types and causes of PH. Subsequent testing determines disease severity and prognosis. A recently developed expert consensus recommendation for required and contingent testing for PAH is shown in Figure 2. A synopsis reflecting this approach is discussed below.

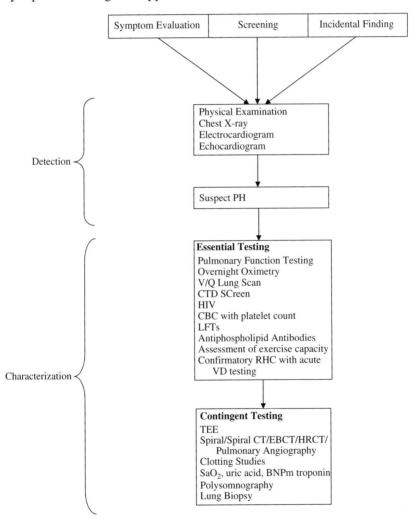

Fig. 2. Required and contingent workup for PAH; CTD = connective tissue disease; EBCT = embolism protocol CT angiogram; HRCT = high resolution CT; LFTs = liver function tests; RHC = right heart catheterization; VD = vasodilator trail; reproduced with permission from Ref. *40.*

4.1. Standard Echocardiography

The most useful initial diagnostic modality used to detect and/or confirm PAH is echocardiography. In PAH, echocardiography correlates well with invasive hemodynamics *(12)*, and it has the advantage of being noninvasive. Because echocardiography can evaluate both right and left heart anatomy and function, it is ideal for evaluating and excluding secondary causes of PH, such as left ventricular failure *(13)*, valvular heart disease, congenital heart disease with systemic-to-pulmonary shunts, and diastolic left ventricular dysfunction. Echocardiography has also been used to determine PAH severity, and is of prognostic utility. A measure of the degree of right ventricular dilation known as the eccentricity index *(14)* (the ratio of the left ventricular anterior-to-posterior dimension to the septal-to-lateral dimension at end diastole) has been shown to track clinical improvement in treated patients with PAH *(15,16)*. The degree of right ventricular systolic impairment, known as the Tei index *(17)*, has also been shown to be of prognostic significance in patients with PAH, as well as indices of left ventricular filling *(18)*. Finally, the presence of a pericardial effusion diagnosed by echocardiography also has prognostic significance *(14,19)*. Despite these attributes, echocardiography alone is inadequate for definitive confirmation of the presence or absence of PAH. For this, cardiac catheterization is required (see below). Table 1 summarizes the echocardiographic measurements that should be obtained in patients with PAH.

Table 1
Echocardiographic Measurements in Patients with PAH*

2D Measurements

Right ventricular size (chamber diameter and volume, and wall thickness)
Right ventricular/left ventricular diastolic volume, eccentricity index
Right ventricular contractility
Pericardial effusion (presence, size)
Inferior vena cava (IVC) size, respiratory variation
Right atrial area/volume

Doppler Measurements

Tricuspid regurgitation (severity and velocity)
Tei index
Left ventricular (LV) early diastolic filling velocity

*Additional measurements must be obtained when secondary pulmonary hypertension is suspected.

4.2. Six-Minute Walk Testing

A simple, inexpensive measure of the functional limitation in PAH patients is the six-minute walk (6MW) distance. This is used as a measure of functional capacity in patients with heart disease (20), has prognostic significance (21–23), and has been used in most randomized controlled trials of PAH therapies as the primary endpoint to demonstrate efficacy (24–30). While useful as a crude measure of aerobic capacity, the 6MW distance does not aid the clinician in confirming the diagnosis of suspected PAH, as it does not differentiate the nature of a patient's exercise limitation.

4.3. Cardiopulmonary Exercise Testing (CPET)

A noninvasive, comprehensive assessment of cardiopulmonary function can be obtained with the use of formal cardiopulmonary exercise testing (CPET). CPET also has prognostic significance (31), because it measures both cardiovascular and ventilatory performance during exercise. It has the advantage of aiding the clinician in determining the physiologic nature of a patient's limitation (i.e., determine the cause of unexplained dyspnea) (32–34). Interestingly, the peak systolic blood pressure (SBP) during CPET has been shown to be an independent predictor of mortality in untreated patients with PAH, with a peak SBP of less than 120 mm Hg correlating with a higher mortality than a peak SBP of more than 120 mm Hg (31).

In patients with PAH, CPET can quantitate PAH severity by assessing cardiovascular impairment and ventilatory inefficiency (35). The reduction in peak oxygen consumption (peak $\dot{V}O_2$) and increased ventilatory inefficiency ($\dot{V}E/\dot{V}CO_2$) are proportional to PAH disease severity, reflecting the inability of PAH patients to adequately increase pulmonary (and therefore systemic) blood flow during exercise (35). Early lactic acidosis in PAH, resulting from impaired blood flow to tissues, causing increased CO_2 output and ventilatory drive, is also best quantitated with CPET, measured as a decrease in the anaerobic threshold, or AT.

Additional useful CPET parameters include O_2 pulse ($\dot{V}O_2/HR$) and the ratio of the change in oxygen consumption with the change in work rate ($\Delta\dot{V}O_2/\Delta WR$). The O_2 pulse reflects the capacity of the heart to deliver oxygen per beat and is equal to the product of stroke volume and arterial-mixed venous O_2 difference. A decreasing O_2 pulse as work rate increases signifies a decreasing stroke volume. In normal patients, $\Delta\dot{V}O_2/\Delta WR$ is approximately 10 ml/min/W. In patients who are unable to increase their cardiac output in response to exercise, this ratio decreases proportional to the severity of the impairment in cardiac output with exercise.

4.4. Pulmonary Function Testing

Measurements of resting forced vital capacity (FVC), forced expiratory volume in 1 second (FEV1), maximum voluntary ventilation (MVV), diffusing capacity for carbon monoxide (DL_{CO}), effective alveolar volume (VA´), and total lung capacity (TLC) are essential components in the workup of PAH, as they can identify significant airway obstruction or mechanical defects as contributing factors to PH.

Pulmonary function testing has also been shown to quantitate the mechanical impairment related to the mild (but statistically significant) reduction in lung volume found in patients with PAH. This reduction in lung volume might be attributed to cardiomegaly and to loss of the normal distensibility of the smaller pulmonary arteries found in patients with PAH (36). The degree of lung volume reduction seen in PAH patients is proportional to the reduction in their peak $\dot{V}O_2$ In addition, DL_{CO} is significantly reduced in patients with PAH, also proportional to their reduction in peak $\dot{V}O_2$ This reduction in DL_{CO} likely reflects obliteration and diminished perfusion of the pulmonary capillary bed in PAH.

4.5. Chest Radiography

Because chest radiography is noninvasive and inexpensive, patients with unexplained dyspnea usually have a screening chest radiograph. Chest radiography is equally important as a first-line screening test in patients with PAH to seek evidence of secondary causes of PH, such as interstitial lung disease and pulmonary venous congestion.

The chest radiograph is often normal in PAH, or it may reveal cardiomegaly and/or an enlarged hilum. Not uncommonly, abnormalities that more specifically indicate the presence of PH are found, such as right ventricular enlargement (lateral view) and/or right atrial enlargement (P/A view), and/or dilated pulmonary arteries (≥ 18 mm Hg diameter in men, ≥ 16 mm Hg in women), occasionally with rapid tapering or "pruning" of the proximal vessels.

4.6. Electrocardiography

The electrocardiograph (ECG) in PAH often shows evidence of right atrial enlargement and right ventricular hypertrophy (3), and has been shown to be of prognostic value (37). ECG abnormalities alone, however, are insensitive indicators of pulmonary vascular disease. The use of serial ECG changes as markers of disease progression and/or response to therapy has not yet been reported. Electrocardiographic studies have been and continue to be collected in most major therapeutic trials for PAH; however, no recent reports of ECG findings in PAH have been reported in the medical literature.

4.7. Sleep Studies

There have been few systematic studies of patients with sleep disorders to evaluate the effect of sleep-disordered breathing on pulmonary hemodynamics. The available evidence suggests that in the absence of underlying respiratory impairment or sustained alveolar hypoxia, PH associated with sleep-disordered breathing is mild to moderate (mean PAP 25–30 mm Hg) *(38)*. Nevertheless, most experts believe that sleep-disordered breathing is an important factor to exclude in the workup of PAH. If the history reveals snoring, daytime hypersomnolence, obesity, or other features suggesting sleep-disordered breathing, screening overnight oximetry or formal polysomnography should be performed.

4.8. Ventilation–Perfusion (V/Q) Lung Scanning

Patients with chronic thromboembolic pulmonary hypertension (CTEPH) represent a significant proportion of PAH patients who have potentially correctable and occasionally curable PH *(39)*. Thus, it is of paramount importance to consider this diagnosis in all patients with documented PH, and to obtain studies to detect or exclude it. Most PAH experts agree that V/Q scanning should be the first-line diagnostic modality for the detection of CTEPH *(40,41)*. Contrast-enhanced, high-resolution computed tomography (CT) of the chest can be safely performed in patients with PAH *(42)*; however, it lacks sensitivity compared to V/Q scanning. It is nevertheless preferred in the presence of substantial underlying parenchymal disease that is likely to render the V/Q indeterminate, or when other etiologies are being considered, such as when there is substantial mediastinal adenopathy. Pulmonary angiography remains the definitive test to confirm the diagnosis of CTEPH, but is reserved for cases when further definition and characterization of suspected lesions are deemed desirable, or the patient is being considered for thromboendarterectomy.

5. INVASIVE TESTING

5.1. Cardiac Catheterization

Right heart catheterization with measurement of pulmonary hemodynamics is the gold standard for confirming and characterizing PAH. By definition, PAH requires demonstration of a mean PAP of ≥25 mm Hg at rest, or ≥30 mm Hg with exercise, and the exclusion of left-sided heart disease (5), i.e., a normal left ventricular end-diastolic pressure (LVEDP) or pulmonary capillary wedge pressure (PCWP). This can only be demonstrated via invasive hemodynamic monitoring, using a balloon flotation catheter to document pulmonary hemodynamics. Careful attention must be given to the PCWP tracing, as the pressure waveforms are often misinterpreted if the catheter is not in proper position. Table 2 lists the essential measurements that should be obtained during right heart catheterization.

Hemodynamics are prognostic in PAH (3,43), but, more importantly, serve to confirm the suspicion of PAH and exclude other secondary etiologies of PH. In particular, echocardiography's inability to measure PCWP (and thus LVEDP) bears important clinical significance, since it is essential to exclude pulmonary venous hypertension when making the diagnosis of PAH. Thus, most PAH experts believe that it is absolutely essential to obtain at least one diagnostic and confirmatory right heart catheterization in PAH patients.

The prognostic value of pulmonary hemodynamic measurements is illustrated by the finding that patients with IPAH whose mean right atrial pressure (RAP) is <10 mm Hg have a median survival of nearly 50

Table 2
Essential Right Heart Catheterization Measurements in Patients with PAH*

Systemic arterial pressure (BP) and heart rate (HR)
Right atrial pressure (RAP)
Right ventricular pressure (RVP)
Pulmonary artery pressure (PAP)
Pulmonary capillary wedge pressure (PCWP)
Cardiac output and index (thermodilution or Fick)
Pulmonary vasoreactivity (see text)
Systemic and pulmonary arterial oxygen saturation (and intracardiac, when intracardiac shunting is suspected)

*If right heart hemodynamics are not significantly abnormal at rest, exercise hemodynamics should be measured whenever possible.

months without pulmonary vasodilator therapy, whereas those with a mean RAP of ≥20 mm Hg survive less than 3 months *(44)*. RAP has also been shown to be prognostic in patients with systemic sclerosis *(45)*.

Realizing that the symptoms of PAH are mainly exertional, investigators have recently begun to focus upon exercise hemodynamics as a measure of hemodynamic exertional impairment *(46–48)*. However, major technical limitations to measuring exercise hemodynamics during catheterization include the lack of a standardized exercise protocol, practical mechanical difficulties in exercising subjects with invasive and intrusive catheters in place, and pressure wave artifacts related to chest wall motion and intrathoracic pressure variations during exercise.

5.2. Vasodilator Testing

During cardiac catheterization, most PAH experts suggest that acute vasodilator testing be performed at least once after PAH is diagnosed to determine pulmonary vascular vasoreactivity. Usually this is done during the confirmatory right heart catheterization. Pulmonary vasoreactivity is loosely defined as a decrease in mean PAP with a concomitant increase in cardiac output, indicating a prominent decrease in PVR after the administration of a selective pulmonary vasodilator (vasodilator "challenge"). Until recently, a "significant" response, one that would suggest clinical benefit from high-dose calcium channel blockers, was defined as a decrease in PAP and/or PVR, usually by at least 20% *(43,49–51)*. However, this practice has recently been challenged in recommendations put forth by the European Society of Cardiology, suggesting that only patients whose PAP drops by ≥10 mm Hg to a target of ≤40 mm Hg (with an increased or unchanged cardiac output) after a vasodilator challenge will benefit from high-dose calcium channel blockers *(52)*. The agents of choice for determining pulmonary vasoreactivity include intravenous epoprostenol, intravenous adenosine, inhaled nitric oxide, and inhaled iloprost. While these agents appear to effect similar responses when used in an acute challenge, they are not identical *(53)*. However, the clinical implications of this variability in vasoreactive responses are unclear. Further discussion of these issues can be found in Chapter 11.

5.3. Ambulatory Hemodynamic Monitoring

Monitoring of ambulatory hemodynamics is a promising but still investigational approach for assessing responses to therapy in PAH patients. One such device, the Chronicle® implantable monitor

(Medtronic, Inc., Minneapolis, MN), measures and stores a multitude of right heart and pulmonary hemodynamic measurements. It may prove useful in monitoring responses to therapy and may also lead to a better understanding of the physiology of PAH.

5.4. Lung Biopsy

Rarely, lung biopsy may be indicated in suspected IPAH patients when standard testing is insufficient to make a definitive diagnosis. As lung biopsy is risky in patients with severe PH (54), it should only be performed when the clinical diagnosis is unclear after an extensive workup (41). Examples of situations warranting a lung biopsy include those in which conditions are suspected such as vasculitis that might respond to immunosuppressives, or pulmonary veno-occlusive disease or pulmonary capillary hemangiomatosis that may have adverse responses to standard vasodilators.

6. LABORATORY TESTING

Patients suspected of PH should have a standard laboratory workup for dyspnea, which should include a full chemistry panel and complete blood count (CBC). In addition, specific laboratory analyses are usually obtained. HIV testing is recommended for patients with risk factors for HIV since the incidence of HIV-associated PAH is over 100-fold greater than that of IPAH (see above), and patients without advanced HIV complications whose PAH is untreated will likely die from PAH before succumbing to their HIV infection.

Thyroid function tests should be obtained because of reports of reversible PH occurring in association with hyperthyroidism (55,56). Liver function tests should also be checked to exclude the presence of significant liver disease, which may be associated with PAH (57,58), and also because specific PAH therapies have the potential for liver toxicity, requiring normal liver function at baseline prior to institution (25). CT scanning or ultrasound of the liver may be helpful if occult liver disease or portal hypertension is suspected.

Finally, screening for incipient autoimmune disease is recommended, including antinuclear antibodies (ANAs), rheumatoid factor, antiphospholipid antibodies, anticentromere antibodies if systemic sclerosis is suspected, and antineutrophil cytoplasmic antibodies (ANCAs) if vasculitis is suspected. Table 3 summarizes standard and optional or investigational laboratory tests that are obtained in patients with PAH.

Table 3
Laboratory Tests in PAH

Essential Testing

CBC
Chemistry panel (includes liver function testing)
HIV
Thyroid-stimulating hormone (TSH)
Antinuclear antibodies (ANAs)
Rheumatoid factor
Antiphospholipid antibody

Optional/Investigational Testing

Anticentromere antibodies
Antineutrophil cytoplasmic antibodies (ANCAs)
Brain natriuretic peptide (BNP)
Troponin T
Uric acid

6.1. Additional Testing

When clinically indicated, additional testing may be required to assist the clinician in confirming, excluding, or characterizing certain diagnoses suggested by standard diagnostic testing. These may include noncontrast, high-resolution CT scanning to assess the lung parenchyma for bronchiectasis, emphysema, or interstitial disease; contrast-enhanced, high-resolution CT scanning to detect and/or characterize pulmonary thromboembolic disease; and exercise echocardiography to elicit evidence of exercise-induced PH *(59)*.

6.2. Future Diagnostic Modalities

Emerging laboratory indicators promise additional utility in detecting or characterizing PAH. B-type natriuretic peptide (BNP) levels correlate with pulmonary hemodynamics and track response to therapy *(60)*, the levels are prognostic *(61)*, and they are also useful in detecting PAH in patients with CTDs and lung fibrosis *(62)*.

Troponin T, a marker of myocardial injury, is detectable in the serum of some patients with PAH. In one study, 7 (14%) of the 51 patients with PAH studied had detectable serum troponin T *(63)*. Of these, 5 (63%) died during the 24-month observation period, and in the 3 survivors troponin T became undetectable during the follow-up period. Troponin T may prove to be a useful indicator of response to therapy, either alone or in combination *(40)*.

Serum uric acid levels correlate with hemodynamics in patients with PAH (64,65), and are also prognostic (31,66); however, the mechanism(s) underlying the association between increased uric acid and PAH severity is unclear. It is thought that either poor tissue perfusion leading to increased tissue (and thus purine) breakdown or reduced glomerular filtration of uric acid may be responsible.

7. SUMMARY

The diagnosis of pulmonary arterial hypertension is complex and involves integrating clinical suspicion, physical findings and required diagnostic tests. These tests initially include noninvasive assessments of cardiopulmonary function and must be followed up with cardiac catheterization. Once PAH is diagnosed, further characterization of the PAH disease process with additional testing can help in assessing PAH severity and response to therapy.

REFERENCES

1. Galiè N, Rubin LJ. New insights into a challenging disease. A review of the Third World Symposium on Pulmonary Arterial Hypertension. J Am Coll Cardiol 2004; 43:1S.
2. Rubin LJ. Diagnosis and management of pulmonary arterial hypertension: ACCP evidence-based clinical practice guidelines. Chest 2004; 126: 7S–10S.
3. Rich S, Dantzker DR, Ayres SM, et al. Primary pulmonary hypertension: A national prospective study. Ann Intern Med 1987; 107:216–23.
4. Gaine SP, Rubin LJ. Primary pulmonary hypertension. Lancet 1998; 352:719–25.
5. Rubin LJ. Primary pulmonary hypertension. N Engl J Med 1997; 336: 111–7.
6. Petitpretz P, Brenot F, Azarian R, et al. Pulmonary hypertension in patients with human immunodeficiency virus infection: Comparison with primary pulmonary hypertension. Circulation 1994; 89:2722–7.
7. de Chadarevian JP, Lischner HW, Karmazin N, et al. Pulmonary hypertension and HIV infection: New observations and review of the syndrome. Mod Pathol 1994; 7:685–9.
8. Abenhaim L, Moride Y, Brenot F, et al. Appetite-suppressant drugs and the risk of primary pulmonary hypertension. International Primary Pulmonary Hypertension Study Group. N Engl J Med 1996; 335:609–16.
9. Thomson JR, Machado RD, Pauciulo MW, et al. Sporadic primary pulmonary hypertension is associated with germline mutations of the gene encoding BMPR-II, a receptor member of the TGF- family. J Med Genet 2000; 37:741–5.

10. Loyd JE, Butler MG, Foroud TM, et al. Genetic anticipation and abnormal gender ratio at birth in familial primary pulmonary hypertension. Am J Respir Crit Care Med 1995; 152:93–7.
11. Simonneau G, Galiè N, Rubin LJ, et al. Clinical classification of pulmonary hypertension. J Am Coll Cardiol 2004; 43:5S–12S.
12. Shapiro SM, Oudiz RJ, Cao T, et al. Primary pulmonary hypertension: Improved long-term effects and survival with continuous intravenous epoprostenol infusion. J Am Coll Cardiol 1997; 30:343–9.
13. Abramson SV, Burke JF, Kelly JJ Jr., et al. Pulmonary hypertension predicts mortality and morbidity in patients with dilated cardiomyopathy. Ann Intern Med 1992; 116:888–95.
14. Ryan T, Petrovic O, Dillon JC, et al. An echocardiographic index for separation of right ventricular volume and pressure overload. J Am Coll Cardiol 1985; 5:918–24.
15. Galiè N, Hinderliter AL, Torbicki A, et al. Effects of the oral endothelin-receptor antagonist bosentan on echocardiographic and doppler measures in patients with pulmonary arterial hypertension. J Am Coll Cardiol 2003; 41:1380–6.
16. Jimenez Lopez-Guarch C, Escribano Subias P, Tello de Meneses R, et al. Efficacy of oral sildenafil as rescue therapy in patients with severe pulmonary arterial hypertension chronically treated with prostacyclin. Long-term results. Rev Esp Cardiol 2004; 57:946–51.
17. Tei C, Dujardin KS, Hodge DO, et al. Doppler echocardiographic index for assessment of global right ventricular function. J Am Soc Echocardiogr 1996; 9:838–47.
18. Yeo TC, Dujardin KS, Tei C, et al. Value of a Doppler-derived index combining systolic and diastolic time intervals in predicting outcome in primary pulmonary hypertension. Am J Cardiol 1998; 81:1157–61.
19. Raymond RJ, Hinderliter AL, Willis PW, et al. Echocardiographic predictors of adverse outcomes in primary pulmonary hypertension. J Am Coll Cardiol 2002; 39:1214–9.
20. Guyatt GH, Sullivan MJ, Thompson PJ, et al. The 6-minute walk: A new measure of exercise capacity in patients with chronic heart failure. Can Med Assoc J 1985; 132:919–23.
21. Miyamoto S, Nagaya N, Satoh T, et al. Clinical correlates and prognostic significance of six-minute walk test in patients with primary pulmonary hypertension: Comparison with cardiopulmonary exercise testing. Am J Respir Crit Care Med 2000; 161,487–92.
22. Sitbon O, Humbert M, Nunes H, et al. Long-term intravenous epoprostenol infusion in primary pulmonary hypertension: Prognostic factors and survival. J Am Coll Cardiol 2002; 40:780–8.
23. Paciocco G, Martinez FJ, Bossone E, et al. Oxygen desaturation on the six-minute walk test and mortality in untreated primary pulmonary hypertension. Eur Respir J 2001; 17:647–52.

24. Channick RN, Simonneau G, Sitbon O, et al. Effects of the dual endothelin-receptor antagonist bosentan in patients with pulmonary hypertension: A randomised placebo-controlled study. Lancet 2001; 358: 1119–23.

25. Rubin LJ, Badesch DB, Barst RJ, et al. Bosentan therapy for pulmonary arterial hypertension. N Engl J Med 2002; 346:896–903.

26. Galiè N, Humbert M, Vachiery JL, et al. Effects of beraprost sodium, an oral prostacyclin analogue, in patients with pulmonary arterial hypertension: A randomized, double-blind, placebo-controlled trial. J Am Coll Cardiol 2002; 39:1496–502.

27. Simonneau G, Barst RJ, Galiè N, et al. Continuous subcutaneous infusion of treprostinil, a prostacyclin analogue, in patients with pulmonary arterial hypertension. A double-blind, randomized, placebo-controlled trial. Am J Respir Crit Care Med 2002; 165:800–4.

28. Barst RJ, McGoon M, McLaughlin V, et al. Beraprost therapy for pulmonary arterial hypertension. J Am Coll Cardiol 2003; 41:2119–25.

29. Olschewski H, Simonneau G, Galiè N, et al. Inhaled iloprost for severe pulmonary hypertension. N Engl J Med 2002; 347:322–9.

30. Langleben D, Christman BW, Barst RJ, et al. Effects of the thromboxane synthetase inhibitor and receptor antagonist terbogrel in patients with primary pulmonary hypertension. Am Heart J 2002; 143:E4.

31. Wensel R, Opitz C, Anker SD, et al. Assessment of survival in patients with primary pulmonary hypertension: Importance of cardiopulmonary exercise testing. Circulation 2002; 106:319–24.

32. Markowitz DH, Systrom DM. Diagnosis of pulmonary vascular limit to exercise by cardiopulmonary exercise testing. J Heart Lung Transplant 2004; 23:88–95.

33. Oudiz RJ. Sun XG. Abnormalities in exercise gas exchange in primary pulmonary hypertension. In K Wasserman, ed. Cardiopulmonary Exercise Testing and Cardiovascular Health. Armonk, NY: Futura Publishing Co., 2002:179–90.

34. Wasserman K, Hansen JE, Sue DY, Casaburi R, Whipp BJ, ed. Principles of Exercise Testing and Interpretation, 4th edn. Philadelphia, PA: Lippincott Williams & Wilkins, 2004.

35. Sun X-G, Oudiz RJ, Hansen JE, Wasserman K. Exercise pathophysiology in primary pulmonary vascular hypertension. Circulation 2001; 104: 429–35.

36. Sun XG, Hansen JE, Oudiz RJ, Wasserman K. Pulmonary function in primary pulmonary hypertension. J Am Coll Cardiol 2003; 41:1028–35.

37. Bossone E, Paciocco G, Iarussi D, et al. The prognostic role of the ECG in primary pulmonary hypertension. Chest 2002; 121:513–8.

38. Bady E, Achkar A, Pascal S, Orvoen-Frija E, Laaban JP. Pulmonary arterial hypertension in patients with sleep apnoea syndrome. Thorax 2000; 55:934–9.

39. Auger WR, Kerr KM, Kim NH, Ben-Yehuda O, Knowlton KU, Fedullo PF. Chronic thromboembolic pulmonary hypertension. Cardiol Clin 2004; 22:453–66.

40. Barst RJ, McGoon M, Torbicki A, et al. Diagnosis and differential assessment of pulmonary arterial hypertension. J Am Coll Cardiol 2004; 43:40S–47S.

41. McGoon M, Gutterman D, Steen V, et al. Screening, early detection, and diagnosis of pulmonary arterial hypertension—ACCP evidence-based clinical practice guidelines. Chest 2004; 126:14S–34S.

42. Oudiz RJ, Budoff MJ, Brundage BH. Safety of EBCT contrast injection studies in severe pulmonary hypertension. Int J Cardiac Imaging 2000; 16:399–403.

43. Sandoval J, Bauerle O, Palomar A, et al. Survival in primary pulmonary hypertension. Validation of a prognostic equation. Circulation 1994; 89:1733–44.

44. D'Alonzo GE, Barst RJ, Ayres SM, et al. Survival in patients with primary pulmonary hypertension. Results from a national prospective registry. Ann Intern Med 1991; 115:343–9.

45. Mukerjee D, St George D, Coleiro B, et al. Prevalence and outcome in systemic sclerosis associated pulmonary arterial hypertension: Application of a registry approach. Ann Rheum Dis 2003; 62:1088–93.

46. Raeside DA, Chalmers G, Clelland J, et al. Pulmonary artery pressure variation in patients with connective tissue disease: 24 hour ambulatory pulmonary artery pressure monitoring. Thorax 1998; 53:857–62.

47. James KB, Maurer J, Wolski K, et al. Exercise hemodynamic findings in patients with exertional dyspnea. Tex Heart Inst J 2000; 27:100–5.

48. Raeside DA, Smith A, Brown A, et al. Pulmonary artery pressure measurement during exercise testing in patients with suspected pulmonary hypertension. Eur Respir J 2000; 16:282–7.

49. Rich S, Kaufmann E, Levy PS. The effect of high doses of calcium-channel blockers on survival in primary pulmonary hypertension. N Engl J Med 1992; 327:76–81.

50. Weir EK, Rubin LJ, Ayres SM, et al. The acute administration of vasodilators in primary pulmonary hypertension. Experience from the National Institutes of Health registry on primary pulmonary hypertension. Am Rev Respir Dis 1989; 140:1623–30.

51. Sitbon O, Humbert M, Jagot JL, et al. Inhaled nitric oxide as a screening agent for sagely identifying responders to oral calcium-channel blockers in primary pulmonary hypertension. Eur Respir J 1998; 12:265–70.

52. Rubin LJ. Diagnosis and management of pulmonary arterial hypertension: ACCP evidence-based clinical practice guidelines. Chest 2004; 126: 4S–6S.

53. Nootens M, Schrader B, Kaufmann E, Vestal R, Long W, Rich S. Comparative acute effects of adenosine and prostacyclin in primary pulmonary hypertension. Chest 1995; 107:54–7.

54. Nicod P, Moser KM. Primary pulmonary hypertension: The risk and benefit of lung biopsy. Circulation 1989; 80:1486–8.

55. Virani SS, Mendoza CE, Ferreira AC, de Marchena E. Graves' disease and pulmonary hypertension: Report of 2 cases. Tex Heart Inst J 2003; 30:314–5.

56. Lozano HF, Sharma CN. Reversible pulmonary hypertension, tricuspid regurgitation and right-sided heart failure associated with hyperthyroidism: Case report and review of the literature. Cardiol Rev 2004; 12:299–305.

57. Schraufnagel DE, Kay JM. Structural and pathologic changes in the lung vasculature in chronic liver disease. Clin Chest Med 1996; 17:1–15.

58. Niemann C, Mandell S. Pulmonary hypertension and liver transplantation. Pulm Perspect 2003; 20:4–6.

59. Bossone E, Rubenfire M, Bach DS, et al. Range of tricuspid regurgitation velocity at rest and during exercise in normal adult men: Implications for the diagnosis of pulmonary hypertension. J Am Coll Cardiol 1999; 33:1662–6.

60. Nagaya N, Nishikimi T, Okano Y, et al. Plasma brain natriuretic peptide levels increase in proportion to the extent of right ventricular dysfunction in pulmonary hypertension. J Am Coll Cardiol 1998; 31:202–8.

61. Nagaya N, Nishikimi T, Uematsu M, et al. Plasma brain natriuretic peptide as a prognostic indicator in patients with primary pulmonary hypertension. Circulation 2000; 102:865–70.

62. Mukerjee D, Yap LB, Holmes AM, et al. Significance of plasma N-terminal pro-brain natriuretic peptide in patients with systemic sclerosis-related pulmonary arterial hypertension. Respir Med 2003; 97: 1230–6.

63. Torbicki A, Kurzyna M, Kuca P, et al. Detectable serum cardiac troponin T as a marker of poor prognosis among patients with chronic precapillary pulmonary hypertension. Circulation 2003; 108:844–8.

64. Hoeper MM, Hohlfeld JM, Fabel H. Hyperuricaemia in patients with right or left heart failure. Eur Respir J 1999; 13:682–5.

65. Voelkel MA, Wynne KM, Badesch DB, Groves BM, Voelkel NF. Hyperuricemia in severe pulmonary hypertension. Chest 2000; 117:19–24.

66. Nagaya N, Uematsu M, Satoh T, et al. Serum uric acid levels correlate with the severity and mortality of primary pulmonary hypertension. Am J Respir Crit Care Med 1999; 160:487–92.

4 Pathophysiology of Pulmonary Arterial Hypertension

Harrison W. Farber

CONTENTS

INTRODUCTION
IMBALANCE OF VASOACTIVE MEDIATORS
ENVIRONMENTAL ASSOCIATIONS WITH
    PULMONARY ARTERIAL HYPERTENSION
CONDITIONS ASSOCIATED WITH PULMONARY
    ARTERIAL HYPERTENSION
GENETIC ABNORMALITIES ASSOCIATED
    WITH PULMONARY HYPERTENSION
CONCLUSIONS
REFERENCES

Abstract

Pulmonary arterial hypertension comprises a group of clinical and patho-physiological entities with similar features but a variety of underlying causes. Genetic polymorphisms, environmental exposures, and acquired disorders predispose patients to PAH, but none of the factors alone is sufficient to cause the disease. PAH is an end-stage phenotype that represents a final common manifestation of multiple preclinical, intermediate phenotypes. Thus, an understanding of the preclinical disease in at-risk populations will be critical for identifying the primary pathogenic mechanisms. Because clinically apparent disease occurs in only a small percentage of carriers of BMPR2, ALK1, and 5HTT mutations, other modifier genes are likely important in the pathogenesis of the disease. Thus, a multiple-hit theory seems to apply, similar to that

From: *Contemporary Cardiology: Pulmonary Hypertension*
Edited by: N. S. Hill and H. W. Farber © Humana Press, Totowa, NJ

often invoked for the development of cancers in which susceptible persons
with a genetic predisposition require additional insults before manifesting the
disease. Expanded natural history studies and further evaluation of persons
at risk for pulmonary arterial hypertension (e.g., those with mutations of the
TGF-β pathway and other identified mutations), as well as a better understanding of the disease-modifying genetic and acquired determinants, will
provide improved insight into the relation between these genotypes and this
complicated phenotype.

Key Words: pulmonary hypertension pathogenesis; genetic mutations;
transformin growth factor beta; serotonin; endothelin; nitric oxide; remodeling.

1. INTRODUCTION

Pulmonary hypertension is defined as the sustained elevation
of mean pulmonary arterial pressure (PAP) ≥25 mm Hg at
rest, ≥30 mm Hg during exercise, or a systolic PAP >45
mm Hg, with a mean pulmonary capillary wedge pressure and
left ventricular end-diastolic pressure of less than 15 mm Hg
(1). Frequently associated with left heart disease, chronic lung
disease complicated by hypoxemia, and recurrent or chronic thromboembolic disease, pulmonary hypertension is less commonly
caused by a primary defect of the pulmonary vasculature *(2)*.
Now known as idiopathic pulmonary arterial hypertension (IPAH;
formerly primary pulmonary hypertension), this condition is characterized by the occlusion of capillary-like channels associated
with intimal fibrosis, increased medial thickness, and plexiform
lesions.

In the past, pulmonary hypertension was classified as either primary
(idiopathic) or secondary to another disease state *(3)*. It is now
clear, however, that within the classification of secondary pulmonary
hypertension, conditions with similar histopathology and response to
treatment as IPAH exist. For this reason, the World Health Organization recently classified pulmonary hypertension in five different
groups based on pathophysiology rather than associated disease
(Table 1). Group 1 is designated pulmonary arterial hypertension
(PAH) and comprises IPAH as well as pulmonary hypertension in
the setting of conditions, such as collagen vascular disease, portal
hypertension, congenital left-to-right shunts, infection with the human
immunodeficiency virus, and persistent pulmonary hypertension of the
newborn. Lung tissue from individuals with each of these entities
demonstrates a very similar histological appearance. The other groups
of pulmonary hypertensive patients in this classification system include

Table 1
WHO Classification of Pulmonary Hypertension

Group 1	Pulmonary arterial hypertension
Group 2	Pulmonary venous hypertension
Group 3	Chronic lung disease
Group 4	Venous thromboembolic disease
Group 5	Miscellaneous disorders

those with pulmonary venous hypertension (group 2), chronic lung diseases (group 3), thromboembolic disease (group 4), and miscellaneous entities such as schistosomiasis or sarcoidosis (group 5).

The pathogenesis of most forms of pulmonary hypertension is unknown; however, there have been many recent developments especially pertaining to the molecular genetics of IPAH. This chapter discusses these developments, with particular reference to IPAH, and relates them to other forms of pulmonary hypertension.

2. IMBALANCE OF VASOACTIVE MEDIATORS

Vascular changes that have been observed in pulmonary hypertension include vasoconstriction, cellular proliferation, and thrombosis, suggesting that an imbalance may exist between vasodilators and vasoconstrictors as well as between growth inhibitors and mitogenic factors.

2.1. Prostacyclin/Thromboxane A_2

Prostacyclin and thromboxane A_2 are major arachidonic acid metabolites of both endothelial cells and smooth muscle cells. Prostacyclin is a potent vasodilator, inhibits platelet aggregation, and has antiproliferative properties; in contrast, thromboxane A_2 is a potent vasoconstrictor *(4,5)*. In pulmonary hypertension, the balance between these two molecules is shifted toward thromboxane A_2 *(6)*. In patients with IPAH and secondary pulmonary hypertension, a decrease in urinary levels of 2,3-dinor-6-keto-prostaglandin $F1_\alpha$, a metabolite of prostacyclin, and an increase in urinary levels in 11-dehydro-thromboxane B_2, a metabolite of thromboxane A_2, have been observed. Furthermore, the expression of prostacyclin synthetase, the enzyme responsible for synthesis of prostacyclin, is decreased in the small and medium-sized pulmonary arteries of patients with pulmonary hypertension, particularly patients with IPAH *(7)*. Transfection of this enzyme in pulmonary artery smooth muscle cells protects against hypoxia-induced pulmonary hypertension in an animal model *(8)*.

2.2. Endothelin-1

Endothelin-1 (ET-1) is a potent vasoconstrictor and has mitogenic activity for pulmonary artery smooth muscle cells *(9)*. Increased levels of ET-1 have been found in rat models of pulmonary hypertension as well as in the plasma and the pulmonary vascular wall of patients with IPAH and other forms of pulmonary hypertension *(10–12)*. This increase in ET-1 levels is proportional to the magnitude of pulmonary blood flow and cardiac output *(13)*.

2.3. Nitric Oxide

Nitric oxide (NO) is a potent vasodilator, an inhibitor of platelet activation, and an inhibitor of vascular smooth muscle cell proliferation; it is synthesized by the NO synthase family of enzymes. Decreased levels of the endothelial isoform of NO synthase have been observed in an animal model of hypoxia-induced pulmonary hypertension *(14)* as well as in pulmonary vascular tissue of patients with pulmonary hypertension, particularly IPAH *(15)*. Endothelial nitric oxide synthase is increased, however, in the plexiform lesions of idiopathic pulmonary arterial hypertension, where it could promote pulmonary endothelial cell proliferation *(16)*.

2.4. Serotonin

Serotonin (5-hydroxytryptamine) is a vasoconstrictor that promotes smooth muscle hypertrophy and hyperplasia *(17)*; multiple abnormalities in the serotonin system have been reported in patients with pulmonary hypertension. Elevated plasma serotonin levels and reduced content of serotonin in platelets have been reported in patients with IPAH; interestingly, these abnormalities persist even after normalization of pulmonary artery pressures following lung transplantation *(18)*. In patients with a platelet storage defect associated with decreased uptake of serotonin (δ storage pool disease), there is a much higher than expected incidence of pulmonary hypertension *(19)*. Exposure to the appetite suppressant medication dexfenfluramine (Redux), which increases platelet serotonin release and inhibits its reuptake, is associated with an increased incidence of pulmonary hypertension *(20)*. In addition, recent reports have described mutations in the serotonin transporter (5HTT) and/or serotonin receptors (5HT) in the platelets and lung tissue from patients with primary and secondary forms of pulmonary hypertension *(21)*. However, the level of serotonin itself is probably not a basic determinant of pulmonary hypertension, since selective serotonin-reuptake inhibitors (SSRIs), which increase serotonin levels but inhibit serotonin transport, are not associated with an increased incidence of pulmonary hypertension and may, in fact, be protective in the setting of hypoxia *(22)*.

2.5. Adrenomedullin

Adrenomedullin dilates pulmonary vessels, increases pulmonary blood flow, and is synthesized by several cell populations in the normal lung. High levels of messenger RNA for adrenomedullin and its receptor in the lungs suggest a regulatory role for the peptide in the pulmonary circulation *(23)*. Plasma levels are elevated in experimental pulmonary hypertension as well as in IPAH and other forms of pulmonary hypertension *(24,25)*. Plasma levels of adrenomedullin have been correlated with mean right atrial pressure, total pulmonary vascular resistance, and mean pulmonary arterial pressure, suggesting that plasma levels of adrenomedullin increase in proportion to the extent of pulmonary hypertension *(26)*. In addition, chronic infusion of adrenomedullin attenuates pulmonary hypertension and medial thickening of pulmonary arteries in rats treated with monocrotaline *(27)*.

2.6. Vasoactive Intestinal Peptide

Vasoactive intestinal peptide (VIP), a potent systemic vasodilator, decreases pulmonary artery pressure and pulmonary vascular resistance in rabbits with monocrotaline-induced pulmonary hypertension *(28)* and in healthy human subjects *(29)*; it also inhibits platelet activation *(30)* and vascular smooth muscle cell proliferation *(31)*. A recent study reported decreased levels of VIP in the serum and lungs of patients with pulmonary arterial hypertension *(32)*.

2.7. Vascular Endothelial Cell Growth Factor

Lungs exposed to acute or chronic hypoxia demonstrate increased expression of vascular endothelial cell growth factor (VEGF) and its receptors, VEGF receptor 1 (KDR/Flk) and VEGF receptor 2 (Flt) *(33)*. Inhibition of VEGF signaling in neonatal rats leads to adult pulmonary hypertension *(34)*, consistent with the normal physiological responses of the VEGF signaling system as an adaptation mechanism for hypoxia. In individuals with IPAH and plexiform lesions, however, disordered angiogenic responses appear to underlie the process. Tuder and colleagues showed that, in plexiform lesions from patients with

IPAH, VEGF mRNA and protein were present; there was also increased expression of VEGF receptor-2, hypoxia inducible factor-alpha, and hypoxia-inducible factor-beta and decreased expression of phosphinositide-3-kinase, Akt, and src, three signaling molecules essential for the angiogenic response to VEGF *(35)*. These data suggest that IPAH patients with established disease have an inadequate molecular angiogenic response to hypoxia because of abnormal signaling intermediates.

2.8. Summary

There is an imbalance of the vascular effectors in PAH that favors vasoconstriction, vascular cell proliferation, and thrombosis. The treatments developed on the basis of these observations (i.e., epoprostenol, nitric oxide, and endothelin-receptor antagonists) have been effective in improving the pulmonary vascular hemodynamics, clinical status, and, in some cases, survival in idiopathic and other forms of pulmonary arterial hypertension. However, none of these vasoactive molecules has yet been conclusively linked to the primary pathogenesis of the disease.

3. ENVIRONMENTAL ASSOCIATIONS WITH PULMONARY ARTERIAL HYPERTENSION

Among the many environmental factors associated with an increased risk for the development of pulmonary hypertension, three—hypoxia, anorexigens, and central nervous system stimulants—have more substantive data (Table 2) than others. The other factors included in this section are based on less substantial evidence.

Table 2
Pulmonary Hypertension:
Environmental Associations

Hypoxia
Anorexigens
Pyrrolizidine alkaloids
Toxic oil syndrome
L-tryptophan
Methamphetamine, cocaine

3.1. Hypoxia

The response of the pulmonary vasculature to hypoxia is distinctly different from that of the systemic circulation. In order to optimize the relationship between ventilation and perfusion, hypoxia induces pulmonary vasoconstriction. This acute effect of hypoxia is regulated by endothelial products, including endothelin-1 and serotonin, and by hypoxia-mediated changes in ion channel activity in pulmonary artery smooth muscle cells (36). Voltage-gated potassium (Kv) channel activity controls the membrane potential, which regulates the intracellular calcium concentration. Acute hypoxia inhibits Kv channel function in pulmonary artery smooth muscle cells, leading to membrane depolarization, a rise in the cytoplasmic calcium concentration, and vasoconstriction (37). Whereas acute hypoxia causes reversible changes in pulmonary vascular tone, chronic hypoxia leads to structural remodeling, vascular smooth muscle cell proliferation and migration, and increased vascular matrix deposition. Chronic responses are likely regulated, in part, by hypoxia-inducible genes (38); some of these genes may also cause neovascularization via elaboration of VEGF (39).

3.2. Anorexigens

Association between anorexigens (appetite suppressants) and pulmonary hypertension was initially observed in the 1960s when an epidemic of IPAH was noted in Europe following the introduction of the anorexigen aminorex fumarate (40). Although this medication was withdrawn from the market, structurally related compounds, such as fenfluramine and dexfenfluramine, were subsequently developed in the 1980s. Use of these agents has also been associated with an increased incidence of IPAH (20). Although the incidence of pulmonary hypertension increases with the duration of use, elevation in pulmonary pressure can occur with as little as four weeks' exposure to these agents (41,42).

3.3. Methamphetamine and Cocaine

Stimulants, including methamphetamine and cocaine, have been associated with an increased incidence of pulmonary hypertension (43). Although it has been suggested that contaminants in illegally synthesized methamphetamine play a major role in causing pulmonary hypertension (44), pulmonary hypertension occurs with use of the contaminant-free amphetamine-like stimulant anorectic drugs fenfluramines and aminorex fumarate. In an autopsy study of 20 heavy smokers of cocaine, the lungs of four (20%) demonstrated medial hypertrophy in the pulmonary arteries, consistent with pulmonary hypertension, without evidence of foreign-particle microembolization *(45)*. Proposed mechanisms include toxic endothelial injury, hypoxic insult, direct vasospasm, vasculitis, and dysregulation of mediators of vascular tone. Use of stimulants and/or exposure to adulterants contaminating them may play an important role in the development of foreign-body granulomas and microembolization that can result in pulmonary hypertension; whether the stimulants by themselves can result in pulmonary hypertension is not yet clear.

3.4. Monocrotaline

Monocrotaline is a pyrrolizidine alkaloid of plant origin that is toxic to the pulmonary vasculature. Monocrotaline must first be oxidized to its pyrrole derivative in the liver to cause pulmonary endothelial cell injury *(46)*. Other members of this family, especially those with unsaturated double bonds in the 1,2 position, are hepatotoxins as well and may account for the hepatic cirrhosis observed with the ingestion of Jamaican bush tea *(47)*. Monocrotaline is principally used to produce pulmonary hypertension in rodent models of the disease.

3.5. Rapeseed oil (Toxic Oil Syndrome)

An epidemic of pulmonary hypertension associated with adulterated cooking oil (rapeseed oil) occurred in Spain in the early 1980s *(48)*. This condition, termed "toxic oil syndrome," was characterized by a respiratory distress syndrome associated with myositis, eosinophilia, widespread vasculitis, and polyneuropathy. Sclerodermiform skin changes and Raynaud's phenomenon were prominent late features that affected women almost exclusively. Pulmonary hypertension developed in ∼20% of the patients; in many, it spontaneously regressed *(49)*. In a small subgroup, however, it progressed rapidly, leading to cor pulmonale and death. The pulmonary hypertension that developed in these individuals was clinically and histologically indistinguishable from IPAH. Although the responsible toxin(s) was never identified conclusively, similar findings were observed in animals fed rapeseed oil, suggesting that direct endothelial injury by the rapeseed oil or possibly oleoanilid contaminants could be the trigger for this type of pulmonary hypertension.

3.6. L-tryptophan

L-tryptophan was prescribed as a treatment for insomnia and neurasthenia and was widely used as a self-medication for improving health in various ways. By 1989, an estimated 2% of Americans were using this agent; however, case reports began to appear of a life-threatening disease seemingly related to tryptophan use: the eosinophilia-myalgia syndrome *(50)*. Approximately 1,500 individuals with the syndrome, characterized by eosinophilia, fasciitis, and, in some cases, sclerodermiform skin changes, Raynaud's phenomenon, and, occasionally, severe pulmonary hypertension, were reported. Interestingly, the pathology resembles the toxic oil syndrome in numerous respects *(51,52)*. Despite a considerable literature on this disease, its cause remains unknown and controversial; both L-tryptophan itself and contaminants of the manufacturing process have been implicated *(53)*.

4. CONDITIONS ASSOCIATED WITH PULMONARY ARTERIAL HYPERTENSION

Several coexisting conditions have been associated with PAH (Table 3). Those with plausible mechanistic links include scleroderma, infection with the human immunodeficiency virus (HIV), human herpesvirus (HHV), portal hypertension, thrombocytosis, hemoglobinopathies, and hereditary hemorrhagic telangiectasia.

4.1. Connective Tissue Diseases

A primary pulmonary arteriopathy occurs most commonly in limited systemic sclerosis (SSc), especially the CREST variant (calcinosis,

Table 3
Pulmonary Hypertension: Associated Disorders

Connective tissue diseases
HIV infection
Portal hypertension
Thrombocytosis
Asplenia
Hemoglobinopathies
Hereditary hemorrhagic telangiectasia

Raynaud's phenomenon, esophageal dysmotility, sclerodactyly, telang-iectasias) *(54–56)*. At autopsy, up to 80% of individuals will have histopathological changes consistent with PAH; however, only 10–15% will develop clinically apparent disease. Histology consistent with PAH has also been observed in systemic lupus erythematosus (SLE), mixed connective tissue disease (MCTD), and rheumatoid arthritis (RA). In all of these disorders, there is a strong association between the presence of pulmonary hypertension and the presence of Raynaud's phenomenon, suggesting that there may be similarities in these vasculopathies *(57)*.

4.2. Infection with the Human Immunodeficiency Virus (HIV)

An association between HIV infection and pulmonary hypertension was first reported in 1991; initial cases occurred primarily in those individuals who acquired HIV infection after receiving blood products for hemophilia *(58,59)*. Since then, almost 150 cases have been reported and have encompassed all etiologies for acquiring HIV infection. Population studies of individuals infected with HIV suggest that the incidence of pulmonary hypertension is approximately 0.5%, or 6–12 times that of the general population. The occurrence of pulmonary hypertension is independent of the CD4 count but appears related to the duration of HIV infection. Many of these patients also have foreign-body emboli from the use of intravenous drugs and/or portal hypertension from a concomitant infection with hepatitis B or C; moreover, both of these entities, intravenous drug use and portal hyper-tension, have been associated with pulmonary hypertension. Because HIV does not directly infect endothelial cells, the mechanism of pulmonary hypertension in HIV infection is unclear.

4.3. Portal Hypertension

Although uncommon, an association between portal hypertension and the development of pulmonary hypertension exists. In a large autopsy series, histological changes consistent with pulmonary hyper-tension occurred in 0.73% of individuals with cirrhosis, six times the prevalence in all autopsies *(60)*. Hemodynamic studies have estimated the prevalence of pulmonary hypertension in these individuals at 2% and 5% *(61)*; however, the prevalence may be higher in patients referred for liver transplantation, ranging from 3.5% to 8.5% *(62)*. In studies using two-dimensional echocardiography of patients under-going evaluation for orthotopic liver transplantation, the incidence of pulmonary hypertension was estimated at 12%; however, this incidence was not confirmed by right heart catheterization (63). With right heart catheterization, the incidence of pulmonary hypertension in these patients is approximately 6% (64). The diagnosis of pulmonary hypertension is usually made four to seven years after the diagnosis of portal hypertension (65) but, in some cases, may precede it. In addition, the risk of developing pulmonary hypertension increases with the duration of portal hypertension. The mechanism of this association is unclear, but cirrhosis without the presence of portal hypertension appears to be insufficient for the development of pulmonary hypertension.

4.4. Thrombocytosis

There is an also association among thrombocytosis, chronic myelodysplastic syndrome, and the development of pulmonary hypertension (66,67). Although there are several case reports and small series of the two entities occurring simultaneously, there is one large reported cohort of 26 patients with chronic myelodysplastic syndrome and unexplained pulmonary hypertension; of these patients, 14 of 26 had elevated platelet counts (median: $\sim600 \times 10^9$) (67). In this group of patients, the incidence of pulmonary hypertension was 5 to 40 times greater than that in the general population, occurred at a much later age than IPAH, and portended a worse prognosis than in IPAH not associated with chronic myelodysplastic syndrome. Possible explanations invoked for the association of the two diseases include the hypermetabolism associated with chronic myelodysplastic syndrome resulting in a chronic high-output state, the chronic disseminated intravascular coagulation associated with CMD leading to the deposition of microthrombi in the pulmonary circulation, and the increased incidence of portal hypertension in these patients.

In many cases, the degree of pulmonary hypertension correlated directly with the platelet count, patients' symptoms mirrored changes in platelet counts, and, in two cases, direct obstruction of pulmonary arteries by circulating megakaryocytes was demonstrated, suggesting that platelets play a central role in the etiology of this process (68). Thus, it is possible that platelet-derived products, such as serotonin or platelet-derived growth factor, are important in the development of pulmonary hypertension in these patients. Platelet-derived growth factor is a strong stimulus for smooth muscle proliferation, and in an animal model of pulmonary hypertension, control of the platelet count retards the development of pulmonary hypertension.

4.5. Asplenia

An increased incidence of asplenia has been reported in patients with pulmonary hypertension *(69,70)*. In one study, the prevalence of postsplenectomy asplenia in patients with pulmonary hypertension was 11.5%; there were no cases of asplenia in the control group (patients without pulmonary hypertension) *(69)*. Lung specimens from postsplenectomy patients with pulmonary hypertension demonstrate abundant thrombotic lesions, intimal fibrosis, and plexiform lesions. It has been speculated that after splenectomy, abnormal erythrocytes remain in the circulatory system longer and trigger platelet activation, leading to thrombi in the pulmonary vascular bed; however, splenectomy can also cause portal hypertension, a risk for the development of pulmonary hypertension *(70)*. In addition, as the spleen buffers circulating platelet counts, asplenia is also associated with significant elevations in circulating platelets. Thus, although it appears that splenectomy is a risk factor for the development of pulmonary hypertension, the pathogenic mechanism(s) is not yet clear and likely complicated.

4.6. Hemoglobinopathies

Several studies have documented pulmonary hypertension and right ventricular dysfunction in patients with thalassemia, particularly homozygous beta-thalassemia *(71,72)*. Although one study found evidence of pulmonary hypertension in 75% of patients with beta-thalassemia, this study and others have relied on echocardiography, not right heart catheterization, for the diagnosis of pulmonary hypertension.

Likewise, in sickle cell anemia, using echocardiography as the diagnostic tool, the estimated incidence of pulmonary hypertension has been variable (8–30%) *(73)*. In a recent catheterization study of 34 adult patients with sickle cell disease *(74)*, 20 patients were diagnosed with pulmonary hypertension (average mean pulmonary artery pressure: 36 mm Hg); several of these patients had elevated pulmonary capillary wedge pressures consistent with a component of left ventricular diastolic dysfunction. Mean pulmonary artery pressure was inversely related to survival: Each increase of 10 mm Hg in mean pulmonary artery pressure was associated with a 1.7-fold increase in the rate of death. More recent data confirm that pulmonary hypertension increases the risk of death in patients with sickle cell disease *(75)*. Historically, recurrent episodes of acute chest syndrome have been considered the most important risk factor for the development of pulmonary hypertension *(76)*; however, recent data suggest this may not be the case. Destruction of bioactive nitric oxide by free hemoglobin *(77)* and an increase in the production of reactive oxygen species *(78,79)* may be more important for the development of pulmonary hypertension in patients with a hemolytic anemia than in those without a hemolytic anemia. For example, in sickle cell anemia, the plasma levels of oxyhemoglobin are high because of intravascular hemolysis; this cell-free hemoglobin can impair responses to intrinsic and exogenously delivered nitric oxide. Likewise, in sickle cell anemia, there are increased circulating and intracellular levels of reactive oxygen species, which can inactivate nitric oxide.

4.7. Hereditary Spherocytosis

Hereditary spherocytosis has been associated with pulmonary hypertension in limited case reports *(80)*. A recent review of the reported cases *(81)* suggests that this association may, in part, be explained by thrombocytosis and chronic thromboembolic disease accompanying the underlying hematological disorder.

4.8. Hereditary Hemorrhagic Telangiectasia

Pulmonary hypertension clinically and histologically indistinguishable from IPAH has been observed in approximately 15% of individuals with hereditary hemorrhagic telangiectasia (HHT; also known as Osler-Weber-Rendu syndrome), an autosomal dominant vascular dysplasia *(82,83)*. Mutations in two genes encoding the TGF-β receptors, endoglin and activin-receptor-like kinase 1 (*ALK1*), have been associated with HHT.

5. GENETIC ABNORMALITIES ASSOCIATED WITH PULMONARY HYPERTENSION

Approximately 100 families worldwide have been identified with a genetic predilection for IPAH *(84–86)*. Familial PAH accounts for at least 6% of all cases and has a similar female-to-male gender ratio, age of onset, and natural history as the sporadic form. Segregation analysis of affected pedigrees demonstrates an autosomal dominant inheritance with markedly reduced penetrance such that only a small percentage of those who inherit the relevant genetic mutation (10–20%) will develop pulmonary hypertension. In addition, the inheritance of the appropriate genetic mutation demonstrates genetic anticipation: In each successive generation in which the disease develops, it occurs at a younger age and is more severe than in the preceding generation.

5.1. TGF-β Receptor Pathway

Two genes in the ubiquitous TGF-β receptor family have been strongly linked to familial PAH *(87)*. The first gene, bone morphogenetic protein receptor type 2 *(BMPR2)*, modulates the growth of vascular cells by activating the intracellular pathways of Smad and LIM (Lin-11, Isl-1, and Mec-3 protein) kinase *(88)*. Under normal conditions, bone morphogenetic proteins 2, 4, and 7 signal through heterodimeric complexes of *BMPR2* and type 1 receptors to suppress the growth of vascular smooth muscle cells. More than 45 different mutations in *BMPR2* have been identified in patients with familial PAH *(85,89)*. Functional studies have shown that point mutations and truncations in the kinase domain exert dominant negative effects on receptor function *(90)*. Because of incomplete penetrance and genetic anticipation, it is probable that *BMPR2* mutations are necessary, but insufficient alone, to account for the clinical expression of the disease.

A rare group of patients with HHT and PAH have been found to harbor mutations in another member of the TGF-β receptor family, *ALK1 (82)*. As with *BMPR2* mutations, mutations in this type 1 receptor are believed to result in growth-promoting, Smad-dependent signaling.

It has been observed that as many as 10–26% of patients with sporadic IPAH also carry a mutation of a member of the TGF-β receptor family *(91)*. Recently, Du et al. *(92)* argued that all forms of PAH also have defects in a common vascular signaling pathway that involves angiopoietin-1 and the phosphorylated form of its endothelial-specific receptor, TIE2. These authors showed that this signaling pathway is upregulated in the lungs of patients with pulmonary hypertension, regardless of the cause of the disease; the increase in angiopoietin signaling is accompanied by a decrease in another member of the TGF-β receptor family, BMPR1A, a complementary type 1 receptor required for normal BMPR2 signaling. Some of these observations, however, run counter to previous findings concerning angiopoietin *(93,94)*; furthermore, if verified, what modulates angiopoietin expression in pulmonary hypertension has not been identified.

5.2. Serotoninergic Pathway

The increased serotonin-dependent proliferation of cultured pulmonary vascular smooth muscle cells in specimens obtained from patients with IPAH is, in part, a consequence of an increase in the serotonin transporter 5-HTT *(21)*. The L-allelic variant of the *5HTT* gene is associated with an increased expression of the transporter and an increase in the growth of vascular smooth muscle cells, and it is more prevalent among patients with IPAH than among controls.

A complementary study by Launay and colleagues *(95)* showed that hypoxia-induced pulmonary arterial hypertension in mice is associated with an increase in the expression of 5-HT2B, resulting in serotonin-dependent vascular remodeling. In addition, they showed that the main metabolite of dexfenfluramine, *nor*-dexfenfluramine, is a potent vascular cell growth-promoting agonist for this receptor, thus linking anorexigenic pulmonary arterial hypertension to signaling pathways in pulmonary vascular cells that are upregulated by hypoxia and activated by serotonin.

6. CONCLUSIONS

Pulmonary arterial hypertension comprises a group of clinical and pathophysiological entities with similar features but a variety of underlying causes. Because of the wide range of medical conditions and environmental exposures associated with PAH, it is difficult to envision a unifying pathogenic mechanism. Although there probably are genetic determinants, environmental exposures, and acquired disorders that predispose patients to PAH, it is clear that none of the factors described in this chapter is sufficient alone to activate the pathways essential to the development of this vascular disease.

It is also likely that clinically apparent PAH is an end-stage phenotype that represents a final common manifestation of multiple preclinical, intermediate phenotypes. For example, some cases of PAH are likely to be a consequence of an initial pathogenic event that involves the pulmonary vascular smooth muscle cell (e.g., familial PAH with *BMPR2* mutations), whereas other cases are likely to be a consequence of an initial pathogenic event that involves the pulmonary endothelial cell (e.g., PAH associated with HHT). Thus, an understanding of the preclinical disease in at-risk populations will be critical for identifying the primary pathogenic mechanisms.

Because clinically apparent disease occurs in only a small percentage of the carriers of the *BMPR2, ALK1,* and *5HTT* mutations, it is probable that there are modifier genes, modifying environmental triggers, or both, and that these genes and environmental factors are important in the pathogenesis of the disease. Thus, a multiple-hit theory has been suggested, similar to that often invoked for the development of cancers in which a susceptible person with a genetic predisposition (i.e., in the form of polymorphisms or mutations) requires additional insults before the disease is manifested.

If a unifying molecular mechanism were involved in the development of PAH, it might involve TGF-β signaling. Because the TGF-β receptors are important in cell proliferation and apoptosis, a decrease in bone morphogenetic protein or in its associated signaling pathways could result in a loss of the antiproliferative or apoptotic mechanisms in the pulmonary vasculature and thereby promote the vascular changes observed in patients with PAH. Expanded natural history studies and further evaluation of persons at risk for pulmonary arterial hypertension (e.g., those with mutations of the TGF-β pathway and other identified mutations) as well as a better understanding of the disease-modifying genetic and acquired determinants will provide improved insight into the relationship between these genotypes and this complicated phenotype.

REFERENCES

1. Gaine SP, Rubin LJ. Primary pulmonary hypertension. Lancet 1998;352:719–25.
2. Rubin LJ. Primary pulmonary hypertension. N Engl J Med 1997;336: 111–7.
3. Simonneau G, Galie N, Rubin LJ, et al. Clinical classification of pulmonary hypertension. J Am Coll Cardiol 2004;43:Suppl S:5S–12S.
4. Gerber JG, Voelkel N, Nies AS, McMurty IF, Reeves JT. Moderation of hypoxic vasoconstriction by infused arachidonic acid: Role of PGI2. J Appl Physiol 1980;49:107–12.
5. Hara S, Morishita R, Tone Y, et al. Overexpression of prostacyclin synthase inhibits growth of vascular smooth muscle cells. Biochem Biophys Res Commun 1995;216:862–7.
6. Christman BW, McPherson CD, Newman JH, et al. An imbalance between the excretion of thromboxane and prostacyclin metabolites in pulmonary hypertension. N Engl J Med 1992;327:70–5.
7. Tuder RM, Cool CD, Geraci MW, et al. Prostacyclin synthase expression is decreased in lungs from patients with severe pulmonary hypertension. Am J Respir Crit Care Med 1999;159:1925–32.
8. Geraci MW, Gao B, Shepherd DC, et al. Pulmonary prostacyclin synthase overexpression in transgenic mice protects against development of hypoxic pulmonary hypertension. J Clin Invest 1999;103:1509–15.
9. Hassoun PM, Thappa V, Landman MJ, Fanburg BL. Endothelin 1 mitogenic activity on pulmonary artery smooth muscle cells and release from hypoxic endothelial cells. Proc Soc Exp Biol Med 1992;199:165–70.
10. Stelzner TJ, O'Brien RF, Yanagisawa M, et al. Increased lung endothelin-1 production in rats with idiopathic pulmonary hypertension. Am J Physiol 1992;262:L614–20.

11. Allen SW, Chatfield BA, Koppenhafer SA, Schaffer MS, Wolfe RR, Abman SH. Circulating immunoreactive endothelin-1 in children with pulmonary hypertension. Association with acute hypoxic pulmonary vasoreactivity. Am Rev Respir Dis 1993;148:519–22.
12. Giaid A, Yanagisawa M, Langleben D, et al. Expression of endothelin-1 in the lungs of patients with pulmonary hypertension. N Engl J Med 1993;328:1732–9.
13. Vincent JA, Ross RD, Kassab J, Hsu JM, Pinsky WW. Relation of elevated plasma endothelin in congenital heart disease to increased pulmonary blood flow. Am J Cardiol 1993;71:1204–7.
14. Giaid A, Saleh D. Reduced expression of endothelial nitric oxide synthase in the lungs of patients with pulmonary hypertension. N Engl J Med 1995;333:214–21.
15. McQuillan LP, Leung GK, Marsden PA, Kostyk SK, Kourembanas S. Hypoxia inhibits expression of eNOS via transcriptional and posttranscriptional mechanisms. Am J Physiol 1994;267:H1921–7.
16. Mason NA, Springall DR, Burke M, et al. High expression of endothelial nitric oxide synthase in plexiform lesions of pulmonary hypertension. J Pathol 1998;185:313–8.
17. Lee SL, Wang WW, Lanzillo JJ, Fanburg BL. Serotonin produces both hyperplasia and hypertrophy of bovine pulmonary artery smooth muscle cells in culture. Am J Physiol 1994;266:L46–52.
18. Herve P, Launay JM, Scrobohaci ML, et al. Increased plasma serotonin in primary pulmonary hypertension. Am J Med 1995;99:249–54.
19. Herve P, Drouet L, Dosquet C, et al. Primary pulmonary hypertension in a patient with a familial platelet storage pool disease: Role of serotonin. Am J Med 1990;89:117–20.
20. Abenhaim L, Moride Y, Brenot F, et al. Appetite-suppressant drugs and the risk of primary pulmonary hypertension. International primary pulmonary hypertension study group. N Engl J Med 1996;335:609–16.
21. Eddahibi S, Humbert M, Fadel E, et al. Serotonin transporter overexpression is responsible for pulmonary artery smooth muscle hyperplasia in primary pulmonary hypertension. J Clin Invest 2001;108:1141–50.
22. Marcos E, Adnot S, Pham MH, et al. Serotonin transporter inhibitors protect against hypoxic pulmonary hypertension. Am J Respir Crit Care Med 2003;168:487–93.
23. Nicholls MG, Lainchbury JG, Lewis LK, et al. Bioactivity of adrenomedullin and proadrenomedullin N-terminal 20 peptide in man. Peptides 2001;22:1745–52.
24. Kakishita M, Nishikimi T, Okano Y, et al. Increased plasma levels of adrenomedullin in patients with pulmonary hypertension. Clin Sci 1999;96:33–9.
25. Shimokubo T, Sakata J, Kitamura K, et al. Augmented adrenomedullin concentrations in right ventricle and plasma of experimental pulmonary hypertension. Life Sci 1995;57:1771–9.

26. Nishikimi T, Nagata S, Sasaki T, et al. Plasma concentrations of adrenomedullin correlate with the extent of pulmonary hypertension in patients with mitral stenosis. Heart 1997;78:390–5.

27. Yoshihara F, Nishikimi T, Horio T, et al. Chronic infusion of adrenomedullin reduces pulmonary hypertension and lessens right ventricular hypertrophy in rats administered monocrotaline. Eur J Pharmacol 1998;355:33–9.

28. Gunaydin S, Imai Y, Takanashi Y, et al. The effects of vasoactive intestinal peptide on monocrotaline induced pulmonary hypertensive rabbits following cardiopulmonary bypass: A comparative study with isoproteronol and nitroglycerine. Cardiovasc Surg 2002;10:138–45.

29. Soderman C, Eriksson LS, Juhlin-Dannfelt A, Lundberg JM, Broman L, Holmgren A. Effect of vasoactive intestinal polypeptide (VIP) on pulmonary ventilation-perfusion relationships and central haemodynamics in healthy subjects. Clin Physiol 1993;13:677–85.

30. Cox CP, Linden J, Said SI. VIP elevates platelet cyclic AMP (cAMP) levels and inhibits in vitro platelet activation induced by platelet-activating factor (PAF). Peptides 1984;5:325–28.

31. Maruno K, Absood A, Said SI. VIP inhibits basal and histamine-stimulated proliferation of human airway smooth muscle cells. Am J Physiol 1995;268:L1047–51.

32. Petkov V, Mosgoeller W, Ziesche R, et al. Vasoactive intestinal peptide as a new drug for treatment of primary pulmonary hypertension. J Clin Invest 2003;111:1339–46.

33. Tuder RM, Flook BE, Voelkel NF. VEGF receptors KDR/Flk and Flt in lungs exposed to acute or chronic hypoxia. Modulation of gene expression by nitric oxide. J Clin Invest 1995;95:1798–807.

34. Le Cras TD, Markham NE, Tuder RM, Voelkel NF, Abman SH. Inhibition of VEGF signalling in pulmonary hypertension. Am J Physiol 2002;283:L555–62.

35. Tuder RM, Charon M, Alger L, Wang J, Taraseciviene-Stewart L, Kasahara Y, Cod CD, Bishop AE, Geraci M, Semenza GL, Yacoub M, Polak JM, Voelkel NF. Evidence of angiogenesis-related molecules in plexiform lesions in severe pulmonary hypertension. Evidence for a process of disordered angiogenesis. J Pathol 2001;195:367–74.

36. Dumas JP, Bardou M, Goirand F, Dumas M. Hypoxic pulmonary vasocon-striction. Gen Pharmacol 1999;33:289–97.

37. Sweeney M, Yuan JX. Hypoxic pulmonary vasoconstriction: Role of voltage-gated potassium channels. Respir Res 2000;1:40–8.

38. Semenza GL, Agani F, Feldser D, et al. Hypoxia, HIF-1, and the pathophysiology of common human diseases. Adv Exp Med Biol 2000;475:123–

39. Voelkel NF, Cool C, Taraceviene-Stewart L, et al. Janus face of vascular endothelial growth factor: The obligatory survival factor for lung vascular endothelium controls precapillary artery remodeling in severe pulmonary hypertension. Crit Care Med 2002;30:S251–6.

40. Gurtner HP. Aminorex and pulmonary hypertension. A review. Cor Vasa 1985;27:160–71.
41. Simonneau G, Fartoukh M, Sitbon O, Humbert M, Jagot JL, Herve P. Primary pulmonary hypertension associated with the use of fenfluramines derivatives. Chest 1998;114:Suppl 3:195S–9S.
42. Mark EJ, Patalas ED, Chang HT, Evans RJ, Kessler SC. Fatal pulmonary hypertension associated with short-term use of fenfluramine and phentermine. N Engl J Med 1997;337:602–6. [Erratum, N Engl J Med 1997;337:1483].
43. Albertson TE, Walby WF, Derlet RW. Stimulant-induced pulmonary toxicity. Chest 1995;108:1140–9.
44. Schaiberger P, Kennedy T, Miller F, Gal J, Petty TL. Pulmonary hypertension associated with long-term inhalation of "crank" methamphetamine. Chest 1993;104:614–6.
45. Murray R, Smialek J, Golle M, Albin RJ. Pulmonary artery medial hypertrophy in cocaine users without foreign particle microembolization. Chest 1989;96:1050–3.
46. Lame MW, Jones AD, Wilson DW, Dunston SK, Segall HJ. Protein targets of monocrotaline pyrrole in pulmonary artery endothelial cells. J Biol Chem 2000;275:29091–9.
47. Williams NA, Lee MG, Hanchard B, Barrow KO. Hepatic cirrhosis in Jamaica. West Indian Med J 1997;46:60–2.
48. Gomez-Sanchez MA, Saenz de la Calzada C, Gomez-Pajuelo C, et al. Clinical and pathologic manifestations of pulmonary vascular disease in the toxic oil syndrome. J Am Coll Cardiol 1991;18:1539–45.
49. Gomez-Sanchez MA, Mestre de Juan MJ, Gomez-Pajuelo C, et al. Pulmonary hypertension due to toxic oil syndrome. A clinicopathologic study. Chest 1989;95:325–31.
50. Sack KE, Criswell LA. Eosinophilia-myalgia syndrome: The aftermath. South Med J 1992;85:878–82.
51. Belongia EA, Gleich GJ. The eosinophilia myalgia syndrome revisited. J Rheumatol 1996;23:1682–4.
52. James TN, Gomez-Sanchez MA, Martinez-Tello FJ, et al. Cardiac abnormalities in the toxic oil syndrome, with comparative observations on the eosinophilia myalgia syndrome. J Am Coll Cardiol 1991;18:1367–79.
53. Silver RM. Pathophysiology of the eosiniphilia-myalgia syndrome. J Rheumatol 1996;46:26–36.
54. Silver RM. Scleroderma. Clinical problems: The lungs. Rheum Dis Clin North Am 1996;22:825–40.
55. Bolster MB, Silver RM. Lung disease in systemic sclerosis (Scleroderma). Baillieres Clin Rheumatol 1993;7:79–97.
56. Battle RW, Davitt MA, Cooper SM, et al. Prevalence of pulmonary hypertension in limited and diffuse scleroderma. Chest 1996;110:1515–9.
57. Peacock AJ. Primary pulmonary hypertension. Thorax 1999;54:1107–18.
58. Speich R, Jenni R, Opravil M, Pfab M, Russi EW. Primary pulmonary hypertension in HIV infection. Chest 1991;100:1268–71.

59. Farber HW. HIV-associated pulmonary hypertension. AIDS Clinical Care 2001;13:53–9.
60. McDonnell PJ, Toye PA, Hutchins GM Primary pulmonary hypertension and cirrhosis: Are they related? Am Rev Respir Dis 1983;127:437–41.
61. Yang YY, Lin HC, Lee WC, et al. Portopulmonary hypertension: Distinctive hemodynamic and clinical manifestations. J Gastroenterol 2001;36:181–6.
62. Castro M, Krowka MJ, Schroeder DR, et al. Frequency and clinical implications of increased pulmonary artery pressures in liver transplant patients. Mayo Clin Proc 1996;71:543–51.
63. Donovan CL, Marcovitz PA, Punch JD, et al. Two-dimensional and dobutamine stress echocardiography in the preoperative assessment of patients with end-stage liver disease prior to orthotopic liver transplantation. Transplantation 1996;61:1180–8.
64. Fallon MB. Portopulmonary hypertension: New clinical insights and more questions on pathogenesis. Hepatology 2003;37:253–5.
65. Hadengue A, Benhayoun MK, Lebrec D, Benhamou JP. Pulmonary hypertension complicating portal hypertension: Prevalence and relation to splanchnic hemodynamics. Gastroenterology 1991;100:520–8.
66. Garcia-Manero G, Schuster SJ, Patrick H, Martinez J. Pulmonary hypertension in patients with myelofibrosis secondary to myeloproliferative diseases. Am J Hematol 1999;60:130–5.
67. Dingli D, Utz JP, Krowka MJ, Oberg AL, Tefferi A. Unexplained pulmonary hypertension in chronic myeloproliferative disorders. Chest 2001;120:801–8.
68. Marvin KS, Spellberg RD. Pulmonary hypertension secondary to thrombocytosis in a patient with myeloid metaplasia. Chest 1993;103:642–4.
69. Hoeper MM, Niedermeyer J, Hoffmeyer F, Flemming P, Fabel H. Pulmonary hypertension after splenectomy? Ann Int Med 1999;130:506–9.
70. Teramoto S, Matsuse T, Ouchi Y. Splenectomy-induced portal hypertension and pulmonary hypertension. Ann Int Med 1999;131:793.
71. Grisaru D, Rachmilewitz EA, Mosseri M, et al. Cardiopulmonary assessment in beta-thalassemia major. Chest 1990;98:1138–42.
72. Koren A, Garty I, Antonelli D, Katzuni E. Right ventricular cardiac dysfunction in beta-thalassemia major. Am J Dis Child 1987;141:93–6.
73. Minter KR, Gladwin MT. Pulmonary complications of sickle cell anemia. A need for increased recognition, treatment, and research. Am J Respir Crit Care Med 2001;164:2016–9.
74. Castro O, Hoque M, Brown BD. Pulmonary hypertension in sickle cell disease: Cardiac catheterization results and survival. Blood 2003;101:1257–61.
75. Gladwin MT, Sachdev V, Jison ML, et al. Pulmonary hypertension as a risk factor for death in patients with sickle cell disease. N Engl J Med 2004;350:886–95.

76. Platt OS, Brambilla DJ, Rosse WF, et al. Mortality in sickle cell disease – life expectancy and risk factors for early death. N Engl J Med 1994;330:1639–44.
77. Reiter CD, Wang X, Tanus-Santos JE, et al. Cell-free hemoglobin limits nitric oxide bioavailability in sickle-cell disease. Nat Med 2002;8: 1383–89.
78. Klings ES, Farber HW. Role of free radicals in the pathogenesis of acute chest syndrome in sickle cell disease. Respir Res 2001;2:280–85.
79. Aslan M, Ryan TM, Adler B, et al. Oxygen radical inhibition of nitric oxide-dependent vascular function in sickle cell disease. Proc Natl Acad Sci USA 2001;98:15215–20
80. Verresen D, DeBacker W, Van Meerback J, Neetens I, Van Varck E, J Vermeire P. Spherocytosis and pulmonary hypertension: Coincidental occurram ence or causal relationship? Eur Resp J 1991;4:629–31.
81. Hayag-Barin JE, Smith RE, Tucker FC Jr. Hereditary spherocytosis, thrombocytosis, and chronic pulmonary emboli: A case report and review of the literature. Am J Hematol 1998;57:82–4.
82. Trembath RC, Thomson JR, Machado RD, et al. NV. Clinical and molecular genetic features of pulmonary hypertension in patients with hereditary hemorrhagic telangiectasia. N Eng J Med 2001;345:325–34.
83. Trell E, Johansson BW, Linell F, Ripa J. Fa9gene milial pulmonary hypertension and multiple abnormalities of large systemic arteries in Osler's disease. Am J Med 1972;53:50–63.
84. Deng Z, Morse JH, Slager SL, et al. Familial pulmonary hypertension (gene PPH1) is caused by mutations in the bone morphogenetic protein receptor-II gene. Am J Hum Genet 2000;67:737–44.
85. Lane KB, Machado RD, Pauciulo MW, et al. Heterozygous germline mutations in BMPR2, encoding a TGF-beta receptor, cause familial pulmonary hypertension. The international PPH consortium. Nature Gen 2000;26:81–4.
86. Machado RD, Pauciulo MW, Thomsom JR, et al. BMPR haploinsufficiency as the inherited molecular mechanism for primary pulmonary hypertension. Am J Hum Genet 2001;68:92–102.
87. Loscalzo J. Genetic clues to the cause of primary pulmonary hypertension. N Engl J Med 2001;345:367–71.
88. Foletta VC, Lim MA, Soosairajah J, et al. Direct signaling by the BMP type II receptor via the cytoskeletal regulator LIMK1. J Cell Biol 2003;162:1089–98. [Erratum, J Cell Biol 2003;163:421.]
89. Newman JH, Wheeler L, Lane KB, et al. Mutation in the gene for bone morphogenetic protein receptor II as a cause of primary pulmonary hypertension in a large kindred. N Engl J Med 2001;345:319–24. [Erratum, N Engl J Med 2001;345:1506, 2002;346:1258.]
90. Newman JH, Trembath RC, Morse JA, et al. Genetic basis of pulmonary arterial hypertension: Current understanding and future directions. J Am Coll Cardiol 2004;43:Suppl S:33S–9S.

91. Liu F, Ventura F, Doody J, Massague J. Human type II receptor for bone morphogenetic proteins (BMPs): Extension of the two-kinase receptor model to the BMPs. Mol Cell Biol 1995;15:3479–86.
92. Du L, Sullivan CC, Chu D, et al. Signaling molecules in nonfamilial pulmonary hypertension. N Engl J Med 2003;348:500–9.
93. Rudge JS, Thurston G, Yancopoulos GD. Angiopoietin-1 and pulmonary hypertension: Cause or cure? Circ Res 2003;92:947–9.
94. Zhao YD, Campbell AI, Robb M, Ng D, Stewart DJ. Protective role of angiopoietin-1 in experimental pulmonary hypertension. Circ Res 2003;92:984–91.
95. Launay JM, Herve P, Peoc'h K, et al. Function of the serotonin 5-hydroxytryptamine 2B receptor in pulmonary hypertension. Nat Med 2002;8:1129–35.

5

Pulmonary Hypertension Genes

Elisabeth Donlevy Willers
and Ivan M. Robbins

CONTENTS

INTRODUCTION
PEDIGREE ANALYSIS
BONE MORPHOGENIC PROTEIN RECEPTOR
 2 GENE (*BMPR2*)
BMPR2 MUTATIONS IN IPAH
BMPR2 IN OTHER PAH COHORTS
BIOLOGY OF *BMPR2*
ALK1 AND HEREDITARY HEMORRHAGIC
 TELANGIECTASIA
MODIFIERS AND TRIGGERS OF PULMONARY
 ARTERIAL HYPERTENSION
SCREENING/COUNSELING
REFERENCES

Abstract

Most of what is known about the genetic basis of pulmonary hypertension (PH) is related to mutations in bone morphogenetic protein receptor 2 (*BMPR2*), which have been identified in patients with pulmonary arterial hypertension (PAH). However, a number of functional polymorphisms in other genes may be associated with the development of PH or may modify disease expression. In particular, polymorphisms in genes encoding serotonin receptors, the serotonin transporter, and nitric oxide synthase may influence the development of PH in the presence or absence of mutations in *BMPR2*. As knowledge of the

From: *Contemporary Cardiology: Pulmonary Hypertension*
Edited by: N. S. Hill and H. W. Farber © Humana Press, Totowa, NJ

genetic basis of PH grows, how to best conduct screening, genetic testing, and genetic counseling will become increasingly important. In the future, identification of specific genotypes associated with response to different therapies (i.e., epoprostenol) or with patterns of disease severity may help tailor therapy and improve the outcome of patients.

Key Words: PPH; PAH; PH; BMPR2; serotonin; nitric oxide; Kv channels; genetic anticipation; incomplete penetrance; epistasis.

1. INTRODUCTION

In 1951, David Dresdale et al. described the pathological, clinical, and hemodynamic characteristics in three patients with unexplained pulmonary hypertension and referred to the disorder as primary pulmonary hypertension (PPH) *(1)*. Pathological changes were found predominantly in the small precapillary pulmonary arteries and included medial hypertrophy, intimal fibrosis, and *in situ* thrombosis. Three years later, he reported the occurrence of PPH in several members of one family, which included a mother, her sister, and her son *(2)*. This report was the first indication that there might be a genetic basis underlying the development of pulmonary hypertension. Over the subsequent 30 years, 14 additional PPH families with two or more affected members were reported *(3)*; however, little progress was made in understanding the genetic basis of PPH until the 1980s.

PPH, now termed either "idiopathic pulmonary arterial hypertension" (IPAH) in sporadic cases or "familial PAH" (FPAH) in inherited disease, most often affects women of childbearing age but has been reported in infants and in patients in the eighth decade of life *(4)*. A National Institutes of Health PPH Registry consisting of 187 patients was established in the 1980s, and 6% of patients were reported to have familial disease *(4)*. In another more recent publication of 485 French patients with pulmonary arterial hypertension (PAH), 7% had FPAH *(5)*. Currently, there is no national registry in the United States. Two registries, one at our institution of 89 families with 299 affected individuals, and one at Columbia University of 100 families, are well established and continue to accrue patients. National PAH registries have also been established in Germany and France.

2. PEDIGREE ANALYSIS

The construction and examination of family pedigrees have revealed a number of important features of FPAH. In 1995, Loyd et al. *(6)* excluded X-linkage as the mode of inheritance for FPAH, as vertical transmission was apparent in many families, with several cases of father-to-son transmission. PAH is transmitted by autosomal dominant inheritance, although there is incomplete penetrance, meaning that many mutation carriers do not develop disease *(3)*. The disease exhibits genetic anticipation, occurring at an earlier age in affected members in subsequent generations *(6)*. In general, more females than males are born in families with FPAH *(6)*. This abnormal gender ratio of progeny suggests male fetal wastage. Familial and sporadic cases share many features: a 2:1 female predominance, mean age at diagnosis in mid-30s, and similar clinical manifestations, including hemodynamic variables, histopathological abnormalities, and response to therapy *(7)*.

The largest reported family with FPAH is originally from Tennessee and was initially thought to be five separate families *(8)* (Fig. 1). This family spans seven generations and has almost 400 members, of which 200 are at-risk or obligate carriers for having a mutation in *BMPR2*. To date, 18 family members have been diagnosed with PAH, and almost half of them were initially misdiagnosed with another cardiopulmonary disease. Evaluation of this superfamily demonstrates how many cases of apparently sporadic PAH may, in fact, be familial and highlights the difficulty in diagnosing FPAH due to incomplete expression within families, skipped generations, and incomplete family pedigrees *(8)*.

3. BONE MORPHOGENIC PROTEIN RECEPTOR 2 GENE (*BMPR2*)

The search for a gene causing PAH began with linkage analysis studies. In 1997, a genome-wide microsatellite marker search using a set of polymorphic short-tandem repeat markers in 19 individuals with PAH from six affected families was performed and all samples linked to a specific area on the long arm of chromosome 2 *(9)*. Genotypes of affected individuals were compared to unaffected family members and revealed several meiotic recombination events, narrowing the region for a candidate gene to a locus on the long arm of chromosome 2 (2q31–33) *(9)*. Evaluation of 81 potential gene prospects at this locus eventually led to the identification of mutations in the *BMPR2* gene in affected individuals *(10)* (Fig. 2). Subsequently, exon-by-exon sequencing of the *BMPR2* gene identified heterozygous mutations in at least 50% of familial cases. This prevalence was recently confirmed in a report of French families that found germline *BMPR2* mutations in 13 of 28 (46%) of families *(11)*. Regardless of the type or presence of a mutation, the age of onset, gender, and disease severity among

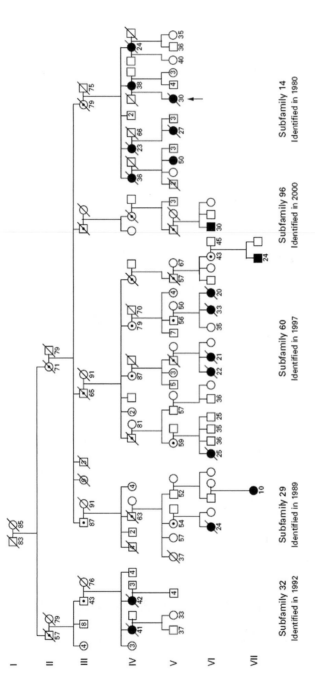

Fig. 1. Abbreviated pedigree of large kindred comprising five subfamilies over seven generations and 394 known descendants of generation I. The propositus (arrow), a woman in generation V of Subfamily 14 who died at the age of 30, received her diagnosis in 1980. There are at least 200 descendants at varying degrees of risk for pulmonary arterial hypertension (PAH). Familial PAH has been diagnosed in 18 members (16 women and 2 men), and at least 23 members (12 women and 11 men, 20 of whom are shown in the figure) are known to carry the gene for the disease. Open symbols indicate unaffected members, solid symbols members with PAH, symbols with dots carriers, squares male family members, circles female family members, and slashes deceased members. Numbers inside the symbols indicate the number of members of that gender; numbers under the symbols indicate the current age or age at death.

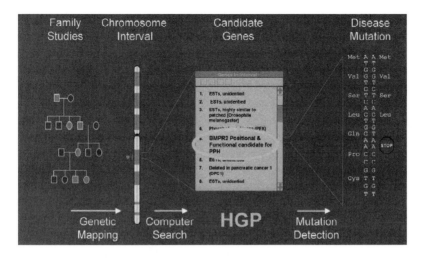

Fig. 2. The process leading to the discovery of mutations in bone morphogenetic protein receptor type-2 (*BMPR2*) as the cause of familial pulmonary arterial hypertension is depicted. Collection of DNA from families with sufficient numbers of affected and unaffected members allowed linkage studies using microsatellite markers that led to identification of a chromosome interval on chromosome 2 at q31–32. Candidate genes known from the Human Genome Project in the interval were then identified and tested by DNA sequencing. Point mutations in exons of the *BMPR2* gene were found that co-segregated with affected individuals known from the family pedigrees. (To view this figure in color, see insert.)

families were similar *(12)*. Most, but not all, families have unique mutations in *BMPR2*, as the same mutation has now been found in three unrelated families (unpublished data from our center).

The *BMPR2* gene is a large gene encoding 13 exons. Exons 1 to 3 encode an extracellular domain, exon 4 encodes a transmembrane domain, exons 5 to 11 encode the serine/threonine kinase domain, and exon 12 encodes a very large intracellular C-terminal domain of unknown function that is unique to *BMPR2*. The protein start codon is in exon 1, and the stop codon in exon 13 *(13)*. To date, over 60 *BMPR2* mutations have been identified in all 13 exons (www.pphgenes.net) *(14)*.

New data from our center suggest that the prevalence of *BMPR2* mutations in PAH may be higher than initially found *(14)*. Using southern blot analysis and reverse transcriptase polymerase chain reaction (RT-PCR) assays to identify large gene rearrangements, *BMPR2* mutations were identified in 4 of 12 families in which *BMPR2* mutations had not been found by exon sequencing. These additional methods of DNA analysis are important in identifying large gene alterations such as insertions, deletions, inversions, and rearrangements not discovered by conventional exon sequencing. These results suggest that the actual prevalence of *BMPR2* mutations in families may actually be as high as 75%. These findings are also consistent with linkage studies, which have linked all mutations in families studied to 2q31–33. However, the existence of other loci in families without a demonstrated *BMPR2* mutation has not been excluded. Investigators in Germany suggest that there may be a second locus near *BMPR2* at 2q31–32, a "PPH2" gene, although mutations in other genes have not been identified in any of their patients, or other patients with FPAH *(15)*.

4. *BMPR2* MUTATIONS IN IPAH

The prevalence of *BMPR2* mutations in IPAH has been studied in several small cohorts of patients. The reported frequency of *BMPR2* mutations in these cohorts ranges from 9–26% *(16,17)*. Some of the reported mutations in IPAH appear to occur *de novo*, whereas others are inherited from an asymptomatic family member and thus are likely to be FPAH. Incomplete family pedigrees make it difficult to accurately ascertain the percentage of *de novo* mutations. In the largest study of IPAH patients, Thompson et al. reported that 13 of 50 unrelated, presumably IPAH patients had 11 heterozygous mutations in *BMPR2*. Parental DNA analysis in five cases showed three occurrences of paternal transmission and two *de novo* mutations. In addition, three patients exhibited an identical mutation, which suggested the possibility of relatedness, although microsatellite markers surrounding the gene were reported to be different in each patient *(17)*. A recent study of 30 IPAH patients from Japan reported a 40% prevalence of *BMPR2* mutations *(18)*. However, no parental DNA was available for testing in 10 of the 12 patients found to have mutations, and so it is quite possible that some of these patients actually had FPAH. These two studies highlight the difficulty of diagnosing or excluding inherited disease. Due to incomplete penetrance demonstrated within families, the accurate classification of IPAH can only be made when the *BMPR2* status of proband and both parents is known.

5. *BMPR2* IN OTHER PAH COHORTS

The general population carrier frequency for *BMPR2* mutations is unknown; however, there have been no exonic *BMPR2* mutations found in the approximately 350 normal control subjects who have been evaluated *(19)*. Therefore, *BMPR2* mutations are unlikely to be present in individuals without disease or who are not related to a family with FPAH. A number of associated conditions and exposures are risk factors for the development of PAH. In a cohort of 33 patients with a history of anorexigen use and the subsequent development of PAH, five were found to have *BMPR2* mutations *(20)*. These patients had a shortened exposure to anorexigens before the onset of illness compared to those without the mutation *(20)*. In addition, two of the five patients were sisters and thus had FPAH, leaving only 9% of patients with anorexigen use with a *BMPR2* mutation. One could argue that anorexigen-associated PAH is identical to IPAH; therefore, the reported prevalence of *BMPR2* mutations in this population may be as low as 9% or as high as 26%.

We have reported a patient with pulmonary veno-occlusive disease (PVOD) who has a *BMPR2* mutation and is part of a family with FPAH, suggesting that *BMPR2* mutations may predispose to either pulmonary arterial or pulmonary venous disease depending upon the interaction with modifying genetic and/or environmental factors *(21)*. A recent study of a cohort of 106 adults and children with a variety of congenital heart defects found *BMPR2* mutations in 6% of patients *(22)*. No *BMPR2* mutations were identified in a cohort of 24 patients with scleroderma, although only exonic genotyping was performed *(23)*. No other negative studies have been reported, and it is unknown whether *BMPR2* mutations occur in PAH associated with portal hypertension, HIV infection, or systemic lupus erythematosus, although analysis of both intronic and exonic DNA with detailed family pedigrees is necessary to accurately determine the prevalence of *BMPR2* mutations in any group.

6. BIOLOGY OF *BMPR2*

BMPR2 is a member of the transforming growth factor beta (TGFβ) receptor superfamily of serine-threonine kinases and interacts with bone morphogenic (BMP) ligands. When BMP binds to *BMPR2*, its kinase domain phosphorylates and activates the *BMPRI* receptor kinase. Accessory binding proteins, betaglycan, and endoglin help facilitate this interaction *(24)*. Subsequently, complex signaling through a series of SMADS, intracellular mediators that translocate from the cytoplasm into the nucleus, ultimately inhibits or activates transcription of target genes. SMADS activate or repress transcription via protein-protein and protein-DNA interactions *(24)* (Fig. 3). There is evidence that other signaling pathways including RAS or mitogen-activated protein kinases (MAPK), most prominently the JNK and p38

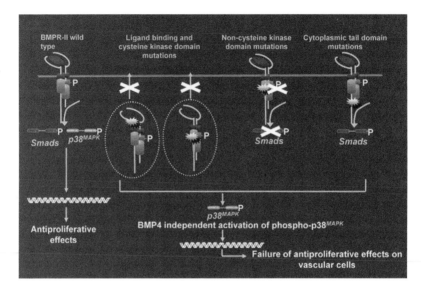

Fig. 3. Consequences of bone morphogenetic protein type-2 receptor (*BMPR2*) mutations on signaling. The mechanism by which *BMPR2* mutants disrupt BMP/Smad signaling is heterogeneous and may be mutation-specific. Thus, substitution of cysteine residues within the ligand binding or kinase domain of *BMPR2* leads to failure of trafficking of the mutant protein to the cell surface, which may interfere with wild-type receptor trafficking. In contrast, noncysteine mutations within the kinase domain reach the cell surface but fail to activate an Smad-responsive gene. However, a feature common to all mutants transfected into normal mouse epithelial cells was ligand-independent activation of p38[MAPK] and enhanced serum-induced proliferation. Based on the results of these studies, it was hypothesized that reduced cell-surface expression of *BMPR2* favors activation of p38[MAPK]-dependent pro-proliferative pathways while inhibiting Smad-dependent signaling in a mutation-specific manner. Thus, a feature common to all mutants is a gain of function involving p38[MAPK] activation. (To view this figure in color, see insert.)

pathways, are activated by TGF-β and BMPs and are also involved in transcriptional regulation *(25)*.

It is uncertain how heterozygous mutations alter signal transduction of *BMPR2* in such a way that would result in pulmonary vascular disease. It is known, however, that BMPs can inhibit cellular proliferation *(26)*. BMP4, in particular, has both antiproliferative and pro-differentiation effects on lung fibroblasts, through both SMAD and MAPK pathways *(27)*. Activation of the TGF-ß/BMPR2 axis leads to suppression of proliferation and activation of apoptosis *(28)*. One hypothesis is that loss of function occurs with *BMPR2* mutations, resulting in unrestrained proliferation of smooth muscle and endothelial cells. Mice that are homozygous for *BMPR2* mutations die shortly after gestation. This finding suggests that *BMPR2* is essential for gastrulation and early development of mouse embryos *(29)*. In addition, TGF-β knockout mice die in utero of multiple abnormalities, including impaired vasculogenesis, hematopoeisis, and cardiac malformations *(30)*. These animal experiments support an important the role for the TGF-β superfamily in a number of vascular growth pathways.

7. *ALK1* AND HEREDITARY HEMORRHAGIC TELANGIECTASIA

Mutations in a second gene, activin receptor-like kinase 1 (*ALK1*), associated with the development of IPAH and FPAH have been found in patients with hereditary hemorrhagic telangiectasia (HHT). HHT is a disease of systemic vascular dysplasia, resulting in mucosal and visceral telangiectasias and bleeding *(31)*. *ALK1* is another member of the TGFβ receptor superfamily. There are 10 reported families with FPAH and HHT type 2, representing 16% of the 61 families with known *ALK1* mutations *(32)*. Such mutations might predispose to the development of PAH, and although *ALK1* mutations are associated with a less common cause of heritable PAH, they likely share signaling abnormalities with the *BMPR2* mutations *(26)*. Endoglin is yet another member of the TGF-β receptor family that has been implicated in the pathogenesis of PAH. A recent study of 11 patients with PAH and HHT found a missense mutation in the *ALK1* gene in 8 patients and a missense mutation in the endoglin gene in 2 additional individuals *(33)*. There is also a case report of a patient with HHT and PAH who was found to have a germline mutation in the endoglin gene *(34)*. How alterations in three different receptors of the TGF-β superfamily lead to identical disease expression in the small precapillary vessels remains unknown.

8. MODIFIERS AND TRIGGERS OF PULMONARY ARTERIAL HYPERTENSION

Since only 15–20% of obligate carriers in families with a *BMPR2* mutation develop PAH, mutations or polymorphisms in other genes and/or environmental factors are necessary for disease expression. A large number of mediator and pathway abnormalities have been described in PAH; however, it is important to consider candidate genes that not only have a role in vascular function but also possess functional polymorphisms. It is also unlikely that a single polymorphism will influence disease expression; rather, groups of polymorphisms in one gene or from multiple loci may be required to satisfy conditions that lead to vascular pathogenesis. Potential modifier genes that have been evaluated in IPAH or other forms of PH include serotonin receptors, the serotonin transporter, nitric oxide synthases, and voltage-gated potassium channels.

8.1. Serotonin Pathway

Serotonin (5HT) is a neurotransmitter that has been extensively studied in neuropsychiatric diseases and is a potent pulmonary vasoconstrictor and pulmonary artery smooth muscle cell (PASMC) mitogen *(5,35)*. In 1990, Herve and colleagues reported elevated plasma 5HT levels in a patient with a platelet storage disease who developed IPAH *(36)*. Five years later, this group of investigators described elevated plasma 5HT levels in 16 patients with PAH of various types which persisted even after bilateral lung transplantation when pulmonary pressures normalized *(37)*. These observations suggested a possible association of 5HT with the development of PAH. More recent studies have shown that cultured PASMCs from IPAH patients demonstrate a greater proliferative response to 5HT in comparison to cells from subjects without PAH and that this proliferation is augmented in the setting of hypoxia *(38)*. 5HT can interact with cells either by binding to specific cell surface receptors that transduce intracellular signaling or via transport into the cell through the serotonin transporter (SERT). The pulmonary vasoconstrictor effects of 5HT are transmitted via binding to receptors, and the mitogenic actions of 5HT are conducted via the SERT pathway *(35,39,40)* (Fig. 4). A number of studies have implicated 5HT in the development of PH via receptor binding or by SERT uptake.

Fourteen classes of 5HT receptors have been identified (www.ncbi.nlm.nih.gov/entrez/query.fcgi?db=OMIM), and there is evidence that the 5HT1B, 5HT2A, and 5HT2B receptors may contribute to the development of pulmonary hypertension. Rats who received a 5HT1B receptor antagonist had decreased right ventricular (RV) hypertrophy and pressure and decreased pulmonary arterial wall thickness when exposed to hypoxia, compared to rats who did not receive the antagonist *(41)*. 5HT1B receptor knockout mice have reduced RV size, decreased pulmonary vasculature remodeling, and less pulmonary artery contraction compared to wild-type mice upon exposure to hypoxia *(41)*. The proliferative effects of 5HT noted in fibroblasts from hypoxic rats were attenuated with the addition of a

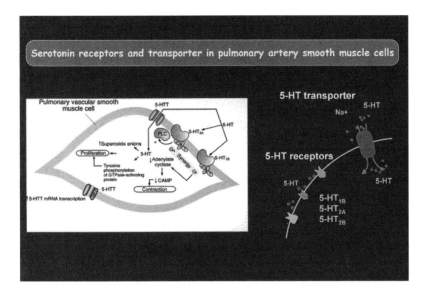

Fig. 4. Serotonin receptors and transporter in pulmonary artery smooth muscle cells. The 5-hydroxytryptamine transporter (5-HTT) expression, activity, or both in pulmonary artery smooth muscle cells contributes to pulmonary vascular remodeling. The 5-hydroxytryptamine (5-HT)$_{1B}$ receptor mediates contraction in human pulmonary artery smooth muscle cells. A role for other 5-HT receptors such as 5-HT$_{2A}$ and 5-HT$_{2B}$ has also been suggested. (To view this figure in color, see insert.)

5HT2A receptor antagonist *(42)*. In addition, the 5HT2B receptor is overexpressed in humans with IPAH and in animal models of PH, and blockade or absence of this receptor leads to inhibition of disease progression in hypoxic mice *(43)*.

Many serotonin receptor polymorphisms have been described in neuropsychiatric diseases, although whether these are functional polymorphisms that influence the development of PAH has yet to be evaluated *(44–46)*. In one study, 10 patients with PAH associated with appetite-suppressant use were genotyped for the 5HT2B receptor, and a mutation causing premature truncation of the protein product was found in one patient *(47)*. This association of PAH with the downregulation of 5HT2B receptor function is difficult to reconcile with previously mentioned cellular and animal data. However, recent in vitro studies of this specific mutation found increased cellular proliferation through MAPK activity and thymidine incorporation, suggesting a gain of function *(48)*. Although 5HT receptor function is potentially important in the development of PH, additional genetic and functional studies are needed to demonstrate their importance in human PAH.

The *SERT* gene is thought to be responsible for the mitogenic effects of 5HT. Increased levels of SERT mRNA have been demonstrated in cultured PASMCs in rats subjected to long-term hypoxia *(39)*. Knockout mice for the SERT gene are protected from developing hypoxia-induced PAH despite greater acute vasoconstriction than wild-type mice *(49)*. Anorexigens, in particular aminorex, fenflumarine, and dexfenfluramine, have been associated with the development of PAH. The metabolites of these drugs bind to the SERT and act as 5HT substrates, which are translocated into smooth muscle cells causing intracellular effects similar to or greater than 5HT itself *(50,51)*.

Several polymorphisms in the *SERT* gene have been described. There is a functional insertion/deletion polymorphism located in the *SERT* promoter region that influences the rate of transcription. The L (long) allele is associated with a two- to threefold higher rate of gene transcription compared to the S (short) allele *(52)*. This polymorphism has been studied in patients with IPAH, and the L allele was found to be more prevalent in IPAH than in control subjects. Homozygosity for the L allele was found in 65% of French IPAH patients ($n = 89$) compared to only 27% of controls ($n = 84$) *(53,54)*. In another study of patients with chronic obstructive pulmonary disease (COPD), 56% of patients had the LL genotype *(55)*, which was associated not only with increased SERT transcription but also with more severe pulmonary hypertension in this cohort *(55)*. Whether polymorphisms in the *SERT* gene correlate with more severe pulmonary hypertension in IPAH is currently being studied.

8.2. Nitric Oxide Pathway

Nitric oxide (NO) is a potent endogenous vasodilator and inhibitor of platelet aggregation that is important in maintaining normal vascular tone in the pulmonary circulation *(56)*. Arginine, a urea-cycle intermediate, is a necessary precursor for the synthesis of NO. Carbamoyl-phosphate synthetase 1 (CPS1) is the first rate-limiting enzyme in the urea cycle, and genetic variations in this enzyme can affect the downstream availability of urea-cycle intermediates *(57)*. A functional single-nucleotide polymorphism (SNP) in the *CPS1* gene, encoded by a C to A transversion, results in the substitution of asparagine for threonine at position 1405 (T1405N) and is predicted to alter the amount of arginine supplied as a precursor for NO synthesis *(57)*.

Pearson et al. genotyped 65 full-term neonates with respiratory distress for the CPS1 T1405N polymorphism. Thirty-one infants had evidence of PH by echocardiography and had significantly lower plasma levels of arginine ($p < 0.001$) and NO metabolites ($p < 0.05$) compared to infants without PH. The AA genotype, associated with the highest levels of arginine, was not found in any of the neonates with PH. Diminished concentrations of precursors and metabolites of NO indicate that inadequate production of NO may be involved in the pathogenesis of neonatal pulmonary hypertension, and the genetically determined efficiency of CPS1 may contribute to the availability of NO precursors *(57)*.

We have also evaluated the CPS1 T1405N polymorphism in 75 individuals from 10 FPAH families with *BMPR2* mutations. The CC genotype was associated with increased penetrance, while the AA genotype was associated with decreased penetrance, suggesting that the CPS1 genotype may affect disease penetrance in those with known *BMPR2* mutations *(58)* (Table 1).

Polymorphisms in NO synthase (NOS), the enzyme that cleaves NO from arginine, may also contribute to disease severity in patients with PAH. Of the three forms of this enzyme, NOS3 is specific to endothelial cells, and polymorphisms in the *NOS3* gene have been shown to affect NO synthesis and development of PH. The BB genotype, also known as the 5/5 genotype, of a polymorphism in intron 4 of the *NOS3* gene has been associated with lower plasma NO metabolites, a marker of NO production *(59)*. COPD patients with this genotype had higher pulmonary artery pressures than those with the non-5/5 genotype *(60)*. Using stepwise linear regression to predict pulmonary artery pressure, partial pressure of oxygen and NOS3 BB genotype were found to be independent variables *(59,60)*. The findings of decreased arginine and NO metabolites, and the association of the certain CPS-1 and NOS3 polymorphisms with pulmonary hypertension, indicate that NO synthesis may modulate the development of PAH.

Table 1
Chi-Square Analysis of CPS-1 Genotypes in 75 FPPH Patients,
Expected Count in Parentheses

Phenotype/Genotype	CC	AC	AA
PPH+/BMPR2+	23 (18)*	16 (19.8)	4 (5.2)
PPH-/BMPR2+	3 (6.3)	6 (6.9)	6 (1.8)*
PPH-/BMPR2-	8 (7.1)	8 (7.8)	1 (2)

* Significantly different from expected count.

8.3. Potassium Channels

Voltage-gated potassium channels (Kv) have been studied in hypoxic pulmonary vasoconstriction. Kv channels allow the efflux of potassium, which establishes the membrane potential of the vascular smooth muscle cell. Kv 1.5 and Kv 2.1, in particular, are thought to account for the majority of the oxygen-sensitive current in PASMCs *(61)*. Inhibition of these Kv channels results in accumulation of intracellular K+ leading to a more positive membrane potential, thereby activating Ca^{2+} influx via voltage gated Ca^{2+} channels and initiating vasoconstriction *(61)* (Fig. 5). Kv1.5 knockout mice have impaired HPV and less hypoxia than control mice *(62)*. Although there is heterogeneity in the various groups of Kvs in pulmonary artery smooth muscle cells, there are no identified polymorphisms for Kv 1.5 or Kv2.1 in pulmonary hypertension *(61)*. K+ channel mutations and polymorphisms have been identified in some inherited cardiac disorders, diabetes, and seizures; however, these genetic variations have not yet been studied in PAH *(63–65)*.

Other polymorphisms in potential modifier genes include endothelin 1 and its receptors, prostacyclin and its receptors, p450 enzymes

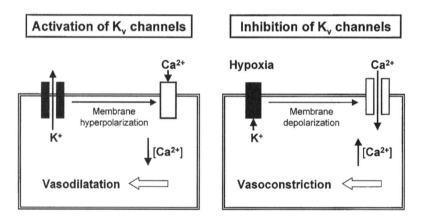

Fig. 5. Role of Kv channels in the regulation of pulmonary vascular tone. Several types of potassium (K^+) channel have been identified in vascular smooth muscle cells, but voltage-gated (Kv) channels are the major subtype implicated in the constrictor response of pulmonary arterial smooth muscle cells (PASMCs) to hypoxia. Inhibition of Kv channel activity reduces K^+ efflux, increases the membrane potential (depolarization), and opens voltage-gated Ca^{2+} channels. This results in a rise in cytosolic Ca^{2+} levels and vasoconstriction, whereas the reverse of this process leads to a fall in the membrane potential (hyperpolarization) and vasodilatation.

(cyp3A and cyp2CA), and plasminogen activator inhibitor-1. It is important to keep in mind that genes do not operate independently of one another, but rather interact with each other. The complexity of the relationship increases geometrically with the number of genes involved. The study of these interactions is called epistasis. Thus, the phenotype of pulmonary hypertension is likely a result of the inter-action among many genes, and most have yet to be determined.

9. SCREENING/COUNSELING

Until more information exists about the role of genetic polymor-phisms in the development of PAH, genetic testing for PAH is limited to the detection of *BMPR2* and *ALK1* mutations. Expert genetic counseling must precede *BMPR2* testing in at-risk individuals, given the complex genetics and severity of PAH. The presence of *BMPR2* mutation alone is not sufficient for the development of PAH since only 20% of obligate carriers of a mutation in FPAH develop disease. If a *BMPR2* mutation is detected in a patient, relatives who also test negative assume the same risk as the general population for developing disease, about one in a million cases per year. There is a chance of discovering nonpaternity when genetic testing is performed, raising potential emotional and perhaps legal issues. The implications of genetic testing, involving life and health insurance, as well as psycho-logical aspects must be thoroughly discussed with a genetic counselor prior to testing. The issue of when and whether to test children remains controversial. Most centers will not test children for a genetic disease unless discovery has therapeutic implications.

At this point there are no adequate clinical screening tests to reliably detect presymptomatic disease. PAH symptoms almost never develop until there is advanced obstruction of the vascular bed with significant pulmonary hypertension and right heart dysfunction *(66)*. Although there are no official recommendations, periodic assessment of individuals at increased risk of developing PAH is suggested. High-risk individuals include those who are known to have a *BMPR2* mutation and those who have a first-degree relative with IPAH with a known *BMPR2* mutation. After a history and physical exam, an electrocardiogram (ECG) may be useful. However, the ECG is not an adequate screening test, as the sensitivity and specificity for PH are 55% and 70%, respectively *(67)*. Exercise Doppler-echocardiography has been suggested as a screening tool, but false-positive results may occur in patients with hypertensive heart disease. In these cases, PH may reflect left ventricular diastolic dysfunction. In addition, healthy athletes can have increased tricuspid regurgitant velocity with exercise *(68)*. The criteria for an abnormal exercise echocardigram have not been established. Thus, an optimal screening method for asymptomatic carriers of the PAH gene has yet to be defined. The natural history of presymptomatic PAH is unknown, and the possibility of disease prevention or alteration of the course of disease with therapy is unexplored.

Research into the genetics of PAH has been helpful in identifying individuals who are at increased risk for the development of disease. In the future, identifying specific genotypes associated with response to different therapies (i.e., epoprostenol) or patterns of disease severity may help tailor therapy and improve the outcome of affected patients.

REFERENCES

1. Dresdale DT. Primary pulmonary hypertension: Clinical and hemodynamic study. Am J Med 1951; 11:686–705.
2. Dresdale DT, Mitchtom RJ, Schultz M. Recent studies in primary pulmonary hypertension, including pharmacodynamic observations on pulmonary vascular resistance. Bull NY Acad Med 1954; 30(3):195–207.
3. Loyd JE, Primm RK, Newman JH. Familial primary pulmonary hypertension: Clinical patterns. Am Rev Respir Dis 1984; 129(1):194–7.
4. Humbert M, Trembath RC. Genetics of pulmonary hypertension: From bench to bedside. Eur Respir J 2002; 20(3):741–9.
5. Morecroft I, Heeley RP, Prentice HM, Kirk A, MacLean MR. 5-Hydroxytryptamine receptors mediating contraction in human small muscular pulmonary arteries: Importance of the 5-HT1B receptor. Br J Pharmacol 1999; 128(3):730–4.
6. Loyd JE, Butler MG, Foroud TM, Conneally PM, Phillips JA, Newman JH. Genetic anticipation and abnormal gender ratio at birth in familial primary pulmonary-hypertension. Am J Respir Crit Care Med 1995; 152(1):93–97.
7. Rich S, Dantzker DR, Ayres SM, et al. Primary pulmonary hypertension. A national prospective study. Ann Intern Med 1987; 107(2):216–23.
8. Newman JH, Wheeler L, Lane KB, et al. Mutation in the gene for bone morphogenetic protein receptor II as a cause of primary pulmonary hypertension in a large kindred. N Engl J Med 2001; 345(5):319–24.
9. Nichols WC, Koller DL, Slovis B, et al. Localization of the gene for familial primary pulmonary hypertension to chromosome 2q31–32. Nat Genet 1997; 15(3):277–80.
10. Lane KB, Machado RD, Pauciulo MW, et al. Heterozygous germline mutations in *BMPR2*, encoding a TGF-beta receptor, cause familial primary pulmonary hypertension. Nat Genet 2000; 26(1):81–4.

11. Sztrymf B, et al. Familial pulmonary arterial hypertension: Genetics, hemodynamics, clinical characteristics, and survival. 2004 Meeting of the American Thoracic Society, 2004.

12. Machado RD, Pauciulo MW, Thomson JR, et al. BMPR2 haploinsufficiency as the inherited molecular mechanism for primary pulmonary hypertension. Am J Hum Genet 2001; 68(1):92–102.

13. Morse JH. Bone morphogenetic protein receptor 2 mutations in pulmonary hypertension. Chest 2002; 121(3 Suppl):50S–3S.

14. Cogan J, Vnencak-Jones CL, Phillips J, et al. Gross *BMPR2* gene rearrangements constitute a new cause for primary pulmonary hypertension. Genet Med; in press.

15. Janssen B, Rindermann M, Barth U, et al. Linkage analysis in a large family with primary pulmonary hypertension: Genetic heterogeneity and a second primary pulmonary hypertension locus on 2q31–32. Chest 2002; 121(3 Suppl):54S–6S.

16. Newman JH, Trembath RC, Morse JA, et al. Genetic basis of pulmonary arterial hypertension: Current understanding and future directions. J Am Coll Cardiol 2004; 43(12 Suppl S):33S–9S.

17. Thomson JR, Machado RD, Pauciulo MW, et al. Sporadic primary pulmonary hypertension is associated with germline mutations of the gene encoding BMPR-II, a receptor member of the TGF-beta family. J Med Genet 2000; 37(10):741–5.

18. Morisaki H, Nakanishi N, Kyotani S, Takashima A, Tomoike H, Morisaki T. *BMPR2* mutations found in Japanese patients with familial and sporadic primary pulmonary hypertension. Hum Mutat 2004; 23(6):632.

19. Loyd J, Newman J, Phillips III J. Respiratory genetics. In E Silverman, S Weiss, J Drazer, eds. Pulmonary Hypertension. London: Arnold and Hodder, 2005.

20. Humbert M, Deng Z, Simonneau G, et al. *BMPR2* germline mutations in pulmonary hypertension associated with fenfluramine derivatives. Eur Respir J 2002; 20(3):518–23.

21. Runo JR, Vnencak-Jones CL, Prince M, et al. Pulmonary veno-occlusive disease caused by an inherited mutation in bone morphogenetic protein receptor II. Am J Respir Crit Care Med 2003; 167(6):889–94.

22. Roberts KE, McElroy JJ, Wong WPK, et al. *BMPR2* mutations in pulmonary arterial hypertension with congenital heart disease. Eur Respir J 2004; 24:371–4.

23. Morse J, Barst R, Horn E, Cuervo N, Deng ZM, Knowles J. Pulmonary hypertension in scleroderma spectrum of disease: Lack of bone morphogenetic protein receptor 2 mutations. J Rheum 2002; 29(11):2379–81.

24. Attisano L, Tuen Lee-Hoeflich S. The Smads. Genome Biol 2001; 2(8):REVIEWS3010.

25. Massague J, Chen YG. Controlling TGF-beta signaling. Genes Dev 2000; 14(6):627–44.

26. Miyazono K, Kusanagi K, Inoue H. Divergence and convergence of TGF-beta/BMP signaling. J Cell Physiol 2001; 187(3):265–76.

27. Jeffery TK, Upton PD, Trembath RC, Morrell NW. BMP4 inhibits prolif-
    eration and promotes myocyte differentiation of lung fibroblasts via
    Smad1 and JNK pathways. Am J Physiol Lung Cell Mol Physiol 2005;
    288:L370–8.

28. Ten DP, Goumans MJ, Itoh F, Itoh S. Regulation of cell proliferation by
    Smad proteins 10. J Cell Physiol 2002; 191(1):1–16.

29. Beppu H, Kawabata M, Hamamoto T, et al. BMP type II receptor is
    required for gastrulation and early development of mouse embryos. Dev
    Biol 2000; 221(1):249–58.

30. Kulkarni AB, Huh CG, Becker D, et al. Transforming growth factor beta
    1 null mutation in mice causes excessive inflammatory response and early
    death. Proc Natl Acad Sci USA 1993; 90(2):770–4.

31. Trembath RC, Thomson JR, Machado RD, et al. Clinical and molecular
    genetic features of pulmonary hypertension in patients with hereditary
    hemorrhagic telangiectasia. N Eng J Med 2001; 345(5):325–34.

32. Abdalla SA, Gallione CJ, Barst RJ, et al. Primary pulmonary hypertension
    in families with hereditary haemorrhagic telangiectasia. Eur Respir J 2004;
    23(3):373–7.

33. Harrison RE, Flanagan JA, Sankelo M, et al. Molecular and functional
    analysis identifies ALK-1 as the predominant cause of pulmonary hyper-
    tension related to hereditary haemorrhagic telangiectasia. J Med Genet
    2003; 40(12):865–71.

34. Chaouat A, Coulet F, Favre C, et al. Endoglin germline mutation in a
    patient with hereditary haemorrhagic telangiectasia and dexfenfluramine
    associated pulmonary arterial hypertension. Thorax 2004; 59(5):446–8.

35. MacLean MR, Sweeney G, Baird M, McCulloch KM, Houslay M,
    Morecroft I. 5-Hydroxytryptamine receptors mediating vasoconstriction
    in pulmonary arteries from control and pulmonary hypertensive rats. Br
    J Pharmacol 1996; 119(5):917–30.

36. Herve P, Drouet L, Dosquet C, et al. Primary pulmonary hypertension in
    a patient with a familial platelet storage pool disease: Role of serotonin.
    Am J Med 1990; 89(1):117–20.

37. Herve P, Launay JM, Scrobohaci ML, et al. Increased plasma serotonin
    in primary pulmonary hypertension. Am J Med 1995; 99(3):249–54.

38. Lee SL, Wang WW, Moore BJ, Fanburg BL. Dual effect of serotonin on
    growth of bovine pulmonary artery smooth muscle cells in culture. Circ
    Res 1991; 68(5):1362–8.

39. Eddahibi S, Fabre V, Boni C, et al. Induction of serotonin transporter by
    hypoxia in pulmonary vascular smooth muscle cells—Relationship with
    the mitogenic action of serotonin. Circ Res 1999; 84(3):329–36.

40. Eddahibi S, Raffestin B, Hamon M, Adnot S. Is the serotonin transporter
    involved in the pathogenesis of pulmonary hypertension? J Lab Clin Med
    2002; 139(4):194–201.

41. Keegan A, Morecroft I, Smillie D, Hicks MN, MacLean MR. Contribution
    of the 5-HT(1B) receptor to hypoxia-induced pulmonary hypertension:

Converging evidence using 5-HT(1B)-receptor knockout mice and the 5-HT(1B/1D)-receptor antagonist GR127935. Circ Res 2001; 89(12):1231–9.

42. Welsh DJ, Harnett M, MacLean M, Peacock AJ. Proliferation and signaling in fibroblasts: Role of 5-hydroxytryptamine2A receptor and transporter. Am J Respir Crit Care Med 2004; 170(3):252–9.

43. Launay JM, Herve P, Peoc'h K, et al. Function of the serotonin 5-hydroxytryptamine 2B receptor in pulmonary hypertension. Nat Med 2002; 8(10):1129–35.

44. Racchi M, Leone M, Porrello E, et al. Familial migraine with aura: Association study with 5-HT1B/1D, 5-HT2C, and hSERT polymorphisms. Headache 2004; 44(4):311–7.

45. Tsai SJ, Hong CJ, Yu YW, Chen TJ, Wang YC, Lin WK. Association study of serotonin 1B receptor (A-161T) genetic polymorphism and suicidal behaviors and response to fluoxetine in major depressive disorder. Neuropsychobiology 2004; 50(3):235–8.

46. Ranade SS, Mansour H, Wood J, et al. Linkage and association between serotonin 2A receptor gene polymorphisms and bipolar I disorder. Am J Med Genet B Neuropsychiatr Genet 2003; 121(1):28–34.

47. Blanpain C, Le PE, Parma J, et al. Serotonin 5-HT(2B) receptor loss of function mutation in a patient with fenfluramine-associated primary pulmonary hypertension. Cardiovasc Res 2003; 60(3):518–28.

48. Deraet M, Manivet P, Janoshazi A, et al. The natural mutation encoding a C-terminus truncated 5-HT$_{2B}$ receptor is a gain of proliferative functions. Mol Pharmacol 2004; 67:983–91.

49. Eddahibi S, Hanoun N, Lanfumey L, et al. Attenuated hypoxic pulmonary hypertension in mice lacking the 5-hydroxytryptamine transporter gene. J Clin Invest 2000; 105(11):1555–62.

50. Rothman RB, Ayestas MA, Dersch CM, Baumann MH. Aminorex, fenfluramine, and chlorphentermine are serotonin transporter substrates. Implications for primary pulmonary hypertension. Circulation 1999; 100(8):869–75.

51. Lee SL, Wang WW, Fanburg BL. Dexfenfluramine as a mitogen signal via the formation of superoxide anion. FASEB J 2001; 15(7):1324–5.

52. Lesch KP, Bengel D, Heils A, et al. Association of anxiety-related traits with a polymorphism in the serotonin transporter gene regulatory region. Science 1996; 274(5292):1527–31.

53. Eddahibi S, Humbert M, Fadel E, et al. Serotonin transporter overexpression is responsible for pulmonary artery smooth muscle hyperplasia in primary pulmonary hypertension. J Clin Invest 2001; 108(8):1141–50.

54. Marcos E, Fadel E, Sanchez O, et al. Serotonin-induced smooth muscle hyperplasia in various forms of human pulmonary hypertension. Circ Res 2004; 94(9):1263–70.

55. Eddahibi S, Chaouat A, Morrell N, et al. Polymorphism of the serotonin transporter gene and pulmonary hypertension in chronic obstructive pulmonary disease. Circulation 2003; 108(15):1839–44.

56. Moncada S, Higgs A. The L-arginine-nitric oxide pathway. N Engl J Med 1993; 329(27):2002–12.
57. Pearson DL, Dawling S, Walsh WF, et al. Neonatal pulmonary hypertension—Urea-cycle intermediates, nitric oxide production, and carbamoyl-phosphate synthetase function. N Engl J Med 2001; 344(24):1832–8.
58. Thomas A, Summar M, Scott N, et al. Penetrance of familial primary pulmonary hypertension (FPPH) may be modified by carbamoyl phosphate synthetase I (CPSI) genotype. Meeting of the American Thoracic Society, 2001.
59. Wang XL, Mahaney MC, Sim AS, et al. Genetic contribution of the endothelial constitutive nitric oxide synthase gene to plasma nitric oxide levels. Arterioscler Thromb Vasc Biol 1997; 17(11):3147–53.
60. Yildiz P, Oflaz H, Cine N, Erginel-Unaltuna N, Erzengin F, Yilmaz V. Gene polymorphisms of endothelial nitric oxide synthase enzyme associated with pulmonary hypertension in patients with COPD. Respir Med 2003; 97(12):1282–88.
61. Archer SL, Wu XC, Thebaud B, et al. Preferential expression and function of voltage-gated, O_2-sensitive K+ channels in resistance pulmonary arteries explains regional heterogeneity in hypoxic pulmonary vasoconstriction: Ionic diversity in smooth muscle cells. Circ Res 2004; 95(3):308–18.
62. Archer SL, London B, Hampl V, et al. Impairment of hypoxic pulmonary vasoconstriction in mice lacking the voltage-gated potassium channel Kv1.5. FASEB J 2001; 15(10):1801–3.
63. Yamada Y, Kuroe A, Li Q, et al. Genomic variation in pancreatic ion channel genes in Japanese type 2 diabetic patients. Diabetes Metab Res Rev 2001; 17(3):213–16.
64. Chioza B, Osei-Lah A, Wilkie H, et al. Suggestive evidence for association of two potassium channel genes with different idiopathic generalised epilepsy syndromes. Epilepsy Res 2002; 52(2):107–16.
65. Bardien-Kruger S, Wulff H, Arieff Z, Brink P, Chandy KG, Corfield V. Characterisation of the human voltage-gated potassium channel gene, *KCNA7*, a candidate gene for inherited cardiac disorders, and its exclusion as cause of progressive familial heart block I (PFHBI). Eur J Hum Genet 2002; 10(1):36–43.
66. Abenhaim L, Moride Y, Brenot F, et al. Appetite-suppressant drugs and the risk of primary pulmonary hypertension. N Engl J Med 1996; 335(9):609–16.
67. Ahearn GS, Tapson VF, Rebeiz A, Greenfield JC, Jr. Electrocardiography to define clinical status in primary pulmonary hypertension and pulmonary arterial hypertension secondary to collagen vascular disease. Chest 2002; 122(2):524–7.
68. Barst RJ, McGoon M, Torbicki A, et al. Diagnosis and differential assessment of pulmonary arterial hypertension. J Am Coll Cardiol 2004; 43(12 Suppl S):40S–7S.

6 The Right Ventricle in Pulmonary Hypertension

Andrew C. Stone
and James R. Klinger

CONTENTS

THE NORMAL RIGHT VENTRICLE AND
  PULMONARY CIRCULATION
RIGHT VENTRICULAR RESPONSE TO
  PULMONARY HYPERTENSION
ADAPTIVE AND MALADAPTIVE CARDIAC
  HYPERTROPHIC RESPONSES
SIGNALING PATHWAYS IN CARDIAC
  HYPERTROPHY
ADAPTIVE HYPERTROPHY
DETERMINANTS OF THE HYPERTROPHIC
  RESPONSE OF THE RIGHT VENTRICLE
RIGHT AND LEFT VENTRICULAR INTERACTIONS
PERICARDIAL EFFUSION
EFFECT OF RIGHT HEART FUNCTION ON
  PATIENT OUTCOME IN PULMONARY
  HYPERTENSION
MONITORING RIGHT VENTRICULAR FUNCTION
CLINICAL APPROACH TO RV DYSFUNCTION
FUTURE DIRECTIONS
ACKNOWLEDGMENTS
REFERENCES

From: *Contemporary Cardiology: Pulmonary Hypertension*
Edited by: N. S. Hill and H. W. Farber © Humana Press, Totowa, NJ

Abstract

The main cause of morbidity and mortality in pulmonary arterial hypertension (PAH) is not injury to the lung, but rather progressive right ventricular (RV) dysfunction. Although the pulmonary vasculopathy associated with PAH can impair gas exchange, patients with PAH suffer most from the inability to adequately increase cardiac output, especially during exercise. RV dysfunction in PAH is typically viewed as a secondary event, an unavoidable consequence of the progressive rise in pulmonary vascular resistance. However, the RV response to increased pulmonary afterload varies considerably between individuals, and those variations may significantly impact functional capacity and survival.

This chapter explores the adaptive and maladaptive responses of the RV to elevated pulmonary arterial pressure (PAP) and the cellular and molecular mechanisms responsible for them. The effect of RV overload on left ventricular (LV) function is also reviewed. New techniques used to monitor RV function at baseline and in response to therapy are presented. Finally, an overview of the management of RV failure in PAH is provided along with a discussion of future therapeutic approaches.

Key Words: right ventricle; right heart; pulmonary hypertension; pulmonary circulation; cardiac hypertrophy; echocardiography; magnetic resonance imaging; natriuretic peptides.

1. THE NORMAL RIGHT VENTRICLE AND PULMONARY CIRCULATION

The right ventricle (RV) differs substantially from the left ventricle (LV) in shape and construction, no doubt due in large part to the marked differences in the functional requirements of these adjacent pumps. Unlike the left chamber, which can be considered a true ventricle, the RV consists essentially of a lateral free wall that is attached, almost as a covering, to the more muscularized medial wall (the interventricular septum) of the LV (Fig. 1). Because the lateral free wall curves in parallel to the intraventricular septum, the cross-section of the RV lumen has a crescent shape as opposed to the circular shape of the LV (Fig. 1). The different shapes of the RV and LV chambers result in considerable differences between how force and wall tension are generated (Fig. 2).

The pulmonary circulation is a low-pressure circuit. Even during periods of heavy exertion, the remarkable ability of the lung to recruit partially collapsed or unused vessels results in only modest increases in PAP despite a three- to fourfold increase in cardiac output *(1)*. As a result, mean PAP (mPAP) is only about one-sixth that of the systemic circulation at rest and one-eighth that of the systemic circulation during exercise. Unlike the muscular LV, which responds well

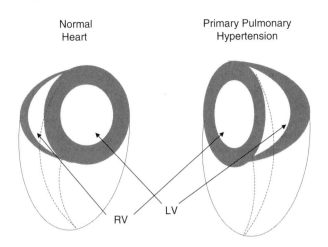

Normal
Heart

Primary Pulmonary
Hypertension

LV
RV

Fig. 1. Illustration comparing heart chamber size and septal positioning in a normal heart and the heart of a patient with pulmonary hypertension. (Adapted from Bristow et al. *(1)*.)

to rapid increases in systemic blood pressure but has difficulty in handling sudden increases in preload, the thin lateral wall of the RV has difficulty in maintaining systolic function in response to elevation in PAP but is capable of accommodating large increases in right-sided return *(1)*. The ability of the RV to function well in response to increased preload is vital for the maintenance of pulmonary blood

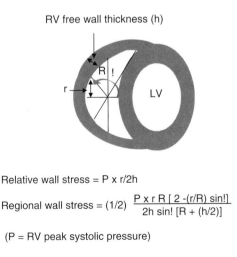

RV free wall thickness (h)

R !
r
LV

Relative wall stress = P x r/2h

Regional wall stress = (1/2) $\dfrac{P \times r \, R \, [\, 2 - (r/R) \sin!\,]}{2h \sin! \, [R + (h/2)]}$

(P = RV peak systolic pressure)

Fig. 2. Illustration demonstrating wall stress proportionality to right ventricular pressure and inverse proportionality to right ventricular wall thickness. The RV hypertrophies in order to reduce wall stress.

flow, as changes in intrathoracic pressure or venous tone can alter the volume of blood returning to the right heart considerably. On the other hand, the lack of significant pulmonary hypertension under normal conditions obviates the need for the RV to sustain cardiac output against elevated systolic pressures.

2. RIGHT VENTRICULAR RESPONSE TO PULMONARY HYPERTENSION

A rapid increase in RV afterload, such as that seen with massive pulmonary embolism, causes global hypokinesis and marked dilation of the RV. However, with a gradual increase in PAP, the RV is capable of substantial hypertrophy with an increase in free wall thickness and contractile force. Under these conditions, the RV may be capable of sustaining marked increases in PAP. For example, the pulmonary hypertension seen in Eisenmenger's syndrome usually develops slowly throughout childhood and is associated with substantial RV hypertrophy and a systolic PA pressure that approaches that of systemic arterial pressure.

In most cases of PAH, PA pressure escalates faster than the RV can adapt. Although many patients develop significant RV hypertrophy, increased myocardial cell size and strength give way to apoptosis, fibrosis, and decreased contractility. The net result is a transition from a hypertrophic RV with preserved systolic function to a dilated, hypokinetic ventricle. As the RV enlarges, wall tension rises and free wall thickness decreases. The expanding RV widens the tricuspid annulus and causes chordal traction and tethering of the tricuspid leaflets, worsening tricuspid regurgitation and further compromising RV function (2). RV end-diastolic pressure rises, forcing the interventricular septum toward the LV during diastole and compromising LV filling (Fig. 1). Increased myocardial oxygen consumption from elevated wall tension and reduced coronary perfusion related to the reduction of the normal driving pressure predispose to increased myocardial ischemia and a falling cardiac output. A pattern of increasing RV failure ensues, ushering in the final stages of clinical deterioration and death.

Recent studies suggest that the nature of the RV response to increased afterload plays an important role in function and survival. Patients who are able to increase RV contractility and maintain systolic function have a greater level of activity and survive longer, whereas those who develop a dilated RV cardiomyopathy do poorly. Determinants of a favorable versus unfavorable RV response are not well understood. A brief discussion of cardiac hypertrophic responses is provided below, but RV response to sustained increases in afterload remains an important area of research.

3. ADAPTIVE AND MALADAPTIVE CARDIAC HYPERTROPHIC RESPONSES

Proliferation of cardiac myocytes generally does not occur after birth. Although recent studies (3) suggest the presence of small populations of cardiac stem cells in the adult heart, the primary mechanism of postnatal cardiac growth is cellular hypertrophy. Enlargement of individual myocytes can increase wall thickness, reduce wall tension, and improve contractility. For example, the increase in LV mass that occurs throughout early development or with repetitive exercise increases cardiac contractility and cardiac output. This type of hypertrophic response is considered beneficial and is termed "adaptive" or "physiologic." In contrast, cardiac hypertrophy induced by sustained increases in LV afterload, such as that seen in systemic hypertension, often results in increased myocardial fibrosis and apoptosis. The shift from synthesis of contractile proteins such as α-skeletal actin to fetal cardiac proteins such as β-myosin heavy chain impairs systolic function. This type of hypertrophic response is considered maladaptive or "pathological" and can adversely affect patient outcome. Epidemiological studies indicate that increased cardiac mass is an independent predictor of mortality in hypertensive cardiovascular disease (4).

A similar association between increased RV mass and worsening survival in PAH has not been shown. In fact, the presence of RV hypertrophy is often considered a favorable finding in patients with PAH. However, the lack of a correlation between RV mass and decreased survival in PAH may be related to the fact that PAH frequently presents with RV dilation and signs of RV failure. In contrast, these findings are usually late manifestations in LV failure. PAH may progress through an initial RV hypertrophic response that is then followed by RV dilation, thinning of the lateral free wall, and hypokinesis. An interesting hypothesis that is badly in need of further investigation is that the presence of RV hypertrophy and preserved systolic function in PAH represent an adaptive response to sustained increase in afterload that avoids or delays the transition to a maladaptive hypertrophic response.

4. SIGNALING PATHWAYS IN CARDIAC HYPERTROPHY

A variety of intracellular signal transduction pathways transfer mechanical or growth factor-mediated signals from the cell surface to the nucleus and thereby modulate synthesis of contractile proteins and the expression of cytokines and other genes that regulate apoptosis and extracellular collagen production. A brief review of the major hypertrophic signaling pathways follows, but the reader is referred to several recent reviews for more details *(5,6)*.

4.1. G Protein-Coupled Receptors

Many hypertrophic stimuli, including adrenergic activation, angiotensin II (AII), and endothelin-1 (ET-1), are mediated by G protein-coupled receptors. The G protein-coupled receptors are a superfamily of receptors characterized by a transmembrane portion comprised of seven alpha-helices linked by three alternating intra- and extracellular loops. Activation of G protein-coupled receptors occurs when ligand binds to the extracellular domain of the receptor, changing the receptor conformation and promoting coupling with an intracellular heterotrimeric guanine nucleotide-binding (G) protein. The activated G protein then dissociates into Gα and Gβγ subunits, each capable of initiating a variety of intracellular signal transduction pathways.

Several subtypes of G protein-coupled receptors have been implicated in cardiac remodeling, including the Gq subtype signal that activates phospholipase C, generating diacylglycerol (DAG) and inositol, 1,4,5-triphosphate (IP3) and, in turn, activating protein kinase C that mobilizes intracellular calcium. Studies in mice have shown that cardiac hypertrophy can be blunted or exaggerated by disruption or overexpression of Gq-coupled receptors, respectively *(7,8)*.

Adrenergic agonists signaling through Gq-coupled receptors can lead to pathological hypertrophy. Indeed, mice with cardiac-directed overexpression of $\alpha 1_B$-adrenergic receptors develop a dilated cardiomyopathy *(9)*. In contrast, G stimulatory (Gs) proteins may mediate a more adaptive cardiac hypertrophy via β-adrenergic stimulation. Both β1- and β2-adrenergic receptors couple Gs-linked receptors and activate adenyl cyclase, thereby increasing intracellular cAMP and activating cAMP-dependent kinase (PKA). Activation of PKA via β1-adrenergic signaling increases cardiac contractility via phosphorylation of L-type calcium channels *(10)*. β2-receptors also couple to G-inhibitory proteins (Gi) that signal through a pertussis toxin-sensitive pathway, inhibiting adenyl cyclase activity and stimulating mitogen activated protein kinase (MAPK). Activation of β-adrenergic receptors also causes a cAMP-dependent inhibition of PKC activation, the pathway that is mediated by Gq-receptors *(11)*. Considerable cross-talk exists between α- and β-adrenergic signal transduction pathways and ultimately determines to what extent catecholamines cause an adaptive or maladaptive hypertrophic response. Of particular interest is the observation that enhanced catecholamine stimulation, as occurs with sustained increases in ventricular afterload, reduces β-adrenergic receptor activity either by receptor desensitization or by decreased receptor expression and thereby reduces the inhibitory effect of β2 activation on α-adrenergic mediated pathological hypertrophic responses (12).

4.2. Angiotensin and Endothelin

Angiotensin-II and ET-1 also signal via Gq receptors to induce pathologic hypertrophy via a PKC-dependent pathway. In addition, AII increases the expression of ET-1 and several cytokines, including TGF-β and TNF-α, that are capable of independently stimulating hypertrophy. Most of the hypertrophic effects of AII are mediated by type 1 receptors (AT$_1$), and AT1 antagonists have been shown to decrease heart mass and improve cardiac function in spontaneously hypertensive rats (13). Activation of type 2 receptors (AT$_2$) may serve to limit some of the pathological hypertrophic responses of AT$_1$, although this theory is controversial (14).

ET-1 has trophic effects in cultured cardiac myocytes (15) and induces and enhances the expression of cytokines (16,17). Plasma levels of ET-1 increase in patients with CHF, as does myocardial expression of endothelin A and B receptors. Recent evidence demonstrating that overexpression of ET-1 is associated with myocardial inflammation and a dilated cardiomyopathy (18) and that cardiac-directed suppression of ET-1 inhibits thyroxin-induced cardiac hypertrophy (19) further strengthens the connection between ET-1 and pathological hypertrophy.

4.3. Cytokines and Growth Factors

The myocardial fibrosis that occurs during the transition from physiological to pathological cardiac hypertrophy may be mediated in part by cytokines, some of which are known to be upregulated by hypertrophic growth factors such as AII and ET-1 as well as by mechanical stretch. Cardiac expression of TGF-β$_1$ is increased in patients with idiopathic hypertrophic cardiomyopathy and dilated cardiomyopathy (20–22). During the transition from stable hypertrophy to heart failure, TGF-β expression is enhanced in the hypertrophic myocardium (23). TGF-β stimulates fibroblast proliferation, increases collagen production by cardiac fibroblasts, and facilitates conversion of fibroblasts to myofibroblasts (24–26). In neonatal cardiac myocytes, TGF-β promotes the expression of fetal genes that serve as a marker of cardiac hypertrophy *(27)*. In rodents, overexpression of TGF-β induces cardiac hypertrophy and fibrosis *(28,29)*, whereas anti-TGF-β antibodies and genetic disruption of TGF-β inhibit the development of cardiac hypertrophy, myocardial fibrosis, and systolic dysfunction *(30,31)*.

TNF-α has also been implicated in the pathogenesis of cardiac hypertrophy. Interaction with its TNF receptors 1 and 2 activates a myriad of signaling pathways with such diverse roles as inflammation, cell growth, and apoptosis. Pressure overload enhances myocardial TNF-α expression *(32)* and, at physiological doses, TNF-α induces hypertrophy in adult cardiocytes *(33,34)*. Moreover, transgenic overexpression of TNF-α induces cardiac hypertrophy in mice *(35)*.

4.4. Mechanical Stretch

Mechanical forces alone are capable of activating many of the signal transduction pathways leading to hypertrophy. This occurs both directly, by physical activation of mechanosensors, and indirectly via the increased synthesis and release of substances known to induce cardiac growth. For example, mechanical stretch directly induces the synthesis and secretion of TGF-β, AII, and ET-1 *(36–38)*. Furthermore, AT1 and ET-1 receptor blockers inhibit many of the hypertrophic signal responses in stretched cardiomyoctes *(37,38)*. However, AII or ET-1 receptor blockade only partially inhibits pressure overload-induced cardiac hypertrophy *(39,40)*, and AT_{1A} knockout mice still develop cardiac hypertrophy in response to pressure overload *(41,42)*. These findings suggest that other mechanisms besides AII or ET-1 expression activate hypertrophic signaling pathways during mechanical stretch.

The mechanosensor mechanism by which stretching of cardiomyocytes invokes hypertrophic responses may act via several mechanisms, chief among them being cell-surface integrins. These transmembrane proteins link the extracellular matrix to the cytoskeleton, a loosely knit structure of scaffolding proteins that support the cell membrane. Although these proteins were first recognized as adhesion molecules, they also act as mechanotransducers by converting physical stimuli at the cell surface into biochemical signals *(43)*. Integrins are associated with G protein-coupled receptors, similar to the types of receptors that mediate α-adrenergic, ATII, and ET-1 signaling, and with nonreceptor-linked intracellular signaling molecules such as focal adhesion kinase (FAK) *(44,45)*. By activating G protein-coupled receptors or FAK through integrins, mechanical stretch can initiate hypertrophic signaling directly.

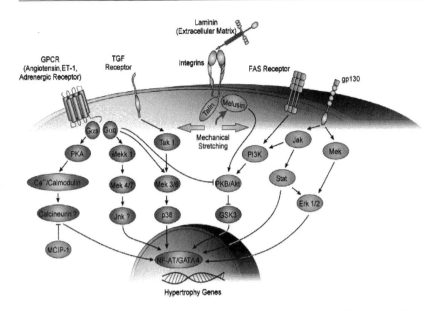

Fig. 3. Adaptive and maladaptive cardiac hypertrophic intracellular signaling pathways. Pathways on the right outlined in red are associated with maladaptive cardiac hypertrophy and those on the left outlined green are associated with a more adaptive hypertrophic response. See text for details. (Reprinted from [5].) (To view this figure in color, see insert.)

In summary, cardiac hypertrophy involves the activation of numerous signal transduction pathways that regulate the expression of numerous proteins needed for cell growth. Many of these pathways induce the synthesis of fetal proteins that better withstand increased wall tension, but at the expense of reduced contractility. Activation of apoptotic pathways and the production of extracellular matrix proteins can lead to cardiocyte death and myocardial fibrosis. To what extent these various pathways are activated determines whether the hypertrophic response will be adaptive or maladaptive (Fig. 3).

5. ADAPTIVE HYPERTROPHY

Adaptive signaling pathways induce cardiac remodeling without decreased systolic function or ventricular dilation. These are not antihypertrophic pathways, but rather pathways that allow myocyte growth to occur without degeneration or reduced contractility. The phosphatidylinositol 3-kinase (P13K) and its downstream serine-threonine kinase effector Akt modulate cellular substrate utilization and play key roles in regulating cardiomyocyte growth. Akt induces hypertrophy in vivo by activating glycogen synthase kinase3-beta (GSK3β) *(46)*. Overexpression of P13K or Akt causes concentric LVH with preservation of systolic function and without the development of cardiac fibrosis *(46–48)*. The lack of deleterious cardiac effects associated with this pathway likely stems from its inhibitory effect on apoptosis *(46)*. Akt has been shown to phosphorylate several modulators of apoptosis, including caspase 9 and nuclear factor (NF)-kB. In addition, activation of GSK3β by the P13K/Akt pathway inhibits the NFAT transcription factor family, a group of transcription factors that activate immune response genes such as interleukin-2 and that have been associated with pathological cardiac hypertrophy via activation by the serine/threonine phosphatase calcineurin *(49)*.

The natriuretic peptides and their guanylyl cyclase-linked receptors are another signaling system that may favor adaptive cardiac hypertrophy. Atrial, brain, and C-type natriuretic peptides (ANP, BNP, CNP) share a 17 amino acid loop that is necessary for their activity. Natriuretic peptides signal via binding to one of two particulate guanylyl cyclase-linked receptors. ANP and BNP preferentially bind to natriuretic peptide receptor-A (NPR-A) and CNP binds to natriuretic peptide receptor-B (NPR-B). A third receptor, NPR-C, binds all three peptides but is not linked to guanylyl cyclase and is thought to function primarily as a clearance receptor *(50)*. Activation of NPR-A or NPR-B increases intracellular cGMP levels, leading to activation of cGMP-related protein kinase (PKG).

The natriuretic peptides relax vascular smooth muscle, inhibit salt and fluid retention, inhibit vascular smooth muscle proliferation and ET-1 synthesis, and antagonize many of the actions of the renin-angiotensin system. Expression of ANP and BNP is upregulated as part of a program of fetal genes that are expressed during cardiac hypertrophy *(51)*. Circulating levels of ANP and BNP correlate directly with the degree of ventricular failure in patients with LV and RV failure (see section on RV monitoring below). Although originally felt to be merely markers of the severity of hypertrophy, these peptides are now thought to be part of a counterregulatory response that limits the degree of hypertrophy and slows the transition from physiological to pathological hypertrophy. All three natriuretic peptides have been shown to inhibit hypertrophy of adult cardiac myocytes in vitro *(52)*. Mice with transgenic overexpression of ANP have smaller RVs and LVs than their nontransgenic littermates, despite only a modest reduction in systemic arterial pressure and no change in PA pressure *(53)*. Targeted disruption of the gene for NPR-A causes severe cardiac hypertrophy, myocardial fibrosis, and early cardiac death *(54)*. Cardiac hypertrophy in NPR-A knockout mice is independent of arterial pressure, as evidenced by studies in which systemic arterial pressure is normalized pharmacologically, with no reduction in LV mass *(55)*. In the same study *(55)*, aortic constriction increased LV mass fivefold more in NPR-A knockout mice than in wild-type mice (55 vs. 11%). Interestingly, LV hypertrophy was associated with a dilated cardiomyopathy and impaired systolic function in the NPR-A knockouts, but not in controls, consistent with the idea that natriuretic peptides protect against maladaptive hypertrophy *(55)*. One mechanism by which BNP limits maladaptive hypertrophic effects in the heart may be its profound inhibitory effect on TGF-β-induced pro-inflammatory, fibrotic, and proliferative effects on cardiac fibroblasts *(56)*.

The natriuretic peptides may play a particularly important role in limiting RV hypertrophic responses during the development of pulmonary hypertension. ANP and BNP are potent pulmonary vasodilators *(57)* and have been shown to blunt hypoxia-induced pulmonary hypertension and RV hypertrophy in animal studies *(58,59)*. Genetic disruption of ANP or NPR-A results in greater pulmonary hypertension and an exaggerated RV hypertrophic response to chronic hypoxia *(60,61)*.

6. DETERMINANTS OF THE HYPERTROPHIC RESPONSE OF THE RIGHT VENTRICLE

There is considerable individual variability in the RV response to pressure overload. The factors that determine a more favorable RV hypertrophic response in PAH are not well understood but likely include differences in the expression of a variety of genes that modulate hypertrophic signaling pathways, synthesis of contractile proteins, and apoptosis. Studies of human endomyocardial biopsies have shown that, compared to normal controls, failing RVs have increased beta-myosin heavy chain (β-MHC) and decreased α-MHC mRNA levels *(62)*. These alterations in MHC expression may allow the RV to better withstand increased wall tension, but at the expense of a reduction in shortening velocity and diminished systolic function. α-MHC mRNA and protein levels are also reduced or absent in patients with biventricular failure presenting for cardiac transplant *(63)*. β-1 adrenergic receptor mRNA is decreased in the failing RVs of patients with PAH, but not in their LVs or in the RVs of normal controls *(62)*. Adenyl cyclase activity and AT_1 receptor density are also decreased in the RVs of PAH patients at the time of transplant, but not in the RVs of patients with biventricular failure or normal hearts *(64)*. These alterations in protein and receptor expression likely contribute to decreased myocardial reserve and exercise capacity and probably represent an adaptive response to counter the overstimulation of adrenergic and angiotensin systems that lead to myocyte dysfunction and apoptosis as well as chamber remodeling.

Chronic adrenergic overdrive may hasten the development of RV failure. A study of 17 patients with PAH and 12 controls found that skeletal muscle sympathetic nerve activity was significantly increased in PAH patients (65). Elevated plasma noradrenaline levels have also been associated with increased mortality in patients with PAH (66). These studies suggest that, similar to left heart failure, PAH causes a pathological increase in sympathetic response that can adversely effect cardiac myocytes and contribute to RV failure.

Genetic differences in ACE activity may also affect RV function in pulmonary hypertension. An insertion/deletion polymorphism in the ACE gene has been identified that enhances ACE activity and increases cardiac tissue ACE levels and circulating AII levels in patients homozygous for the deletion polymorphism (D/D) (67,68). One study (69) found that the frequency of the ACE D/D genotype was nearly twice as high in patients with PAH as in healthy controls or heart organ donors (45% vs. 24% and 28%, respectively). However, in the same study (69), the ACE D/D genotype was also associated with significantly better cardiac output, lower RAP, and better NYHA functional class than ACE I/D or I/I genotype. These studies suggest that the ACE D/D genotype or increased ACE activity may predispose to PAH but also promote a more adaptive RV response. However, the favorable hemodynamic effect of ACE D/D could not be identified in another, smaller study of PAH patients (70).

7. RIGHT AND LEFT VENTRICULAR INTERACTIONS

Pressure overload of the RV can influence LV performance in two ways. The most obvious is series interaction: the interdependency between two pumps connected in series. Decreased output of the RV diminishes flow to the LV, leading to a global low-output state. The second mechanism, known as "ventricular interdependence," refers to interference with LV diastolic filling by RV pressure transmitted via the interventricular septum. Normally, the lower end-diastolic pressure (EDP) in the RV results in the interventricular septum moving toward it during diastole. The compliant RV free wall permits expansion of the RV during diastole despite the inward shift of the septum. As PAH develops, however, RVEDP rises, eventually exceeding LVEDP, and the interventricular septum bows toward the LV during diastole. This

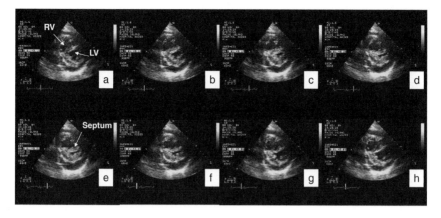

Fig. 4. Echocardiogram of patient with pulmonary arterial hypertension from early systole (a) to end diastole (h). Note the enlarged right ventricle, septal bowing at end diastole (h) and the eccentric shape of the LV due to the enlarged septum.

paradoxical septal motion can easily be detected on an echocardiogram and is often described as "septal flattening" (Fig. 4). The relatively stiff LV free wall cannot accommodate this intrusion as well as the RV free wall. LV filling is impeded and cardiac output falls. The pericardium may contribute to ventricular interdependence by limiting ventricular free wall distension, and pericardiectomy has been shown to improve cardiac output, in animal models of acute RV pressure overload *(71–73)*.

The combination of reduced pulmonary venous return from decreased RV output and diminished filling capacity from ventricular interdependence greatly impairs LV performance. Unfortunately, the reduction in LV preload arising from this situation may be difficult to improve by intravascular volume expansion, as raising the central venous pressure will only increase RVEDP more and further compromise LV filling. In one study of COPD patients with chronic pulmonary hypertension *(74)*, volume loading was shown to actually decrease LVEDV despite an increase in LVEDP.

8. PERICARDIAL EFFUSION

Pericardial effusions are often seen in patients with PAH. Normally, pericardial fluid drains through the cardiopericardial lymphatics in the subepicardium into mediastinal nodes and, ultimately, via the thoracic duct, back into the venous system *(75)*. Although the mechanism for pericardial effusion in PAH is uncertain, one study found a correlation between RAP and effusion size *(76)*, suggesting that the pericardial effusion in patients with severe PAH may be due to impaired venous and lymphatic drainage.

The presence of a pericardial effusion in PAH is associated with a worse clinical outcome. Two studies with 26 and 81 patients, respectively, found that the severity of pericardial effusion was an independent predictor of mortality (77,78). In another study, Hinderliter et al. (76) found that pericardial effusion was associated with reduced exercise tolerance, more severe right heart failure, and a one-year mortality that was 2.5-fold higher than in patients with trace or undetectable pericardial effusion.

Tamponade physiology is unusual with PAH-associated pericardial effusions, probably because the elevated RVEDP prevents collapse of the RV during diastole. Occasionally, a large pericardial effusion might reduce LV transmural filling pressure enough to decrease cardiac output. Pericardiocentesis is usually not helpful, although it was thought to be life-saving in at least one reported case (79). The authors suggested that if the clinical suspicion for tamponade is high, pericardiocentesis should be considered in PAH patients, even in the absence of echocardiographic signs of RV collapse.

9. EFFECT OF RIGHT HEART FUNCTION ON PATIENT OUTCOME IN PULMONARY HYPERTENSION

As mentioned at the beginning of this chapter, mortality in PAH is related mainly to loss of cardiac output. Patients do not often die from respiratory failure, but rather from progressive circulatory collapse, explaining why numerous studies in PAH patients have found RV function to be a greater predictor of death than PAP. The first large-scale evaluation of prognostic indicators in PAH came from the NIH Registry in the 1980s. Data from that registry showed that mPAP, RAP, and cardiac index all affected survival by univariate and multivariate analysis (80). However, the odds ratio for elevated mPAP (1.19) was relatively small compared to the elevated RAP (1.99) or decreased cardiac index (1.62). At least one study (81) found mPAP to be a better predictor of mortality in PAH than the cardiac index, but most studies (82–84) have found baseline indices of RV function such as mRAP, cardiac index, RVEDP, or mixed venous oxygen saturation to be better prognostic indicators. In fact, one study (85) found that lower mPAP was associated with a worse survival by univariate analysis. This finding may reflect the possibility that a fall in mPAP is a consequence of worsening RV function in patients with advanced disease.

Thus, monitoring of RV function in PAH patients is at least as important as monitoring PA pressure. Previous studies examining the effect of RV function on outcome relied on right heart catheterization, but this test is simply too invasive and expensive for intermittent monitoring. More recently, noninvasive tests that assess RV function have been used to follow RV failure and response to treatment. Although the best test and the frequency for monitoring have yet to be determined, a number of approaches are currently available, as discussed in the next section.

10. MONITORING RIGHT VENTRICULAR FUNCTION

10.1. Chest Radiograph

Early RV changes are often difficult to recognize on a traditional plain chest radiograph (CXR). Due to its position directly in front of the LV, moderate increases in RV volume are not easily detectable on a posterior-anterior projection. As the RV enlarges, straightening of the left heart border occurs that is often misidentified as LV dilation on the anterior view (Fig. 5). Only when RV dilation becomes severe and RA enlargement develops does the right heart border become more rounded and protrude into the right hemithorax. A better assessment of RV dilation can be obtained from the lateral chest film, where an enlarging RV is seen to occupy more of the retrosternal airspace and push the posterior border of the LV closer to the spine (Fig. 5). Although these findings may be helpful in identifying RV failure in PAH patients as part of their initial evaluation, the CXR is too

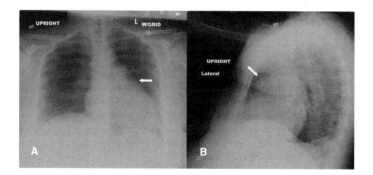

Fig. 5. Posterior-anterior (a) and lateral (b) chest radiograph of patient with idiopathic pulmonary arterial hypertension. Note flattening of the left heart border (a) and loss of retrosternal air space (b) due to the right ventricle enlargement.

insensitive to monitor changes in RV size or function during disease progression or in response to treatment.

10.2. Electrocardiography

Most PAH-related ECG abnormalities reflect the development of RV hypertrophy or ischemia. In one study (86), 78% of PAH patients had right-axis deviation defined as frontal plane QRS axis > 90°. A qR and rSR' pattern in V1 was seen in 18% and 20% of patients, respectively, whereas complete right bundle branch block (RBBB) was seen in only two patients. Markers of RV ischemia, such as T-wave inversion in II, III, or aVF, or ST-T segment depression in the prechordial leads, were seen in 68% and 28% of patients, respectively. The sensitivity of the ECG to predict RV hypertrophy in PAH patients varied from 38–96% depending on the criteria used. One set of ECG criteria, developed in an autopsy series of 51 patients with isolated RV hypertrophy (12 patients), biventricular hypertrophy (14 patients), and no hypertrophy of either ventricle (24 patients), consist of four criteria that detect RV hypertrophy with a sensitivity of 63% and a specificity of 96% (Table 1) (87). ECG changes may be helpful in the initial evaluation of patients with PAH but are too insensitive for ongoing monitoring.

10.3. Echocardiography

Two-dimensional transthoracic echocardiography with Doppler ultrasound (TTE) has become the key screening tool for PAH (see Chapter 3). In addition to estimating systolic PA pressure, the

Table 1
Electrocardoigraphic Criteria to Identify Right Ventricular Hypertrophy

1) Right axis deviation > 110 degrees (in absence of RBBB)
2) R or R' amplitude $\geq$ S amplitude in V1 or V2
3) R amplitude $\leq$ S amplitude in V6 (in absence of anterior infarct)
4) A + R – PL $\geq$ 0.7 mV
   Where:
   A = maximal R or R' in amplitude in V1 or V6
   R = maximal S in lead 1 or V6
   PL = minimal S in V1 or minimal R in lead I or V6

Any one of the above four criteria indicates right ventricular hypertrophy with a specificity of 96% (from reference 87 with permission).

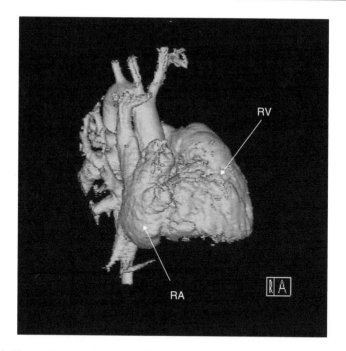

Fig. 6. Three-dimensional magnetic resonance image reconstruction demonstrating enlarged right atrium and ventricle in a 35 year old about to undergo tetralogy of Fallot repair.

echocardiogram provides a useful assessment of LV function and can exclude significant valvular disease or intracardiac shunting. Echocardiography also assesses RA and RV size as well as RV function and thereby provides important information on how the RV is compensating for the sustained increase in afterload (Fig. 4). Finally, this noninvasive test is readily accepted by most patients and allows the clinician to obtain repeated measurements over time.

An estimate of RV contractility can be obtained by measuring RV end-diastolic and end-systolic dimensions (RVEDD, RVESD). Fractional shortening of the RV chamber can then be calculated as

$$\text{fractional shortening} = \text{RVEDD-RVESD/RVEDD}.$$

Unfortunately, the irregular shape of the RV makes accurate measurement of RV dimensions difficult. Interobserver and interexam variability is high and this index cannot be used as a reliable estimation of RV ejection fraction. Another assessment of RV function, the

Doppler RV index or Tei index, assesses RV function by isovolumetric contraction time *(88)*:

Tei index $=$ $\dfrac{\text{isovolumetric contraction time} + \text{isovolumetric relaxation time}}{\text{ejection time.}}$

Ejection time is defined as the duration of pulmonic outflow *(88)*. In one study *(89)*, the Tei index was threefold higher in PAH patients (indicating deterioration of RV performance), and an index ≥ 0.83 portended a poor prognosis. In fact, the Tei index was a stronger predictor of mortality than hemodynamic variables obtained at right heart catheterization *(89)*.

The echocardiogram can also be used to assess disease progression or regression. Increases in the severity of tricuspid regurgitation correlate with worsening exercise capacity as measured by the six-minute walk test *(2)*. Echocardiographic measurements have been used to demonstrate a decrease in RV size in selected patients with favorable responses to calcium channel blockers, prostacyclin, lung transplant, or thromboendarterectomy *(90–93)*. Decreases in right ventricular end-systolic (RVES) area, RV dilatation, the Tei index, and the degree of septal flattening have also been associated with clinical improvements in patients treated with prostacyclin infusions or bosentan *(94,95)*. However, the echocardiagram does not provide reliable information on cardiac output, and its ability to direct therapeutic decisions in individual patients has not been established.

10.4. Magnetic Resonance Imaging

Magnetic resonance imaging (MRI) is a promising new tool for assessing the RV function in PAH. In addition to producing more accurate and consistent determinations of RVED and RVES dimensions than echocardiography, it is capable of measuring ventricular volumes and mass by computer processing of multiple cross-sectional areas (Fig. 7). These measurements can then be used to calculate RV ejection fraction, PAP, cardiac output, and RV hypertrophy.

The RV ejection fraction can be calculated by the formula

$$\text{RVEDV-RVESV}/\text{RVEDV} \times 100\%.$$

An assessment of RV stroke volume can be determined via volumetric flow in the PA, and RV output can be calculated from the product of RV stroke volume and heart rate. Maximal systolic cross-sectional area and mean systolic blood flow velocity through the main pulmonary artery can be used to calculate the mPAP. Finally, RV

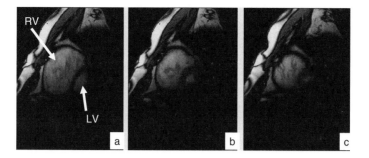

Fig. 7. Magnetic resonance images of right ventricle at end diastole (a), mid systole (b), and end systole (c) in the same patient as figure 3. Note extremely large right ventricle (RV) and septal bowing at end diastole (a).

hypertrophy can be assessed by measuring RV mass and comparing it to that of the LV.

Measurements of mPAP calculated by MRI agree well with mPAP measured simultaneously by pulmonary artery catheter in patients with PAH. In one study *(96)*, the mean difference between measurements was only 5.4 mm Hg *(96)*. The ventricular mass index (VMI), calculated by dividing the RV mass (RVM) by the LV mass (LVM), is nearly twofold greater in patients with PAH than in patients with normal mPAP *(97)*, and a threshold value for the VMI of 0.6 has been shown to identify PAH with a sensitivity of 84% and a specificity of 71% *(97)*. Ventricular volumes and myocardial mass from cine MRI can be used to calculate RV pressure-volume loops. The slope of the end-systolic pressure-volume relationship (E_{max}) is a load-independent parameter of myocardial contractility *(98)*.

Indices of RV function determined by serial MRIs correlate well with changes in functional capacity in patients being treated for PAH. In nine patients treated with epoprostenol *(99)*, MRI showed no significant changes in RVEDV or RVESV, but RV stroke volume and functional capacity both increased in close parallel (Fig. 8). Repeated right heart catheterization revealed no change in mPAP but detected a significant increase in cardiac output, suggesting that epoprostenol improved RV performance by increasing RV contractility and reducing pulmonary vascular resistance. These findings suggest that MRI might be a useful tool for following RV function in patients with PAH and for monitoring response to therapy.

10.5. Biomarkers of RV Failure

Another approach to assessing RV function in PAH is to monitor circulating levels of biomarkers such as BNP and troponin. As

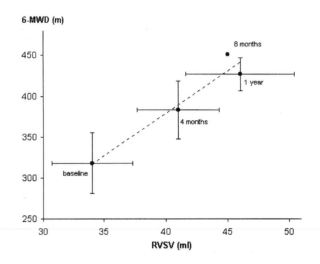

Fig. 8. Relationship between six minute walking distance (6 MWD) and right ventricular stroke volume (RVSV) in patients with pulmonary arterial hypertension treated for 12 months with epoprostenol. (Reprinted from *(99)*.)

discussed earlier in this chapter, the natriuretic peptides appear to play an important role in blunting the development of maladaptive cardiac hypertrophy. ANP and BNP are released by the cardiac atria and ventricles in response to several stimuli including myocardial distension, tachycardia, and hypoxia. Elevated plasma BNP levels are negative prognostic indicators in patients with left-sided heart failure *(100)*, and decreases in plasma BNP in such patients correlate with improvement in NYHA functional class *(101)*. In acute respiratory failure, plasma BNP has been shown to discriminate accurately between cardiac and noncardiac causes *(102)*. The same principal of using elevated circulating BNP levels as an indicator of ventricular overload in CHF applies to patients with PAH and RV failure.

Pulmonary hypertension increases RV mRNA and circulating levels of both ANP and BNP *(57)*. Furthermore, circulating BNP levels correlate directly with PAP, pulmonary vascular resistance, and right atrial pressure and inversely with cardiac index, six-minute walk distance, and peak oxygen uptake *(103)*. Elevated BNP at presentation is a poor prognostic indicator in PAH patients, as is failure to reduce plasma BNP levels during treatment. A plasma BNP level under 150 pg/ml at presentation predicts a better two-year survival than higher BNP levels *(104)*. Furthermore, failure of therapy to lower plasma BNP levels below a median value of 180 pg/ml was associated with a fourfold increase in two-year mortality *(104)*. These findings suggest that plasma BNP can serve as a biomarker of RV overload and as a useful tool to monitor RV function in patients with PAH. In the authors' experience, low plasma BNP levels (<100 pg/ml) are common in patients with preserved functional capacity (NYHA Class II-III) despite gross dilatation and hypokinesis of the RV on echocardiogram. Furthermore, a progressive rise in plasma BNP may indicate impending RV failure, even before patients become overtly symptomatic. In these patients, a rising BNP level may signal a need for more aggressive therapy or consideration of lung transplantation.

Cardiac troponin, a sensitive indicator of myocardial ischemia in coronary artery disease, is another biomarker that holds promise for assessing RV function in PAH. Small increases in plasma troponin levels are commonly seen in clinical situations where myocardial oxygen demand exceeds supply without acute obstruction to coronary blood flow. A rising RV pressure in PAH patients with progressive disease increases RV wall tension and oxygen demand. At the same time, reduced systemic blood pressure combined with a falling cardiac output compromises RV coronary perfusion. Under these conditions, the imbalance of oxygen supply and demand renders the RV ischemic, promoting troponin release. In 7 (14%) of 56 patients with PAH (105), cardiac troponin T levels were elevated above the detectable range of 0.1 ng/ml. These patients had higher heart rates, lower mixed venous oxygen saturations, and 98 meters fewer on a six-minute walking distance, compared to patients in whom troponin T was undetectable. Although the elevation in troponin level tended to be small (mean value: 0.034 ± 0.022 ng/ml), cumulative 24-month survival was only 29% in patients who had a positive troponin test compared to 81% in troponin-negative patients.

11. CLINICAL APPROACH TO RV DYSFUNCTION

Details regarding the symptomatic and physical manifestations of RV dysfunction are found in Chapter 3. In brief, these symptoms are attributable to the failure of the RV to adequately increase cardiac output during exercise, leading to exertional dyspnea, dizziness, or even syncope. The latter is an alarming symptom and demands prompt intervention. Terminally, patients often develop delirium and obtundation related to their low-flow state. Physical findings of RV dysfunction reflect hypertrophy, dilatation, and, eventually, failure of the RV.

Therapeutic interventions are aimed at preserving RV function, increasing exercise capacity, and relieving the discomfort of chronic fluid overload. The mainstay of treatment is relief from pressure overload by reducing PAP. The role of pulmonary vasodilators and other agents that help to remodel the pulmonary vasculature is discussed in other chapters. There are, however, several additional therapies that should be considered for aiding the failing RV. Foremost is the relief of the chronic hypoxia that hastens the progression of pulmonary vascular disease by enhancing pulmonary vasoconstriction and vascular remodeling. Hypoxia has been shown to increase the synthesis of several growth factors implicated in pulmonary hypertension such as endothelin-1 *(106)* and to increase muscle sympathetic nerve activity *(65)* while possibly suppressing NO synthesis *(107)*. In addition, hypoxia compromises RV contractility by depriving the myocardium of its most important energy source. Although the impact of reversing hypoxia on RV function has not been well studied in PAH, improvements in RV function, exercise capacity, and fluid retention have been demonstrated with oxygen therapy used to treat RV failure associated with chronic lung disease *(108)*.

A particular consideration for patients with RV failure is to exclude obstructive sleep apnea (OSA) and nocturnal hypoxemia. Transient episodes of hypoxia during sleep increase catecholamine levels and reduce vasodilatory responses in systemic arterioles *(109,110)*. Although the contributory role of transient hypoxia to the development of pulmonary hypertension is not well established, it is reasonable to speculate that a condition known to cause congestive heart failure and systemic hypertension in normal individuals will abet RV failure in patients with PAH. Furthermore, treatment with continuous positive airway pressure (CPAP) has been shown to normalize PAP in some OSA patients with pulmonary hypertension *(111)*. Therefore, OSA should be excluded by a formal sleep study in patients with suggestive findings and, if found, should be treated with CPAP or other methods that prevent nocturnal hypoxia.

Diuretics are indicated when peripheral edema, hepatic congestion, or ascites become uncomfortable in patients with advanced PAH, but their use must be balanced against the need to maintain adequate RV preload. Patients with advanced RV failure may require higher filling pressures to maintain cardiac output and often will need to tolerate some degree of volume overload. Judicious diuresis may improve RV function by returning the RV to a more favorable position on its Starling curve. In addition, adequate diuresis may dramatically improve symptoms of discomfort in the legs and abdomen swelling even without altering the severity of the pulmonary hypertension. On the other hand, overzealous diuresis can reduce cardiac output and systemic blood pressure by excessively lowering intravascular volume. Some patients may become refractory to diuretics due to decreased cardiac output; under these circumstances, sodium and fluid restriction become important. Potassium sparing diuretics, such as spirinolactone, may be useful in treating patients with chronic ascites.

Natriuretic peptides also hold promise as a therapy for right ventricular hypertrophy and volume overload in patients with RV failure and PAH, by virtue of their antihypertrophic, vasodilator, and natriuretic actions. Plasma levels of both ANP and BNP are elevated in PAH, probably due to a combination of increased synthesis and decreased clearance, the latter related to the downregulation of endocardial natriuretic peptide receptor density *(112)*. Interestingly, binding affinity for radio-labeled ANP is normally greater in the RV than in the LV but decreases to nearly undetectable levels in rats with monocrotaline-induced pulmonary hypertension *(112)*. Both ANP and BNP have been shown to decrease pulmonary arterial pressure in patients with cor pulmonale *(113)*. Presently, the only commercially available natriuretic peptide is BNP. It's use in PAH remains investigational.

Ideally, the strategy for improving RV function should be not only to reduce afterload but also to increase contractility. However, the role of positive inotropic agents in RV failure associated with PAH is limited due to a fixed myocardial oxygen supply and a reduction of functional myocardial tissue from myocardial fibrosis and apoptosis. Nevertheless, some studies have been able to demonstrate acute improvements in cardiac output with the use of cardiac inotropes in patients with RV failure from PAH. Cardiac output improved acutely from 3.49 ± 1.2 to 3.81 ± 1.2 L/min ($p = 0.028$) in 16 PAH patients 2 hours after receiving 1 mg of intravenous digoxin *(114)*. Prostacyclin derivatives are potent pulmonary vasodilators, and chronic administration improves pulmonary vascular remodeling, but these agents also cause an acute increase in cardiac output that can be attributed at least partially to improvements in cardiac contractility. In end-stage RV, dobutamine and milrinone have been used to augment RV function as rescue therapies *(115,116)*.

In advanced disease, atrial septostomy has been used successfully to unload the failing RV *(117)*. This technique creates an alternative pathway, permitting a portion of the RV preload to reach the left heart without transversing the pulmonary circulation. The resultant right-to-left shunt reduces RV work, but at the cost of greater arterial hypoxemia due to venous blood reaching the left atrium. Hypoxia due to right-to-left shunting across the septostomy is essentially irreversible and does not respond to supplemental oxygen. Thus, the size of the septostomy must be limited. In experienced hands, the technique improves clinical symptoms, cardiac index, systemic oxygen transport, and exercise capacity in PAH patients with advanced RV failure *(118,119)*. This procedure is typically used in parts of the world where therapeutic options are limited or as a bridge to a more definitive procedure such as heart-lung transplantation.

12. FUTURE DIRECTIONS

Decades of research have yielded new insight into the etiology and treatment of PAH. Recent therapies have dramatically changed the outcome of these patients, with improvements in both survival and functional class. Unfortunately, PAH remains a progressive and usually fatal disease. Research continues to explore new ways to reverse the pulmonary vascular remodeling that is responsible for the intolerable afterload that the RV eventually faces. In the meantime, investigators are beginning to appreciate that RV adaptation to chronic pressure overload is vital to the maintenance of performance and prolonged survival. Although this concept has became fairly well appreciated among clinicians and investigators alike, there remains a general lack of knowledge on how the RV adapts (or fails to adapt) to the increase in workload on a molecular and cellular level. Future studies aimed at identifying these mechanisms may lead to new strategies for preserving RV function in high-impedance states. A similar line of research has been ongoing for many years in the study of LV failure. These studies strongly indicate that survival in CHF can be improved by inhibition of the renin-angiotensin and alpha-adrenergic systems and that these beneficial effects are not related solely to decreased LV afterload *(120,121)*. The same therapeutic approach that targets inhibition of maladaptive hypertrophic responses in the LV needs to be applied to the RV in patients with PAH. Now that patients with PAH are living longer, the number of patients with progressive RV failure is likely to increase. In addition to treatments aimed at reducing PA pressure, new treatments aimed primarily at improving RV function are needed.

ACKNOWLEDGMENTS

This work was supported by American Heart Association Established Investigator Award 0240190N (J. R. Klinger).

REFERENCES

1. Bristow MR, Zisman LS, Lowes BD, et al. The pressure-overloaded right ventricle in pulmonary hypertension. Chest 1998; 114(1 Suppl):101S–106S.
2. Hinderliter AL, Willis PW 4th, Long WA, et al. PPH Study Group. Frequency and severity of tricuspid regurgitation determined by Doppler echocardiography in primary pulmonary hypertension. Am J Cardiol 2003; 91(8):1033–7, A9.
3. Anversa P, Nadal-Ginard B. Myocyte renewal and ventricular remodelling. Nature 2002; 415(6868):240–3.
4. de Simone G, Verdecchia P, Pede S, Gorini M, Maggioni AP. Prognosis of inappropriate left ventricular mass in hypertension: the MAVI Study. Hypertension 2002; 40(4):470–6.
5. Selvetella G, Hirsch E, Notte A, Tarone G, Lembo G. Adaptive and maladaptive hypertrophic pathways: points of convergence and divergence. Cardiovasc Res 2004; 63(3):373–80.
6. Ross RS. Molecular and mechanical synergy: cross-talk between integrins and growth factor receptors. Cardiovasc Res 2004; 63(3):381–90.1
7. Milano CA, Dolber PC, Rockman HA, et al. Myocardial expression of a constitutively active alpha 1B-adrenergic receptor in transgenic mice induces cardiac hypertrophy. Proc Natl Acad Sci USA 1994; 91(21):10109–13.
8. Akhter SA, Luttrell LM, Rockman HA, Iaccarino G, Lefkowitz RJ, Koch WJ. Targeting the receptor-Gq interface to inhibit in vivo pressure overload myocardial hypertrophy. Science 1998; 280:574–7.
9. Lemire I, Ducharme A, Tardif JC, et al. Cardiac-directed overexpression of wild-type alpha1B-adrenergic receptor induces dilated cardiomyopathy. Am J Physiol Heart Circ Physiol 2001; 281(2):H931–8.
10. Xiao RP, Cheng H, Zhou YY, Kuschel M, Lakatta EG. Recent advances in cardiac beta(2)-adrenergic signal transduction. Circ Res 1999; 85(11):1092–100.
11. Schafer M. Ponicke K. Heinroth-Hoffmann I. Brodde OE. Piper HM. Schluter KD. Beta-adrenoceptor stimulation attenuates the hypertrophic effect of alpha-adrenoceptor stimulation in adult rat ventricular cardiomyocytes. Journal of the American College of Cardiology 2001; 37(1):300–7.
12. Bristow MR. Why does the myocardium fail? Insights from basic science. Lancet 1998; 352 (Suppl 1):SI8–14.
13. Kaneko K, Susic D, Nunez E, Frohlich ED. Losartan reduces cardiac mass and improves coronary flow reserve in the spontaneously hypertensive rat. J Hypertens 1996; 14(5):645–53.
14. Opie LH, Sack MN. Enhanced angiotensin II activity in heart failure: reevaluation of the counterregulatory hypothesis of receptor subtypes. Circ Res 2001; 88(7):654–8.
15. Ito H, Hirata Y, Hiroe M, et al. Endothelin-1 induces hypertrophy with enhanced expression of muscle-specific genes in cultured neonatal rat cardiomyocytes. Circ Res 1991; 69(1):209–15.

16. Shubeita HE, McDonough PM, Harris AN, et al. Endothelin induction of inositol phospholipid hydrolysis, sarcomere assembly,and cardiac gene expression in ventricular myocytes. A paracrine mechanism for myocardial cell hypertrophy. J Biol Chem 1990; 265(33):20555–62.

17. McMillen MA, Huribal M, Cunningham ME, Kumar R, Sumpio BE. Endothelin-1 increases intracellular calcium in human monocytes and causes production of interleukin-6. Crit Care Med 1995; 23(1):34–40.

18. Yang LL, Gros R, Kabir MG, Sadi A, Gotlieb AI, Husain M, et al. Conditional cardiac overexpression of endothelin-1 induces inflammation and dilated cardiomyopathy in mice. Circulation 2004; 109(2):255–61.

19. Shohet RV, Kisanuki YY, Zhao XS, Siddiquee Z, Franco F, Yanagisawa M. Mice with cardiomyocyte-specific disruption of the endothelin-1 gene are resistant to hyperthyroid cardiac hypertrophy. Proc Natl Acad Sci USA 2004; 101(7):2088–93.

20. Pauschinger M, Knopf D, Petschauer S, et al. Dilated cardiomyopathy is associated with significant changes in collagen type I/III ratio. Circulation 1999; 99(21):2750–6.

21. Li G, Li RK, Mickle DA, et al. Elevated insulin-like growth factor-I and transforming growth factor-beta 1 and their receptors in patients with idiopathic hypertrophic obstructive cardiomyopathy. A possible mechanism. Circulation 1998; 98(19 Suppl):II144–9.

22. Li RK, Li G, Mickle DA, et al. Overexpression of transforming growth factor-beta1 and insulin-like growth factor-I in patients with idiopathic hypertrophic cardiomyopathy. Circulation 1997; 96(3):874–81.

23. Boluyt MO, L O'Neill, AL Meredith, et al. Alterations in cardiac gene expression during the transition from stable hypertrophy to heart failure: marked upregulation of genes encoding extracellular matrix components. Circ Res 1994; 75:23–3.

24. Villarreal FJ, Lee AA, Dillmann WH, Giordano FJ. Adenovirus-mediated overexpression of human transforming growth factor-beta 1 in rat cardiac fibroblasts, myocytes and smooth muscle cells. J Mol Cell Cardiol 1996; 28(4):735–42.

25. Heimer R, Bashey RI, Kyle J, Jimenez SA. TGF-beta modulates the synthesis of proteoglycans by myocardial fibroblasts in culture. J Mol Cell Cardiol 1995; 27(10):2191–8.

26. Eghbali M, Tomek R, Sukhatme VP, Woods C, Bhambi B. Differential effects of transforming growth factor-beta 1 and phorbol myristate acetate on cardiac fibroblasts. Regulation of fibrillar collagen mRNAs and expression of early transcription factors. Circ Res 1991; 69(2):483–90.

27. Parker TG, Packer SE, Schneider MD. Peptide growth factors can provoke "fetal" contractile protein gene expression in rat cardiac myocytes. J Clin Invest 1990; 85(2):507–14.

28. Rosenkranz S, Flesch M, Amann K, et al. Alterations of beta-adrenergic signaling and cardiac hypertrophy in transgenic mice overexpressing TGF-beta(1). Am J Physiol Heart Circ Physiol 2002; 283(3):H1253–62.

29. Nakajima H, Nakajima HO, Salcher O, et al. Atrial but not ventricular fibrosis in mice expressing a mutant transforming growth factor-beta(1) transgene in the heart. Circ Res 2000; 86(5):571–9.
30. Brooks WW, Conrad CH. Myocardial fibrosis in transforming growth factor beta(1)heterozygous mice. J Mol Cell Cardiol 2000; 32(2):187–95.
31. Kuwahara F, Kai H, Tokuda K, et al. Transforming growth factor-beta function blocking prevents myocardial fibrosis and diastolic dysfunction in pressure-overloaded rats. Circulation 2002; 106(1):130–5.
32. Kapadia SR, Oral H, Lee J, Nakano M, Taffet GE, Mann DL. Hemodynamic regulation of tumor necrosis factor-alpha gene and protein expression in adult feline myocardium. Circ Res 1997; 81(2):187–95.
33. Yokoyama T, Nakano M, Bednarczyk JL, McIntyre BW, Entman M, Mann DL. Tumor necrosis factor-alpha provokes a hypertrophic growth response in adult cardiac myocytes. Circulation 1997; 95(5):1247–52.
34. Nakamura K, Fushimi K, Kouchi H, et al. Inhibitory effects of antioxidants on neonatal rat cardiac myocyte hypertrophy induced by tumor necrosis factor-alpha and angiotensin II. Circulation 1998; 98(8):794–9.
35. Kubota T, McTiernan CF, Frye CS, Demetris AJ, Feldman AM. Cardiac-specific overexpression of tumor necrosis factor-alpha causes lethal myocarditis in transgenic mice. J Card Fail 1997; 3(2):117–24.
36. Villarreal FJ, Dillmann WH. Cardiac hypertrophy-induced changes in mRNA levels for TGF-beta 1, fibronectin, and collagen. Am J Physiol 1992; 262:H1861–6.
37. Miyata S, Haneda T, Osaki J, Kikuchi K. Renin-angiotensin system in stretch-induced hypertrophy of cultured neonatal rat heart cells. Eur J Pharmacol 1996; 307:81–8.
38. Yamazaki T, Komuro I, Kudoh S, et al. Endothelin-1 is involved in mechanical stress-induced cardiomyocyte hypertrophy. J Biol Chem 1996; 271:3221–28.
39. Yamazaki T, Komuro I, Kudoh S, et al. Angiotensin II partly mediates mechanical stress-induced cardiac hypertrophy. Circ Res 1995; 77: 258–65.
40. Ito H, Hiroe M, Hirata Y, et al. Endothelin ETA receptor antagonist blocks cardiac hypertrophy provoked by hemodynamic overload. Circulation 1994; 89(5):2198–203.
41. Harada K, Komuro I, Zou Y, et al. Acute pressure overload could induce hypertrophic responses in the heart of angiotensin II type 1a knockout mice. Circ Res 1998; 82(7):779–85.
42. Harada K, Komuro I, Shiojima I, et al. Pressure overload induces cardiac hypertrophy in angiotensin II type 1A receptor knockout mice. Circulation 1998; 97(19):1952–9.
43. Ingber D. Integrins as mechanochemical transducers. Curr Opin Cell Biol 1991; 3(5):841–8.
44. Lewis JM, Schwartz MA. Mapping in vivo associations of cytoplasmic proteins with integrin beta 1 cytoplasmic domain mutants. Mol Biol Cell 1995; 6(2):151–60.

45. Dominguez-Jimenez C, Yanez-Mo M, Carreira A, et al. Involvement of alpha3 integrin/tetraspanin complexes in the angiogenic response induced by angiotensin II. FASEB J 2001; 15(8):1457–9.
46. Matsui T, Nagoshi T, Rosenzweig A. Akt and PI 3-kinase signaling in cardiomyocyte hypertrophy and survival. Cell Cycle 2003; 2(3):220–3.
47. Condorelli G, Drusco A, Stassi G, et al. Akt induces enhanced myocardial contractility and cell size in vivo in transgenic mice. Proc Natl Acad Sci USA 2002; 99(19):12333–338.
48. Matsui T, Li L, Wu JC, Cook SA, Nagoshi T, Picard MH, Liao R, Rosenzweig A. Phenotypic spectrum caused by transgenic overexpression of activated Akt in the heart.J Biol Chem 2002; 277(25):22896–901.
49. Zhou P, Sun LJ, Dotsch V, Wagner G, Verdine GL. Solution structure of the core NFATC1/DNA complex. Cell 1998; 92(5):687–96.
50. Maack T, Suzuki M, Almeida FA, et al. Physiological role of silent receptors of atrial natriuretic factor. Science 1987; 238(4827):675–8.
51. Chien KR, Knowlton KU, Zhu H, Chien S. Regulation of cardiac gene expression during myocardial growth and hypertrophy: molecular studies of an adaptive physiologic response. FASEB J 1991; 5(15):3037–46.
52. Rosenkranz AC, Woods RL, Dusting GJ, Ritchie RH. Antihypertrophic actions of the natriuretic peptides in adult rat cardiomyocytes: importance of cyclic GMP. Cardiovasc Res 2003; 57(2):515–22.
53. Klinger JR, Petit RD, Curtin LA, et al. Cardiopulmonary responses to chronic hypoxia in transgenic mice that overexpress ANP. J Appl Physiol 1993; 75(1):198–205.
54. Oliver PM, Fox JE, Kim R, et al. Hypertension, cardiac hypertrophy, and sudden death in mice lacking natriuretic peptide receptor A. Proc Natl Acad Sci USA 1997; 94(26):14730–5.
55. Knowles JW, Esposito G, Mao L, et al. Pressure-independent enhancement of cardiac hypertrophy in natriuretic peptide receptor A-deficient mice. J Clin Invest 2001; 107(8):975–84.
56. Kapoun AM, Liang F, O'Young G, et al. B-type natriuretic peptide exerts broad functional opposition to transforming growth factor-beta in primary human cardiac fibroblasts: fibrosis, myofibroblast conversion, proliferation, and inflammation. Circ Res 2004; 94(4):453–61
57. Hill NS, Klinger JR, Warburton RR, Pietras L, Wrenn DS. Brain natriuretic peptide: possible role in the modulation of hypoxic pulmonary hypertension. Am J Physiol 1994; 266(3 Pt 1):L308–15.
58. Klinger JR, Warburton RR, Pietras L, Hill NS. Brain natriuretic peptide inhibits hypoxic pulmonary hypertension in rats.J Appl Physiol 1998; 84(5):1646–52.
59. Jin H, Yang RH, Chen YF, Jackson RM, Oparil S. Atrial natriuretic peptide attenuates the development of pulmonary hypertension in rats adapted to chronic hypoxia. J Clin Invest 1990; 85(1):115–20.
60. Klinger JR, Warburton RR, Pietras L, et al. Targeted disruption of the gene for natriuretic peptide receptor-A worsens hypoxia-induced cardiac hypertrophy. Am J Physiol 2002; 282(1):H58–65.

61. Klinger JR, Warburton RR, Pietras LA, Smithies O, Swift R, Hill NS. Genetic disruption of atrial natriuretic peptide causes pulmonary hypertension in normoxic and hypoxic mice. Am J Physiol 1999; 276(5 Pt 1):L868–74.

62. Lowes BD, Minobe W, Abraham WT, et al. Changes in gene expression in the intact human heart. Downregulation of alpha-myosin heavy chain in hypertrophied, failing ventricular myocardium. J Clin Invest 1997; 100(9):2315–24.

63. Miyata S, Minobe W, Bristow MR, Leinwand LA. Myosin heavy chain isoform expression in the failing and nonfailing human heart. Circ Res 2000; 86(4):386–90.

64. Bristow MR, Minobe W, Rasmussen R, et al. Beta-adrenergic neuroeffector abnormalities in the failing human heart are produced by local rather than systemic mechanisms. J Clin Invest 1992; 89(3):803–15.

65. Velez-Roa S, Ciarka A, Najem B, Vachiery JL, Naeije R, van de Borne P. Increased sympathetic nerve activity in pulmonary artery hypertension. Circulation 2004; 110(10):1308–12.

66. Nootens M, Kaufmann E, Rector T, et al. Neurohormonal activation in patients with right ventricular failure from pulmonary hypertension: relation to hemodynamic variables and endothelin levels. J Am Coll Cardiol 1995; 26(7):1581–5.

67. Tiret L, Rigat B, Visvikis S, et al. Evidence, from combined segregation and linkage analysis, that a variant of the angiotensin I-converting enzyme (ACE) gene controls plasma ACE levels. Am J Hum Genet 1992; 51(1):197–205.

68. Danser AH, Schalekamp MA, Bax WA, et al. Angiotensin-converting enzyme in the human heart. Effect of the deletion/ insertion polymorphism. Circulation 1995; 92(6):1387–8.

69. Abraham WT, Raynolds MV, Badesch DB, et al. Angiotensin-converting enzyme DD genotype in patients with primary pulmonary hypertension: increased frequency and association with preserved haemodynamics. J Renin Angiotensin Aldosterone Syst 2003; 4(1):27–30.

70. Hoeper MM, Tacacs A, Stellmacher U, Lichtinghagen R. Lack of association between angiotensin converting enzyme (ACE) genotype, serum ACE activity, and haemodynamics in patients with primary pulmonary hypertension. Heart 2003; 89(4):445–6.

71. Belenkie I, Smith ER, Tyberg JV. Ventricular interaction: from bench to bedside. Ann Med 2001; 33(4):236–41.

72. Belenkie I, Dani R, Smith ER, Tyberg JV. Ventricular interaction during experimental acute pulmonary embolism. Circulation 1988; 78(3):761–8.

73. Belenkie I, Dani R, Smith ER, Tyberg JV. Effects of volume loading during experimental acute pulmonary embolism. Circulation 1989; 80(1):178–88.

74. Jardin F, Gueret P, Prost JF, Farcot JC, Ozier Y, Bourdarias JP. Two-dimensional echocardiographic assessment of left ventricular function

in chronic obstructive pulmonary disease. Am Rev Respir Dis 1984; 129(1):135–42.

75. Miller AJ, Pick R, Johnson PJ. The production of acute pericardial effusion: the effects of various degrees of interference with venous blood and lymph drainage from the heart muscle in the dog. Am J Cardiol 1971; 28: 463.

76. Hinderliter AL, Willis PW 4th, Long W, et al. Frequency and prognostic significance of pericardial effusion in primary pulmonary hypertension. PPH Study Group. Primary pulmonary hypertension. Am J Cardiol 1999; 84(4):481–4, A10.

77. Eysmann SB, Palevsky HI, Reichek N, Hackney K, Douglas PS. Two-dimensional and Doppler-echocardiographic and cardiac catheterization correlates of survival in primary pulmonary hypertension. Circulation 1989; 80(2):353–60.

78. Raymond RJ, Hinderliter AL, Willis PW, et al. Echocardiographic predictors of adverse outcomes in primary pulmonary hypertension. J Am Coll Cardiol 2002; 39(7):1214–9.

79. Akinci SB, Gaine SP, Post W, Merrit WT, Tan HP, Winters B. Cardiac tamponade in an orthotopic liver recipient with pulmonary hypertension. Crit Care Med 2002; 30(3):699–701.

80. D'Alonzo GE, Barst RJ, Ayers SM, et al. Survival in patients with primary pulmonary hypertension: results from a national prospective registry. Ann Intern Med 1991; 115:343–49.

81. Okada O, Tanabe N, Yasuda J, et al. Prediction of life expectancy in patients with primary pulmonary hypertension. A retrospective nationwide survey from 1980–1990. Internal Medicine 1999; 38(1):12–6.

82. Sandoval J, Bauerle O, Palomar A, et al. Survival in primary pulmonary hypertension: validation of a prognostic equation. Circulation 1994; 89:1733–44.

83. Rajasekhar D, Balakrishnan KG, Venkitachalam CG, et al. Primary pulmonary hypertension: natural history and prognostic factors. Indian Heart Journal 1994; 46(3):165–70.

84. Glanville AR, Burke CM, Theodore J, Robin ED. Primary pulmonary hypertension. Length of survival in patients referred for heart-lung trans-plantation. Chest 1987; 91(5):675–81.

85. Sitbon O, Humbert M, Nunes H, et al. Long-term intravenous epoprostenol infusion in primary pulmonary hypertension: prognostic factors and survival. J Amer Coll of Cardiol 2002; 40(4):780–8.

86. Bossone E, Paciocco G, Iarussi D, et al. The prognostic role of the ECG in primary pulmonary hypertension. Chest 2002; 121(2):513–8.

87. Lehtonen J, Sutinen S, Ikaheimo M, Paakko P. Electrocardiographic criteria for the diagnosis of right ventricular hypertrophy verified at autopsy. Chest 1988; 93(4):839–42.

88. Kim W, Otsuji Y, Seward J, Tei C. Estimation of Left Ventricular Function in Right Ventricular Volume and Pressure Overload; Detection

of Early Left Ventricular Dysfunction by the Tei Index. Japanese Heart Journal 1999; 40(2):145–54.

89. Yeo T, Dujardin K, Tei C, Mahoney D, McGoon M, and Seward J. Value of a Doppler Derived Index Combining Systolic and Diastolic Time Intervals in Predicting Outcomes in Primary Pulmonary Hypertension. Amer J Cardiol 1998; 81:1157–61.

90. Rich S, Brundage BH. High-dose calcium channel-blocking therapy for primary pulmonary hypertension: evidence for long-term reduction in PAP and regression of right ventricular hypertrophy. Circulation 1987; 76(1):135–41.

91. Barst RJ. Pharmacologically induced pulmonary vasodilatation in children and young adults with primary pulmonary hypertension. Chest 1986; 89(4):497–503.

92. Ritchie M, Waggoner AD, Davila-Roman VG, Barzilai B, Trulock EP, Eisenberg PR. Echocardiographic characterization of the improvement in right ventricular function in patients with severe pulmonary hypertension after single-lung transplantation. J Am Coll Cardiol 1993; 22(4):1170–4.

93. Menzel T, Kramm T, Bruckner A, Mohr-Kahaly S, Mayer E, Meyer J. Quantitative assessment of right ventricular volumes in severe chronic thromboembolic pulmonary hypertension using transthoracic three-dimensional echocardiography: changes due to pulmonary thromboendarterectomy. Eur J Echocardiogr 2002; 3(1):67–72.

94. Hinderliter AL, Willis PW 4th, Barst RJ, et al. Effects of long-term infusion of prostacyclin (epoprostenol) on echocardiographic measures of right ventricular structure and function in primary pulmonary hypertension. Primary Pulmonary Hypertension Study Group. Circulation 1997; 95(6):1479–86.

95. Galie N, Hinderliter AL, Torbicki A. et al. Effects of the oral endothelin-receptor antagonist bosentan on echocardiographic and doppler measures in patients with pulmonary arterial hypertension. J Am Coll Cardiol 2003; 41(8):1380–6.

96. Laffon E, Vallet C, Bernard V, et al. A computed method for noninvasive MRI assessment of pulmonary arterial hypertension. J Appl Physiol 2004; 96(2):463–8.

97. Saba TS, Foster J, Cockburn M, Cowan M, Peacock AJ. Ventricular mass index using magnetic resonance imaging accurately estimates pulmonary artery pressure. Eur Respir J 2002; 20(6):1519–24.

98. Kuehne T, Yilmaz S, Steendijk P, et al. Magnetic resonance imaging analysis of right ventricular pressure-volume loops: in vivo validation and clinical application in patients with pulmonary hypertension. Circulation 2004; 110(14):2010–6.

99. Roeleveld RJ, Vonk-Noordegraaf A, Marcus JT, et al. Effects of epoprostenol on right ventricular hypertrophy and dilatation in pulmonary hypertension. Chest 2004; 125(2):572–9.

100. Tsutamoto T, Wada A, Maeda K, et al. Attenuation of compensation of endogenous cardiac natriuretic peptide system in chronic heart failure:

prognostic role of plasma brain natriuretic peptide concentration in patients with chronic symptomatic left ventricular dysfunction. Circulation 1997; 96(2):509–16.

101. Lee SC, Stevens TL, Sandberg SM, et al. The potential of brain natriuretic peptide as a biomarker for New York Heart Association class during the outpatient treatment of heart failure. J Card Fail 2002; 8(3):149–54.

102. Maisel AS, Krishnaswamy P, Nowak RM, et al.; Breathing Not Properly Multinational Study Investigators. Rapid measurement of B-type natriuretic peptide in the emergency diagnosis of heart failure. N Engl J Med 2002; 347(3):161–7. 1

103. Leuchte HH, Holzapfel M, Baumgartner RA, et al. Clinical significance of brain natriuretic peptide in primary pulmonary hypertension. J Am Coll Cardiol 2004; 43(5):764–70.

104. Nagaya N, Nishikimi T, Uematsu M, et al. Plasma brain natriuretic peptide as a prognostic indicator in patients with primary pulmonary hypertension. Circulation 2000; 102(8):865–70.

105. Torbicki A, Kurzyna M, Kuca P, et al. Detectable serum cardiac troponin T as a marker of poor prognosis among patients with chronic precapillary pulmonary hypertension. Circulation 2003; 108(7):844–8.

106. Elton TS, Oparil S, Taylor GR, et al. Normobaric hypoxia stimulates endothelin-1 gene expression in the rat. Am J Physiol 1992; 263(6 Pt 2):R1260–4.

107. Berkenbosch JW, Baribeau J, Perreault T. Decreased synthesis and vasodilation to nitric oxide in piglets with hypoxia-induced pulmonary hypertension. Am J Physiol Lung Cell Mol Physiol 2000; 278(2):L276–83.

108. Long term domiciliary oxygen therapy in chronic hypoxic cor pulmonale complicating chronic bronchitis and emphysema. Report of the Medical Research Council Working Party. Lancet 1981; 1(8222):681–6.

109. Fletcher EC. Sympathetic over activity in the etiology of hypertension of obstructive sleep apnea. Sleep 2003; 26(1):15–9.

110. Fletcher EC. Invited review: Physiological consequences of intermittent hypoxia: systemic blood pressure. J Appl Physiol 2001; 90(4):1600–5. Review.

111. Sajkov KD, Wang T, Saunders NA, Bune AJ, McEvoy RD. Continuous positive airway pressure treatment improves pulmonary hemodynamics in patients with obstructive sleep apnea. Am J Respir Crit Care Med 2002; 165:152–158.

112. Kim SZ, Cho KW, Kim SH. Modulation of endocardial natriuretic peptide receptors in right ventricular hypertrophy. Am J Physiol 1999; 277(6 Pt 2):H2280–9.

113. Cargill RI, Lipworth BJ. Atrial natriuretic peptide and brain natriuretic peptide in cor pulmonale. Hemodynamic and endocrine effects. Chest 1996; 110(5):1220–5.

114. Rich S, Seidlitz M, Dodin E, et al.. The short-term effects of digoxin in patients with right ventricular dysfunction from pulmonary hypertension. Chest 1998; 114(3):787–92.

115. Wittwer T, Pethig K, Struber M, et al. Aerosolized iloprost for severe pulmonary hypertension as a bridge to heart transplantation. Ann Thorac Surg 2001; 71(3):1004–6.
116. Nelson DM, Main E, Crafford W, Ahumada GG. Peripartum heart failure due to primary pulmonary hypertension. Obstet Gynecol 1983; 62(3 Suppl):58s-63s.
117. Chau EM, Fan KY, Chow WH. Combined atrial septostomy and oral sildenafil for severe right ventricular failure due to primary pulmonary hypertension. Hong Kong Med J 2004; 10(4):281–4.
118. Sandoval J, Gaspar J, Pulido T, et al. Graded balloon dilation atrial septostomy in severe primary pulmonary hypertension. A therapeutic alternative for patients nonresponsive to vasodilator treatment. J Am Coll Cardiol 1998; 32(2):297–304.
119. Kerstein D, Levy PS, Hsu DT, Hordof AJ, Gersony WM, Barst RJ. Blade balloon atrial septostomy in patients with severe primary pulmonary hypertension. Circulation 1995; 91(7):2028–35.
120. Swedberg K, Kjekshus J, Snapinn S. Long-term survival in severe heart failure in patients treated with enalapril. Ten year follow-up of CONSENSUS I. Eur Heart J 1999; 20(2):136–9.
121. Packer M, Bristow MR, Cohn JN, et al. The effect of carvedilol on morbidity and mortality in patients with chronic heart failure. U.S. Carvedilol Heart Failure Study Group. N Engl J Med 1996; 334(21): 1349–55.

7 Congenital Heart Disease Associated with Pulmonary Arterial Hypertension

Michael J. Landzberg

CONTENTS

INTRODUCTION
DYNAMIC PAH
IMMEDIATE-POSTOPERATIVE "REACTIVE"
   PULMONARY HYPERTENSION
LATE-POSTOPERATIVE PULMONARY
   HYPERTENSION
NORMAL TO MILDLY ABNORMAL PVR STATES
EISENMENGER PHYSIOLOGY
CONCLUSIONS
REFERENCES

Abstract

Pulmonary arterial hypertension (PAH) associated with congenital heart disease (CHD) is common among the subtypes of PAH. It is quite variable in terms of clinical manifestations, severity of associated PAH, response to therapy, and outcomes, depending on the anatomy of the specific lesion, pulmonary circulatory flows and pressures, and other factors. Genetic predisposition likely plays a role, but no specific genetic abnormality has yet been identified for this form of PAH. Patients with CHD-PAH should undergo a careful evaluation that includes imaging of the defect as well as catheterization to characterize the severity and nature of pulmonary hemodynamic abnormalities. Surgical correction is desirable as long as the chances of reversibility are sufficient, but this may be difficult to ascertain preoperatively in marginal cases. Many patients

From: *Contemporary Cardiology: Pulmonary Hypertension*
Edited by: N. S. Hill and H. W. Farber © Humana Press, Totowa, NJ

now respond to pulmonary hypertension therapies if they are not surgical candidates or fail to improve after surgery, and lung or heart/lung transplantation remains an option for selected recalcitrant patients.

Key Words: congenital heart disease; Eisenmenger's syndrome; tetralogy of Fallot; Fontan procedure; Glenn procedure.

1. INTRODUCTION

Congenital heart disease (CHD) is currently the world's leading birth defect. In North America, it occurs in some eight of every one thousand live births, and an estimated one million or more adults and a similar number of children are living with CHD. Survival for affected individuals is increasing due to advances in detection, diagnostics, monitoring, pharmacotherapeutics, and surgical and transcatheter techniques. However, the functional capacity of CHD patients often remains limited when compared to age-matched controls, in large part because of nonreparable defects, postoperative cardiac and noncardiac residuae, and medical comorbidities.

Pulmonary arterial hypertension (PAH) associated with CHD (CHD-PAH) is one of the most common causes of severe morbidity and premature mortality in CHD patients *(1)*. Without surgery, PAH will develop in an estimated 30% of CHD patients *(2)*. With indicated surgery, epidemiological studies estimate that 15% of all CHD survivors will develop PAH *(3)*.

CHD-PAH occurs in a number of different scenarios, including

- "dynamic" PAH related to high shunt flow and responding to control of the shunt,
- immediate postoperative or "reactive" PAH,
- late, postoperative PAH,
- normal or mild elevation of pulmonary vascular resistance with unusual congenital defects, and
- shunt reversal (Eisenmenger physiology).

These forms of CHD-PAH are discussed separately in the chapter.

In addition, it should be emphasized that conceptions about CHD-PAH are evolving. In the past, CHD-PAH was classified directly within the "primary pulmonary hypertension" category (now referred to as idiopathic). More recently, CHD-PAH has been thought to have potentially differing pathogenetic mechanisms, therapeutic goals, treatment plans, and outcomes compared to IPAH. Hence, during the Third World Symposium on Pulmonary Arterial Hypertension held in Venice in 2003 *(4)*, CHD-PAH was categorized as a unique entity within the more global PAH (Group 1) category. Subcategories were also designated, based on the complexity and size of the defect, the association with additional extracardiac anomalies, as well as the status of anatomical repair. More recently, an expansion of the subcategorization has been proposed, allowing for further classification based on anatomy (defects above and below the tricuspid valve as well as clarification of specific types of complex disease), the presence of myocardial restriction as evidenced by equalization of pressure between chambers, and the direction of shunt (left-to-right, right-to-left, balanced) *(5)*.

2. DYNAMIC PAH

The original descriptions of PAH associated with systemic-to-pulmonary arterial shunts demonstrated that both the type and size of the underlying anatomical defect, as well as the magnitude of shunt flow, are risk factors for the development of PAH *(6)*. The pulmonary vascular histology resembled that described in IPAH, with medial thickening and plexiform lesions in severe cases *(7)*. Animal studies of surgically induced shunts to increase pulmonary blood flow and/or pulmonary arterial pressure suggest that both contribute to increased shear stress and structural changes *(8,9)*. In addition, increased expression of numerous mediators and receptors has been observed in the pulmonary arteries of shunted animals including endothelin-1 and ETB receptors with or without increased expression of ETA receptors *(10)*, angiotensin-II and the angiotensin A and B receptors *(11)*, VEGF with or without its Flk-1/KDR receptors *(12)*, and TGFβ-1 with the ALK1 receptor *(13)* (Table 2). Expression of signaling molecules such as calcium-dependent K+ channels *(14)*, phosphodiesterase 5 *(15)*, inducible NO synthase, angiopoietin-1, MCP-1, ICAM, and tenascin is also increased, and that of BMPR1A,

Table 1
Risk Factors for the Development of
Pulmonary Arterial Hypertension in
Patients with Congenital Heart Disease

Type of defect
  High risk: Truncus arteriosus
  Moderate risk: Ventricular septal defect
  Low risk: Atrial septal defect
Size of defect
Flow rate of shunt

BMPR2, and N-cGMP is decreased in animal models of pulmonary overcirculation *(16–18)*. The experimental studies as well as recent evidence in humans (BREATHE-5) suggest that endothelin plays a key pathogenetic role in the development and sustenance of CHD-PAH *(19–22)*.

Clinically, the development of PAH also depends on the specific anatomical lesion (Table 1). Individuals with an unrepaired truncus arteriosus are at a very high risk of developing PAH, whereas those with ventricular septal defects and atrial septal defects are at a moderate and relatively low risk, respectively. Whether the variation in these risks is related to shunt flow or to an underlying genetic predisposition, such as an abnormality in *BMPR2 (23)*, is unknown. The nature of the anatomic abnormality also determines the age at presentation. Patients with atrioventricular septal defects, truncus arteriosuses, transpositions of the great vessels, large patent ductus arteriosuses, and ventricular septal defects present earliest.

Surgical experience has suggested that the changes occurring with shunt-mediated PAH are reversible, as long as the surgery is performed before pulmonary vascular changes are "fixed." The determination of when lesions are "fixed" is more of an art than a science, however. Catheterization-based calculations of pulmonary blood flow (Qp) with isolation of all sources of Qp, individualized measurements of resistance in isolated lung segments, and direct measurement of pulmonary

Table 2
Vasoactive Mediators and Signaling Molecules Implicated in the Pathogenesis of CHD-PAH

Vasoactive mediators
    Endothelin-1 and endothelin receptors A and B
    Angiotensin II and angiotensin receptors
    Vascular endothelial growth factor and the flk1/tdr receptor
Signaling pathways
    Calcium-dependent K+ channels
    Increased phosphodiesterase-5 activity
    Decreased nitric oxide synthase activity
    Angiopoietin 1
    Tenascin
    Diminished function of
        BMPR1A
        BMPR2

BMPR = bone morphogenic protein receptor.

venous pressure are sometimes used to assess PAH reversibility and the likelihood of surgical success *(24)*. However, studies have not been performed that establish the pressures, flows, and resistances that define reversibility. Many centers use a preoperative PVR < 15 Wood units and pulmonary/systemic resistance ratio ≤ 2/3 as thresholds associated with better surgical outcomes *(25)*, but individual institutions vary on these thresholds, often modifying them according to the specific anatomical lesion and responses to acute vasodilator testing.

Patients with advanced disease deemed to be at a high surgical risk may still be considered for staged procedures. Either aggressive pharmacotherapy (i.e., infused prostacyclins) or catheter-based interventions (or both) can be used in an attempt to halt the progression of the pulmonary vascular disease. The choice depends on whether the pulmonary vascular disease or shunt is thought to be more detrimental. Patients are then reassessed periodically; if the functional or hemodynamic status improves, surgery can be reconsidered.

Occasionally, a reduction in pulmonary blood flow and pressure may be advantageous to unload a failing right ventricle. This can be achieved by creating or enlarging an intra-atrial shunt (graded atrial septostomy) at the expense of increased shunt and systemic cyanosis *(26)*. This procedure can improve functional status and probably increases survival in selected cases, although this has yet to be established in controlled trials. In addition, some patients achieve sufficient hemodynamic stabilization, perhaps related to some reversal of the vascular remodeling, so that further surgical repair may be contemplated.

An important concept with regard to predicting the outcome of surgery, especially in borderline cases, is that PVR is flow-dependent. Thus, it should not be assumed that PVR will necessarily fall in proportion to the reduction in shunt and pulmonary blood flow. High shunt flows can recruit pulmonary vasculature (thereby reducing PVR). With the elimination of the shunt, these additionally recruited vascular beds may "derecruit," no longer accommodating the increased blood flow, and PVR (and hence PA pressure) may fall less than would be predicted based on the reduction of blood flow alone.

3. IMMEDIATE-POSTOPERATIVE "REACTIVE" PULMONARY HYPERTENSION

Pulmonary vascular reactivity may be heightened in the immediate postoperative phase of cardiopulmonary surgery. This can precipitate marked increases in pulmonary vascular resistance leading to acute right heart syndrome, with the attendant decrease in cardiac output, systemic hypotension, metabolic acidemia, and right heart ischemia. In addition, airway resistance increases related to peribronchial edema and bronchoconstriction, and gas exchange suffers due to worsening ventilation–perfusion matching. Alveolar edema and cardiovascular collapse mark the end stages of this process *(27)*. Interestingly, perioperative acute increases in pulmonary resistance that precipitate a "crisis" tend to occur in individuals with more "dynamic" and less "fixed" resistance. Preoperatively, these individuals have dynamic flow-mediated increases in pulmonary vascular resistance that may be detected by exercise or vasodilator testing.

Perioperative endothelial cell dysfunction is thought to be central in the pathogenesis of immediate-postoperative pulmonary hypertension, leading to an imbalance in eicosenoid production *(28)* and impaired nitric oxide synthesis *(29)*, favoring vasoconstriction and vascular proliferation. Increased synthesis and decreased clearance of endothelin are also thought to contribute *(30)*.

The increasing knowledge of such processes has led to management strategies aimed at lowering PA pressure and reducing RV afterload while optimizing fluid balance. Reduction of adrenergic tone may also be helpful. Enhancing postoperative RV function and atrio-ventricular valve function and optimizing medical management (including the use of appropriate sedation agents and treatment of painful stimuli, avoidance of respiratory or metabolic acidosis, overcoming alveolar hypoxia or mechanical atelectasis, and correcting anemia or myocardial demand abnormalities) may reverse the crisis, but potential residual anatomical abnormalities that could be corrected surgically should also be sought.

Standard vasodilator agents such as ACE inhibitors or beta blockers are rarely helpful in this situation because they are not pulmonary-selective, and calcium channel blockers should be avoided because of their negative inotropic effects. Newer vasodilators such as epoprostenol and phosphodiesterase inhibitors (III and V) have been tried with some success, and inhaled vasodilators like inhaled nitric oxide or inhaled epoprostenol have piqued particular interest because they are more pulmonary-selective than systemically administered vasodilators and may also improve gas exchange by improving ventilation–perfusion matching.

The support of systemic blood pressure is critically important to maintain coronary perfusion in the acute right heart syndrome, necessitating the use of agents like norepinephrine. Low cardiac output states may be treated with the addition of dobutamine or a similar drug. An aggressive approach like that described has nearly eliminated mortality related to postoperative pulmonary hypertension in most large centers, but morbidity and duration of mechanical ventilation, ICU stay, and hospitalization are all still increased (27,28).

4. LATE-POSTOPERATIVE PULMONARY HYPERTENSION

Late-postoperative pulmonary hypertension may be the least well understood of all CHD-PAH syndromes. This is distinguished from the "reactive" type in that it refers to the development or persistence of pulmonary hypertension after the immediate postoperative period despite what appears to be an adequate surgical repair. Typically, this is attributed to timing of an anatomical shunt correction that is too late, miscalculation of the likelihood of surgical correction, or longstanding effects of stable but elevated right ventricular afterload that leads to recalcitrant remodeling. Therapeutic options are either to focus on chronic use of pulmonary vasoactive agents such prostacyclins, endothelin-receptor antagonists, or phosphodiesterase V inhibitors or to proceed to lung (or heart-lung) transplantation.

However, individuals with congenital cardiac defects harbor multiple additional factors contributing to their pulmonary hypertension depending on the specific intrinsic physiology of the cardiac defect. Such factors include long-term increases in systemic afterload that contribute to LV hypertrophy and left atrio-ventricular diastolic dysfunction, valvular abnormailities, or pulmonary venous hypertension or obstruction. In addition, restrictive pulmonary disease may be a complicating factor in patients with longstanding congenital heart disease, as may hypercoagulable states in patients with chronic liver disease due to longstanding cardiac congestion. Aggressive medical therapy of these factors with diuretics, agents that reduce cardiac remodeling (ACE inhibitors or calcium channel blockers), pulmonary hypertension therapies, and anticoagulation can conceivably promote reversal of remodeling changes over subsequent months.

5. NORMAL TO MILDLY ABNORMAL PVR STATES

This refers to conditions that depend on low PVR for continued survival. Examples include individuals with tricuspid atresia or similar single-ventricle physiologies who undergo surgical creation of cavopulmonary anastamoses (Glenn shunt and its variants or Fontan palliation and its variants). The surgery creates a unique pulmonary circulation that lacks pulsatile flow and connects directly to the systemic venous circulation. With the Glenn shunt, the superior vena cava communicates directly with the pulmonary arteries, whereas with the Fontan anastamosis, the inferior vena cava is separated from the superior vena cava anastomosis via construction of a baffle. Because the right ventricle has been bypassed and circulation of blood relies solely on left ventricular function, any increase in pulmonary vascular impedance can interfere with left ventricular filling. Thus, maintenance of a low PVR is critically important.

An interesting physiological aspect of these anatomoses is that the pulmonary and systemic circulations respond differently to vasoactive triggers, leading to the redistribution of blood flow within the anastomoses. For example, hypercapnia, acidemia, and hypoxia lower the cerebral vascular resistance, thereby raising the cerebral blood flow while lowering the pulmonary blood flow. On the contrary, hypocapnia, alkalosis, and hyperoxia raise the cerebral vascular resistance and decrease the pulmonary vascular resistance, causing a redistribution of blood flow from the brain to the lungs *(31,32)*.

Although effective in bypassing the obstructive lesions, the Glenn and Fontan procedures are still associated with functional impairment because of the limitations of a single-ventricular system. Whether long-term pulmonary vasoactive therapy to maintain low PVR improves outcomes in these patients remains controversial *(32–34)*.

A similar controversy exists regarding the potential benefits of administering pulmonary vasoactive agents to individuals with defects such as Ebstein's anomaly or tetralogy of Fallot that depend on the functional status of the right ventricle. Given the increasing morbidities seen with aging in patients with these defects, a further study of such potential therapies would be welcomed.

6. EISENMENGER PHYSIOLOGY

Eisenmenger physiology refers to the development of bidirectional or a predominant right-to-left shunt accompanied by oxygen-unresponsive hypoxemia and PAH in patients born with large systemic-to-pulmonary shunts *(35)*. This was first reported in "simple lesions" such as atrial and ventricular septal defects and patent ductus arteriosus but is also seen in more "complex lesions" such as atrio-ventricular septal defects, conoventricular defects including truncus arteriosus and tetralogy of Fallot and its variants, and single-ventricle variants. In patients with medium- or large-sized septal defects, Eisenmenger physiology may appear later in life and first be recognized during the changes in hemodynamic loading that occur with pregnancy. Whether additional triggers of PAH other than intravascular shunt are required for the development of Eisenmenger physiology remains debated.

Dyspnea on exertion is the most common presenting symptom of patients with Eisenmenger physiology, followed by palpitations, edema and fluid retention, hemoptysis, and syncope *(6)*. Eisenmeger patients encounter increasing morbidity through the third decade of life. Eisenmenger physiology is also associated with additional complications as compared to patients with idiopathic or other forms of secondary PAH. Hypoxemia-related secondary erythrocytosis (frequently associated with iron deficiency due to increased red cell turnover) leads to increased blood viscosity and intravascular "sludging." Additional damage to the cerebrovasculature, kidneys (glomerular, tubular, and interstitial function may be altered) and lungs (in the form of *in situ* thromboses or frank pulmonary emboli) can occur.

Intravascular fluid retention and elevated systemic venous pressure may alter hepatic function. Hyperuricemia may cause gout. The occurrence of clinical bleeding disorders is debated. Concomitant congenital skeletal abnormalities and restrictive thoracic disease may contribute to hypoxemia. True cardiac ischemic chest pain, usually due to right ventricular ischemia caused by excessive right ventricular tension, coronary arterial compression by a dilated pulmonary artery, or atherosclerosis, may occur with exertion or at rest. Progressive right ventricular failure and premature death are the rule. The immediate causes of death include sudden death (likely due to tachy- or brady-arrhythmias), recalcitrant right ventricular failure, hemoptysis (typically due to bronchial arterial rupture or pulmonary infarction), and complications during pregnancy. Because of the direct communication of the systemic venous and arterial circulations, strokes caused by systemic "paradoxical" embolization and brain abscesses also contribute to morbidity and mortality *(36–38)*. Poor functional class is a significant predictor of mortality for Eisenmenger physiology patients *(39)*.

The diagnosis of Eisenmenger physiology requires a detailed history to inquire about all other possible forms of associated PAH, a thorough understanding of the anatomical abnormalities, and knowledge of all prior interventions. Imaging techniques such as "bubble" echocardiograms, radionuclide studies, CT angiograms, and magnetic resonance imaging studies are used to establish the level of intravascular shunting: atrial, ventricular, or great arterial. Cardiac catheterization is mandatory to establish the severity of pulmonary arterial hypertension and quantify shunting. This can be established by right heart catheterization in many cases, but left heart catheterization may be needed to better define the anatomy, accurately measure left ventricular end-diastolic pressure, and assess the coronary arteries in older patients who are at risk for atherosclerosis.

In the past, the lack of safe and effective therapies for Eisenmenger physiology led many clinicians to advocate a "noninterventional approach" to diagnosis. The emphasis was on "educated consumerism" with avoidance of destabilizing situations like large fluid shifts, alterations in catecholamines, extreme fatigue, high altitude, cigarette and other smoke exposures, changes in renal or hepatic function, and pregnancy. Reversible contributing factors such as anemia related to iron deficiency, electrolyte disorders, arrhythmias, and infection were (and still are) treated aggressively (Table 3).

All procedures in Eisenmenger physiology patients require careful "team planning" because patients are at increased risk for morbidity and mortality even with the "simplest" of interventions. The type and mode of anesthetic administration should be optimized for individual patients by those skilled in treating Eisenmenger physiology patients. Air filters are generally used on all venous catheters to minimize the risk of cerebral air embolism, although controversy exists regarding the benefit of this approach compared to meticulous guarding of all intravenous administration systems.

Table 3
Potentially Preventable or Reversible Factors Contributing to the Deterioration of Pulmonary Hypertension in Eisenmenger Physiology

Pregnancy
Increased fluid volume
Increased left-sided filling pressure
    Left ventricular diastolic dysfunction
    Obstructive congenital lesion
    Myocardial restriction with diastolic equalization of intrachamber pressures
    Systemic hypertension with increased left ventricular afterload
Erythrocytosis and increased blood viscosity
Hypercoagulability
Acute infection
Arrhythmias

Erythrocytosis tends to remain stable in cyanotic patients, and alterations in serum hemoglobin more often reflect other problems such as infection, malnutrition, or changes in fluid volume (see section on cyanosis). Prophylactic phlebotomy and erythropheresis have no role in patient management. Studies that determine the role of iron store repletion and optimization of serum hemoglobin and blood viscosity (with or without phlebotomy) in lowering the occurrence of other organ system damage or thrombosis have not been performed (40,41).

Pregnancy is risky for persons with Eisenmenger physiology, with earlier case series reporting high maternal and fetal mortality rates (both up to 50%), particularly in the first several days after delivery (42). Therapeutic termination of pregnancy during the second and third trimesters precipitates fluid volume and hormonal fluctuations and is similarly risky. More recently, case series have reported successful pregnancy, labor, and delivery with concomitant use of medical therapies (see below). Whether pregnancy is any more or less risky in persons with Eisenmenger physiology compared to those with other forms of PAH is unclear. However, because there are no reliable ways to predict its outcome, even with medical therapy, pregnancy remains absolutely contraindicated for adults with Eisenmenger physiology. Birth control counseling is strongly advised, although the preferred method of contraception has not been established. Maternal sterilization carries a risk of mortality, hormonal therapies increase the risk for thrombosis, barrier methods have a higher failure rate than other methods, and intrauterine device implantation carries an infection risk. Double-barrier methods, such as condoms with spermicidal foam, may reduce failure rates, but comparative studies among the various methods have not been performed in Eisenmenger physiology patients.

The improving understanding of pulmonary arteriolar hypertension and subpulmonary ventricular failure in Eisenmenger physiology patients has led to recognition that therapy should include efforts to modulate pulmonary vascular inflammation and its ramifications. Until recently, therapies for adults with shunt-associated pulmonary hypertension have consisted of supplemental oxygen, anticoagulation, diuretics, high-dose calcium channel blocker therapy, and lung or lung/heart transplantation. The benefit of supplemental oxygen administration in Eisenmenger physiology patients has been debated. Patients with large shunts often remain severely hypoxemic, even with high-flow supplemental oxygen. The same guidelines used to provide oxygen to COPD patients are applied to those with Eisenmenger physiology, but clinical trials to systematically assess the benefit of oxygen supplementation in these patients have not been performed (43,44).

Likewise, calcium channel blockers and transplantation have shown limited benefit or even subjective deterioration *(45)*. Transplant-free survival in Eisenmenger physiology is difficult to predict, with some patients having long survivals despite severe hypoxemia. Also, perioperative transplant mortality is higher in this cohort of patients, though some individuals do very well after transplantation *(46)*.

Anticoagulation with warfarin is widely employed in patients with CHD-PAH. In adults with Eisenmenger physiology, increasing recognition of in vivo prothrombotic states *(47)* and in vitro abnormalities of coagulation in persons with cyanosis *(48)* has supported the anticoagulation of patients despite the lack of randomized studies to support the practice.

The medical therapy of Eisenmenger physiology has raised concerns about worsening of right-to-left shunting and the safety of using pulmonary arterial modulating therapies that also have systemic vasodilator potential. Nevertheless, some of these agents (intravenous prostacyclin, subcutaneously administered treprostinil, inhaled iloprost, and oral beraprost, bosentan, or sildenafil) have improved the hemodynamics and exercise capacity in case series of CHD-PAH patients *(49–55)*. Randomized controlled trials showing the benefit of many of these agents in PAH patients (IV prostacyclin, subcutaneously administered treprostinil, and oral beraprost and sitaxsentan) have included smaller numbers of persons with Eisenmenger physiology. However, the utility of these trials in guiding therapy for persons with Eisenmenger physiology is limited because the trials were not designed prospectively to test hypotheses within the congenital heart disease subgroup *(53–57)*.

The BREATHE-5 trial of bosentan for congenital heart disease, thus far only reported preliminarily, was the first randomized controlled trial of an agent specifically for individuals affected by Eisenmenger physiology. It compared oral bosentan to placebo *(58)* and found that in short-term follow-up, bosentan was not only safe but led to improvement in pulmonary hemodynamics as well as in both six-minute walk distance and WHO/NYHA functional class *(58)*. The positive findings of this trial justify the use of bosentan as a first-line therapy in patients with CHD-PAH to improve functional capacity and potentially to prolong survival. In view of this favorable response to medical therapy, further studies of pulmonary vasoactive agents, both alone and in combination in individuals with CHD-PAH, are strongly encouraged.

7. CONCLUSIONS

Pulmonary arterial hypertension associated with congenital heart disease is common among the subtypes of PAH. It is quite variable in terms of clinical manifestations, severity of associated PAH, response to therapy, and outcomes, depending on the anatomy of the specific lesion, pulmonary circulatory flows and pressures, and other factors. Genetics likely play a role, but no specific genetic abnormality has yet been associated with this form of PAH. Patients with CHD-PAH should undergo a careful evaluation that includes imaging of the defect as well as catheterization to characterize the severity and nature of pulmonary hemodynamic abnormalities. Surgical correction is desirable as long as the chances of reversibility are sufficient, but this may be difficult to ascertain preoperatively in marginal cases. Many patients now respond to pulmonary hypertension therapies if they are not surgical candidates or fail to improve after surgery, and lung or heart/lung transplantation remains an option for selected recalcitrant patients.

REFERENCES

1. Diller GP, Dimopoulis K, Okonko D, et al. Exercise intolerance in adult congenital heart disease: comparative severity, correlates, and prognostic implication. Circulation 2005; 112:828–835.
2. Friedman WF. Proceedings of national heart, lung and blood institute pediatric cardiology workshop: pulmonary hypertension. Pediatr Res 20:811–824.
3. Kidd L, Driscoll DJ, Gersony WM, et al. Second natural history study of congenital heart defects: results of treatment of patients with ventricular septal defects. Circulation 1993; 87:138–151.
4. Simonneau G, Galie N, Rubin LJ, et al. Clinical classification of pulmonary hypertension. J Am Coll Cardiol 2004; 43(suppl):5S–12S.
5. Galie N, "Classification of patients with congenital systemic-to-pulmonary shunts associated with pulmonary arterial hypertension: current status and future directions." *Pulmonary Arterial Hypertension Related to Congenital Heart Disease*. Ed Maurice Beghetti. Munich, Elsevier GmbH, 2006, 11–17.
6. Wood P. The Eisenmenger syndrome or pulmonary hypertension with reversed central shunt. Br Med J 1958; 46:701–709.
7. Rabinovitch M, Haworth SG, Castaneda AR, Nadas AS, Reid LR. Lung biopsy in congenital heart disease: a morphometric approach to pulmonary vascular disease. Circulation 1978; 58:1107–1122.
8. Fratz S, Geiger R, KResse H, et al. Pulmonary blood pressure, not flow, is associated with net endotehlin-1 production in the lungs of patients with congenital heart disease and normal pulmonary vascular resistance. J Thorac Cardiovasc Surg 2003; 126:1724–1729.

9. van Albada ME, Shoemaker RG, Kemna MS, et al. The role of increased pulmonary blood flow in pulmonary arterial hypertension. Eur Respir J. 2005; 26:487–493.

10. Black SM, Bekker JM, Johengen MJ, et al. Altered regulation of the ET-1 cascade in lambs with increased pulmonary blood flow and pulmonary hypertension. Pediatr Res 2000; 47:97–106.

11. Fratz S, Meyrick B, Ovadia B, et al. Chronic endothelin A Receptor blockade in lambs with increased pulmonary blood flow and pressure. Am J Physiol Lung Cell Mol Physiol 2004; 287:L592–L597.

12. Mata-Greenwood E, Meyrick B, Soifer SJ, Fineman JR, Black SM. Expression of VEGF and its receptors Flt-1 and Flk-1/KDR is altered in lambs with increased pulmonary blood flow and pulmonary hypertension. Am J Physiol Lung Cell Mol Physiol 2003; 285:L222–L231.

13. Mata-Greenwood E, Meyrick B, Steinhorn RH, Fineman JR, Black SM. Alterations in TGF-beta1 expression in lambs with increased pulmonary blood flow and pulmonary hypertension. Am J Physiol Lung Cell Mol Physiol. 2003; 285:L209–L221.

14. Cornfield DN, Resnik ER, Herron JM, Reinhartz O, Fineman JR. Pulmonary vascular K+ channel expression and vasoreactivity in a model of congenital heart disease. Am J Physiol Lung Cell Mol Physiol 2002; 283:L1210–L1219.

15. Black SM, Sanchez LS, Mata-Greenwood E, et al. sGC and PDE5 are elevated in lambs with increased pulmonary blood flow and pulmonary hypertension. Am J Physiol Lung Cell Mol Physiol 2001; 281:L1051–L1057.

16. Van Beneden R, Rondelet B, Kerbaul F, Ray L, Naeje R. Ang-1/BMPR2 signalling and the expression of MCP-1 and ICAM in overcirculation-induced experimental pulmonary hypertension. Eur Respir J 2004; 24:533 S.

17. Rondelet B, Kerbaul F, Motte S, et al. Bosentan for the prevention of overcirculation-induced experimental pulmonary arterial hypertension. Circulation 2003; 107:1329–1335.

18. Rondelet B, Kerbaul F, Van Beneden R, et al. Signalling molecules in overcirculation-induced pulmonary hypertension in piglets: effects of sildenafil therapy. Circulation 2004; 110:2220–2225.

19. Bolger AP, Sharma R, Li W, et al. Neurohormonal activation and the chronic heart failure syndrome in adults with congenital heart disease. Circulation 2002; 106:92–99.

20. Cacoub P, Dorent R, Maistre G, et al. Endothelin-1 in primary pulmonary hypertension and the Eisenmenger syndrome. Am J Cardiol 1993; 71: 448–450.

21. Ishikawa S, Miyauchi T, Sakai S, et al. Elevated levels of plasma endothelin-1 in young patients with pulmonary hypertension caused by congenital heart disease are decreased after successful surgical repair. J Thorac Cardiovasc Surg 1995; 110:271–273.

22. Cacoub P, Dorent R, Nataf P, et al. Endothelin-1 in the lungs of patients with pulmonary hypertension. Cardiovasc Res 1997; 33:196–200.

23. Roberts KE, McElroy JJ, Wong WP, et al. BMPR2 mutations in pulmonary arterial hypertension with congenital heart disease. Eur Respir J 2004; 24:371–374.

24. Steele PM, Fuster V, Cohen M, Ritter DG, McGoon DC. Isolated atrial septal defect with pulmonary vascular obstructive disease—long-term follow-up and prediction of outcome after surgical correction. Circulation 1987; 76:1037–1042.

25. Batista RJ, Santos JL, Takeshita N, et al. Successful reversal of pulmonary hypertension in Eisenmenger complex. Arq Bras Cardiol. 1997 Apr; 68(4):279–280.

26. Bando K, Turrentine MW, Sharp TG, et al. Pulmonary hypertension after operations for congenital heart disease: analysis of risk factors and management. J Thorac Cardiovasc Surg 1996; 112:1600–1607.

27. Schulze-Neick I, Li J, Penny DJ et al. Pulmonary vascular resistance after cardiopulmonary bypass in infants: effect on postoperative recovery. J Thorac Cardiovasc Surg 2001; 121:1033–1039.

28. Adatia I, Barrow S, Stratton P, et al. Effect of intracardiac repair on biosynthesis of thromboxane A2 and prostacyclin in children with a left to right shunt. Br Heart J 1994; 72:452–456.

29. Schulze-Nieck I, Penny DJ, Rigby ML, et al. L-arginine and substance P reverse the pulmonary endothelial dysfunction caused by congenital heart surgery. Circulation 1999; 100:749–755.

30. Hiramatsu T, Imai Y, Takanishsi Y, et al. Time course of endothelin-1 and nitrate anion levels after cardiopulmonary bypass in congenital heart defects. Ann Thorac Surg 1997; 63:648–652.

31. Bradley SM, Simsic JM, Mulvihill DM. Hypoventilation improves oxygenation after bidirectional superior cavopulmonary connection, J Thorac Cardiovasc Surg 2003; 126:1033–1039.

32. Hoskote A, Li J, Hickey C, et al. The effects of carbon dioxide on oxygenation and systemic, cerebral and pulmonary vascular hemody-namics after the bidirectional superior cavopulmonary anastomosis. J Am Coll Cardiol 2004; 44:1501–1509.

33. Guadagni G, Bove EL, Migliavacca F, Dubini G. Effects of pulmonary afterload on the hemodynamics after the hemi-Fontan procedure. Med Eng Phys 2001; 23:293–298.

34. Ikai A, Shirai M, Nishimura K, et al. Hypoxic pulmonary vasoconstriction disappears in a rabbit model of cavopulmonary shunt. J Thorac Cardiovasc Surg 2004; 127:1450–1457.

35. Simsic JM, Bradley SM, Mulvihill DM. Sodium nitroprusside after bidirectional superior cavopulmonary connection: preserved cerebral blood flow velocity and systemic oxygenation. J Thorac Cardiovasc Surg 2003; 126:186–190.

36. Daliento L, Somerville J, Presbitero P, et al. Eisenmenger syndrome. Factors relating to deterioration and death. Eur Heart J 1998; 19:1845–1855.

37. Saha A, Balakrishnan K, Jaiswal P, et al. Prognosis for patients with Eisenmenger syndrome of various aetiology. Int J Cardiol 1994; 45: 199–207.
38. Vongpatanasin W, Brickner ME, Hillis LD, et al. The Eisenmenger syndrome in adults. Ann Int Med 1998; 128:745–755.
39. Cantor WJ, Harrison DA, Moussadji JS, et al. Determinants of survival and length of survival in adults with Eisenmenger syndrome. Am J Cardiol 1999; 84:677–681.
40. Sondel PM, Tripp ME, Ganick DJ, Levy JM, Shahidi NT. Phlebotomy with iron therapy to correct the microcytic polycythemia of chronic hypoxia. Pediatrics 1981; 67:667–670.
41. Perloff JK, Marelli AJ, Miner PD. Risk of stroke in adults with cyanotic congenital heart disease. Circulation 1993; 87:1954–1959.
42. Jones P, Patel A. Eisenmenger's syndrome and problems with anaesthesia. Br J Hosp Med 1996; 54(5):214–219.
43. Bowyer JJ, Busst CM, Denison DM, Shinebourne EA. Effect of long-term oxygen treatment at home in children with pulmonary vascular disease. Br Heart J 1986; 55:385–390.
44. Sandoval J, Aguirre JS, Pulido T, et al. Nocturnal oxygen therapy in patients with the Eisenmenger Syndrome. Am J Respir Crit Care Med 2001; 164:1682–1687.
45. Gildein HP, Wildberg A, Moellin R. Comparative studies of hemodynamics under prostacyclin and nifedipine in patients with Eisenmenger syndrome. Z Kardiol (Germany) 1995; 84:55–63.
46. Trulock EP. Lung transplantation for primary pulmonary hypertension. Clin Chest Med 2001; 22:583–593.
47. Silversides CK, Granton JT, Konen T, et al. Pulmonary thrombosis in adults with Eisenmenger syndrome. J Am Coll Cardiol 2003; 42:1982–1987.
48. Rosove MH, Hocking WG, Harwig SS, Perloff JK. Studies of beta-thromboglobulin, platelet factor 4, fibrinopeptide-A in erythrocytosis due to cyanotic congenital heart disease. Thromb Res 1983; 29:225–235.
49. Rosenzweig EB, Kerstein D, Barst RJ. Long-term prostacyclin for pulmonary hypertension with associated congenital heart defects. Circulation 1999; 99:1858–1865.
50. McLaughlin VV, Genthner DE, Panella MM, et al. Compassionate use of continuous prostacyclin in the management of secondary pulmonary hypertension: As case series. Ann Intern Med 1999; 130:740.
51. Ferndandes SM, Newburger JW, Lang P, Pearson DD, Feinstein JA, Gauvreau KK, Landzberg MJ. Usefulness of epoprostenol therapy in the severely ill adolescent/adult with Eisenmenger physiology. Am J Cardiol 2003; 91:46–49.
52. Olschewski H, Simonneau G, Galie N, et al. Inhaled iloprost for severe pulmonary hypertension. N Engl J Med 2002; 347:322–329.
53. Barst RJ, Rubin LJ, Long WA, et al. A comparison of continuous intravenous epoprostenol (prostacyclin) with conventional therapy for primary

pulmonary hypertension. The Primary Pulmonary Hypertension Study Group. N Engl J Med 1996; 334:296–302.

54. Simonneau G, Barst RJ, Galie N, et al. Continuous subcutaneous infusion of treprostinil, a prostacyclin analogue, in patients with pulmonary arterial hypertension: a double-blind, randomized, placebo-controlled trial. Am J Respir Crit Care Med 2002; 165:800–804.

55. Galie N, Humbert M, Vachiery JL, et al. Effects of beraprost sodium, an oral prostacyclin analogue, in patients with pulmonary arterial hypertension: a randomized, double-blind, placebo-controlled trial. J Am Coll Cardiol 2002; 39:1496–502.

56. Rubin LJ, Badesch DB, Barst RJ, et al. Bosentan therapy for pulmonary arterial hypertension. N Engl J Med 2002; 346:896–903.

57. Barst RJ, Langleben D, Frost A, Horn EM, et al. Sitaxsentan therapy for pulmonary arterial hypertension. Am J Respir Crit Care Med 2004; 169:441–447.

58. Galie N, Beghetti M, Gatzoulis MA, et al. Bosentan therapy in patients with Eisenmenger syndrome: a multicenter, double-blind, randomized, placebo-controlled study. Circulation 2006; 114:48–54.

Color Plates

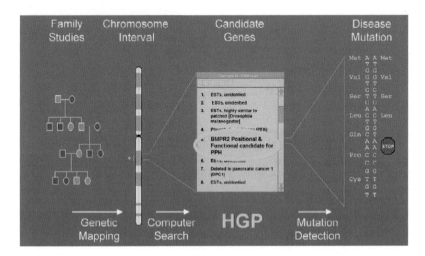

Color Plate 1. The process leading to the discovery of mutations in bone morphogenetic protein receptor type-2 (*BMPR2*) as the cause of familial pulmonary arterial hypertension is depicted. (Fig. 2, Chapter 5; *See* complete caption on p. 77)

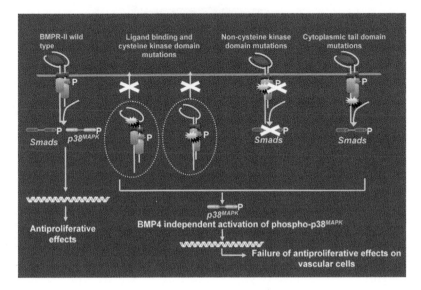

Color Plate 2. Consequences of bone morphogenetic protein type-2 receptor (*BMPR2*) mutations on signaling. (Fig. 3, Chapter 5; *See* complete caption on p. 80)

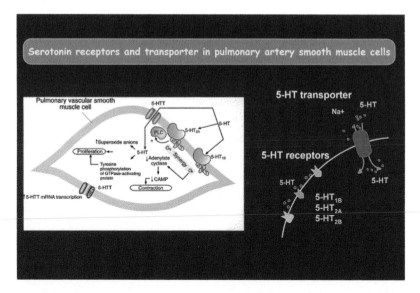

Color Plate 3. Serotonin receptors and transporter in pulmonary artery smooth muscle cells. (Fig. 4, Chapter 5; *See* complete caption on p. 83)

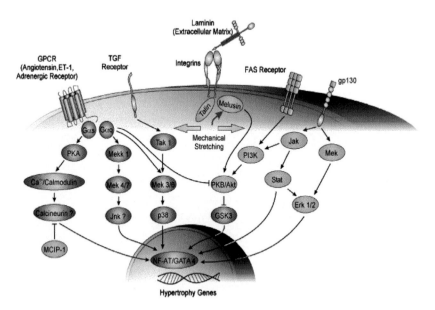

Color Plate 4. Adaptive and maladaptive cardiac hypertrophic intracellular signaling pathways. (Fig. 3, Chapter 6; *See* complete caption on p. 101)

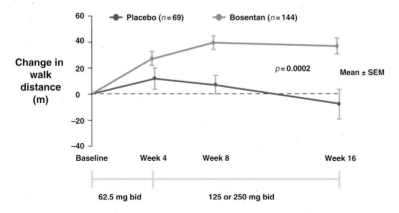

Color Plate 5. Increase in six-minute walk distance (m) in BREATHE-1, the major outcome variable in the pivotal trial testing the clinical efficacy of bosentan in PAH. (Fig. 1, Chapter 13; *See* complete caption on p. 288)

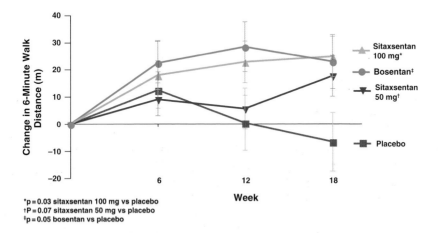

Color Plate 6. Increase in six-minute walk distance, the major outcome variable in the STRIDE-2 study. (Fig. 2, Chapter 13; *See* complete caption on p. 293)

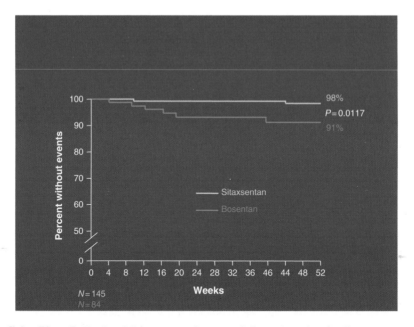

Color Plate 7. Kaplan–Meier curves for rate of discontinuation for liver enzyme elevations (larger than fivefold elevation over normal) in the STRIDE-2X study. (Fig. 3, Chapter 13; *See* complete caption on p. 294)

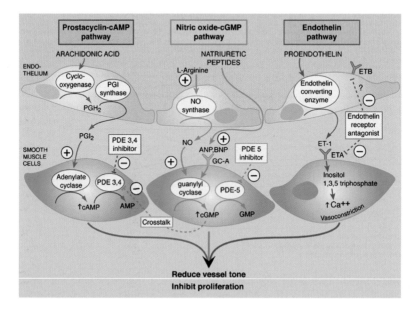

Color Plate 8. The three main therapeutic pathways currently targeted in the treatment of PAH are schematized. (Fig. 1, Chapter 16; *See* complete caption on p. 346)

8 Connective Tissue Disease Associated Pulmonary Hypertension

Kimberly A. Fisher, Nicholas S. Hill, and Harrison W. Farber

CONTENTS

INTRODUCTION
EPIDEMIOLOGY
PATHOPHYSIOLOGY
CLINICAL PRESENTATION AND DIAGNOSIS
THERAPY OF SSc-PH
SURGICAL TREATMENTS
SUMMARY
REFERENCES

Abstract

Pulmonary hypertension is a common complication of connective tissue disease (CTD) and confers a worse prognosis. Connective tissue disease associated pulmonary hypertension (CTD-PH) occurs most often with systemic sclerosis (SSc) but may also complicate mixed connective tissue disease (MCTD), systemic lupus erythematosus (SLE), and, rarely, rheumatoid arthritis, dermatomysositis/polymyositis, and Sjogren's syndrome. Although the pathogenesis leading to CTD-PH may vary, the clinical presentation, treatment, and pathological lesions are often similar to those observed in idiopathic pulmonary arterial hypertension (IPAH). This chapter examines the epidemiology, pathophysiology, clinical presentation, and diagnosis of CTD-PH and the evidence supporting the available treatment options.

From: *Contemporary Cardiology: Pulmonary Hypertension*
Edited by: N. S. Hill and H. W. Farber © Humana Press, Totowa, NJ

Key Words: pulmonary hypertension; connective tissue disease; Lupus erythematosis; Dermatomyositis; rheumatoid arthritis; Sjogren's syndrome.

1. INTRODUCTION

Pulmonary hypertension, defined as increased mean pulmonary arterial pressure (mPAP, $\geq$ 25 mm Hg at rest; $\geq$ 30 mm Hg with exercise), with a normal pulmonary arterial wedge pressure (PAWP, $\leq$ 15 mm Hg), is a well-known complication of connective tissue diseases (CTD). The clinical presentation, treatment, and pathological lesions of CTD-associated pulmonary hypertension are typically similar to those observed in idiopathic pulmonary arterial hypertension (IPAH; formerly primary pulmonary hypertension). Thus, although various pathophysiological mechanisms may contribute to CTD-associated pulmonary hypertension, the 2003 Consensus Conference in Venice considered it a form of pulmonary arterial hypertension (PAH) in the revised clinical classification of pulmonary hypertension (see Chapter 2) *(1)*. This chapter reviews the epidemiology, pathophysiology, diagnosis, and treatment of CTD-associated PAH.

2. EPIDEMIOLOGY

2.1. Systemic Sclerosis

Scleroderma [also known as systemic sclerosis (SSc)], a systemic disease characterized by widespread vascular lesions and organ fibrosis, is the CTD most commonly associated with pulmonary hypertension. Pathologically, patients with SSc-associated pulmonary hypertension (SSc-PH) develop a pulmonary arteriopathy primarily characterized by intimal fibrosis and microvascular obliterative lesions similar to those seen in the kidneys and digits of scleroderma patients; however, plexiform lesions similar to those of IPAH are also seen *(2,3)*. Rarely, the histopathology of SSc-PH may reveal pulmonary veno-occlusive disease or pulmonary capillary hemangiomatosis *(4–6)*.

Estimates of the incidence of SSc-PH vary from 6–60%, depending on the SSc population and the method for diagnosing pulmonary hypertension *(7)*. When right heart catheterization (RHC) is used, which is the gold standard for diagnosing pulmonary hypertension, the incidence among patients with limited SSc [formerly known as the CREST (calcinosis, Raynaud's, esophageal dysmotility, sclerodactyly, and telangiectasias) syndrome] ranges from 12% to 16% *(8,9)*. Patients with diffuse SSc (based on the pattern of cutaneous involvement) are less likely to have pulmonary hypertension and more likely to have pulmonary fibrosis than those with the limited form *(10)*. Among SSc patients with isolated pulmonary hypertension (i.e., without accompanying pulmonary fibrosis), 78% to 90% have limited SSc *(10–13)*.

When limited SSc patients have been screened for pulmonary hypertension using echocardiography, up to 50% have elevation of the estimated pulmonary arterial systolic pressure *(10–13)*. Autopsy studies have revealed evidence of pulmonary arteriopathy in as many as 65% of limited SSc patients *(14)*. All groups of SSc patients (including those without clinical pulmonary hypertension) have greater luminal occlusion and intimal proliferation than nonscleroderma autopsy controls *(15)*. Thus, pathological pulmonary vascular involvement is highly prevalent and often not accompanied by clinically detectable disease.

Advanced age is another risk factor for developing PAH among SSc patients. The estimated increase in the risk of developing pulmonary hypertension among SSc patients is 22% for every 10 years of age, with the highest risk being in patients who develop SSc during the seventh decade of life *(13)*. Pulmonary hypertension is also a late complication of SSc, developing an average of 14.4 years after disease onset *(16)*. Raynaud's phenomenon may also be a risk factor; in a study of 673 patients with SSc, 100% of patients with pulmonary hypertension had Raynaud's phenomenon as the initial CTD symptom as compared to 68% without pulmonary hypertension *(17)*. In contrast, Steen and Medsger found that SSc patients with and without pulmonary hypertension had similar frequencies of Raynaud's phenomenon, but patients with pulmonary hypertension had significantly higher severity scores for Raynaud's phenomenon and digital tip ulcers *(16)*.

With the introduction of angiotensin converting enzyme (ACE) inhibitors as effective therapy for scleroderma renal crisis, pulmonary complications of systemic sclerosis have become the leading cause of mortality in patients with limited SSc. Specifically, the presence of pulmonary hypertension greatly worsens the prognosis in SSc patients (Fig. 1) *(12,16,18)*. Untreated, SSc patients with pulmonary hypertension have a two-year survival rate of 40% to 50% as compared to 80% to 88% for those without pulmonary hypertension *(16,17)*. Patients with SSc-PH also appear to have a worse outcome than idiopathic PAH patients (Fig. 2). In a retrospective analysis of 55 patients, those with SSc-PH (33 patients) had a significantly shorter survival and increased unadjusted risk of death than those with idiopathic PAH (hazard ratio 2.9; 95% CI 1.1–7.8) *(19)*.

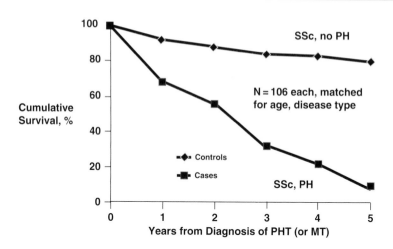

Fig. 1. Cumulative survival curves showing worse survival of scleroderma patients with pulmonary hypertension (SSc, PH) than those without pulmonary hypertension (SSc, no PH) from time of diagnosis of pulmonary hypertension (PHT) or matching time (MT) and without major organ involvement. [Adapted with permission from *(12)*.]

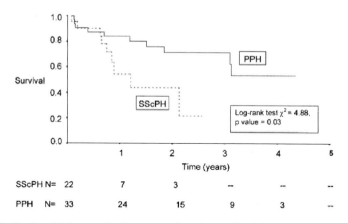

Fig. 2. Kaplan–Meier survival curves of patients with idiopathic PAH (PPH – solid line) showing better survival than patients with scleroderma associated pulmonary hypertension (SSc-PH – interrupted line). [Adapted with permission from *(19)*.]

2.2. Mixed Connective Tissue Disease

Mixed connective tissue disease (MCTD) combines clinical features of several different connective tissue diseases including systemic lupus erythematosus (SLE), SSc, and polymyositis-dermatomyositis *(20)*.

The pathological findings of pulmonary hypertension in association with MCTD are similar to those of other forms of PAH, with intimal and medial thickening in small and medium-sized pulmonary arteries and plexiform lesions in some cases *(21)*. Fewer studies have examined the occurrence of pulmonary hypertension complicating MCTD, but one study with 26 patients found pulmonary hypertension in 7 patients (27%) on the basis of RHC *(22)*. Others have found evidence of pulmonary hypertension in as many as 75% of patients with MCTD *(23)*. Pulmonary hypertension has also been reported as the most frequent disease-associated cause of death in patients with MCTD *(24)*.

2.3. Rheumatoid Arthritis

Pulmonary hypertension is a rare complication of rheumatoid arthritis, with most descriptions being case reports *(25–29)*. Among 146 unselected patients with rheumatoid arthritis screened echocardiographically for pulmonary hypertension, 30 cases (21%) had "pulmonary hypertension" in the absence of other significant cardiac or pulmonary disease. However, the majority of cases (97%) were mild, with estimated systolic pulmonary artery pressure (PASP) between 30 and 39, which does not meet current standards for the echocardiographic definition of pulmonary hypertension (PASP > 35–40 mm Hg) *(30)*. Furthermore, none of these was confirmed by right heart catheterization. Pathological findings in RA-associated pulmonary hypertension include intimal proliferation, medial hypertrophy, and plexogenic arteriopathy similar to idiopathic PAH *(26,27)*. The occurrence of vasculitis has also been reported in several cases *(28,31)*.

2.4. Systemic Lupus Erythematosus

The reported occurrence of pulmonary hypertension in systemic lupus erythematosus (SLE) ranges from 4% to 21% *(32–36)*. Most of these cases had mild pulmonary hypertension, diagnosed only by echocardiography, and often associated with restrictive lung disease or thromboembolic disease. Severe isolated pulmonary hypertension complicating SLE is uncommon *(37–41)*. Among 70 consecutive patients with SLE screened for pulmonary hypertension using echocardiography, 15 (21%) patients had estimated pulmonary artery systolic pressure $\geq$ 30 mm Hg. Of these, 12 (80%) had mild pulmonary hypertension with PASP between 31 and 50 mm Hg (again, many of these not meeting current definitions of echocardiographic pulmonary hypertension) *(36)*. Only 3 of 70, or 4%, had moderate to severe pulmonary hypertension. Mortality rates as high as 25% to 50% have been reported two years after the diagnosis of SLE-related pulmonary hypertension *(7)*, but it is unclear that these mortalities are attributable entirely to the increased pulmonary arterial pressure. Pathological changes of pulmonary hypertension in SLE may be isolated and due to direct involvement of the pulmonary circulation, resembling those of idiopathic PAH, or may be secondary to interstitial lung disease or thromboembolic disease *(7,37,38,40)*.

2.5. Dermatomyositis/Polymyositis and Sjogren's Syndrome

Pulmonary hypertension is a known but unusual complication of dermatomyositis/polymyositis and Sjogren's syndrome, and little is known about its pathology in these entities *(7,42)*.

3. PATHOPHYSIOLOGY

3.1. Mediators of CTD-PH

Consistent with the shared pathological features of CTD-PH and idiopathic PAH, pathophysiological mechanisms overlap as well. These include increased expression of angiopoietin-1 and TIE2 phosphorylation as well as decreased bone morphogenic protein receptor 1A (BMPR1A) expression *(43)*. As in idiopathic PAH, abnormalities in nitric oxide (NO) synthesis and release have been described in patients with SSc-PH *(44–46)*, including decreased NO/endothelin-1 (ET-1) ratios. In addition, nitric oxide synthase 2 (NOS2) haplotypes associated with decreased transcriptional activity are more prevalent in patients with SSc-PH than in SSc patients without PH *(46)*. However, the genetics of CTD-PH and idiopathic PAH appear to differ because mutations of the *BMPR2* gene that occur in at least 50% of patients with familial PAH have not been found in patients with SSc-PH *(47)*.

Endothelin-1 (ET-1) has also been implicated in the development of both CTD-PH and idiopathic PAH. Endothelin-1 levels are increased in the plasma and sera of patients with SSc and SLE *(46,48–51)* and in the fibroblasts *(52)*, alveolar macrophages *(53)*, and lung tissue isolated from patients with SSc-associated pulmonary fibrosis *(54)*. The link between ET-1 perturbations and the clinical development of PAH has not been clarified though, because several studies have failed to demonstrate a difference in ET-1 levels between CTD patients with and without pulmonary hypertension *(49,50)*. Higher serum ET-1 levels in PAH compared to non-PAH patients have been found in the limited SSc subgroup *(49)*, however, and because most of the studies based the diagnosis of PAH on echocardiographic findings, some patients may have been misclassified. Thus, ET-1 is considered an important molecule in the pathogenesis of CTD-PH, providing a rationale for endothelin-receptor antagonism as a therapeutic approach in CTD-PH *(55)*.

3.2. Autoantibodies

A distinct feature of CTD-PH compared to the idiopathic form is the association of specific autoantibodies with disease phenotypes. For example, anti-topoisomerase I (Scl-70) has been associated with diffuse SSc, whereas anti-centromere antibody (ACA) has been associated with limited SSc, pulmonary hypertension, better survival, and a decreased incidence of interstitial lung disease *(56,57)*. Whether these autoantibodies are markers of disease activity or play a role in disease pathogenesis is as yet unknown.

Although a positive ACA is known to be associated with limited SSc and pulmonary hypertension, studies looking within the subset of patients with limited SSc have not found an association between ACA and pulmonary hypertension *(13,58,59)*. Furthermore, only 17% of SSc patients with PAH are ACA-positive *(13)*, suggesting that other factors must be contributing to the development of pulmonary hypertension in many of these patients.

Other autoantibodies have been associated with PAH in specific CTD populations, including anti-U3RNP *(16,60)*, anti-B23 *(61)*, antiendothelial cell antibodies (AECA) *(62,63)*, and anti-U1 ribonucleoprotein (U1RNP) *(64)*. Antibodies against U1RNP upregulate adhesion molecules on pulmonary artery endothelial cells in vitro *(65)*, suggesting a mechanism by which these autoantibodies may play a pathogenic role in the development of CTD-PH.

The role of AECA is of particular mechanistic interest in the development of CTD-PH. AECA derived from the sera of six patients with diffuse SSc induce human umbilical endothelial cell apoptosis in a Fas-independent manner *(66)*. Studies of both avian and human skin SSc lesions suggest that endothelial cell apoptosis is the earliest pathogenic event *(67)*. Additionally, conditioned media from apoptotic endothelial cells stimulates vascular smooth muscle cell proliferation in vitro *(68)*. Taken together, these data suggest that AECA-mediated endothelial cell apoptosis may be an early mechanism of vascular injury in SSc, contributing to vascular smooth muscle hypertrophy. AECA derived from patients with SLE-related PAH stimulate ET-1 release from endothelial cells in vitro *(62)*, and AECA in patients with MCTD may contribute to elevated serum ET-1 levels *(69)*. These observations indicate that AECA may also contribute to the development of CTD-PH related PAH via the stimulation of ET-1 release.

A final possible mechanism by which autoantibodies may play a mechanistic role in the genesis of CTD-PH involves platelet-derived growth factor (PDGF), a potent smooth muscle mitogen implicated in the development of pulmonary hypertension *(70,71)*. Inhibition of PDGF with imatinib mesylate reversed pulmonary hypertension in two animal models of pulmonary hypertension and in two case reports in humans *(72–74)*. Patients with SSc have PDGFR-activating autoantibodies that induce collagen gene expression *(75)*. Further investigation is needed, but these studies suggest that PDGFR-activating autoantibodies may mediate SSc-PH and raise the possibility that imatinib mesylate may be uniquely suited as a treatment for patients with SSc-PH.

4. CLINICAL PRESENTATION AND DIAGNOSIS

4.1. Symptoms and Signs

The clinical presentation and diagnosis of connective tissue disease-related pulmonary hypertension are similar to those of idiopathic PAH. Dyspnea is the most common presenting symptom and is generally insidious in onset. An early manifestation on physical examination is an increased intensity of P2, the sound of pulmonic valve closure, which intensifies as pulmonary artery pressure rises. Depending on the extent of right heart involvement, a right ventricular (RV) heave, murmur of tricuspid regurgitation, and evidence of right heart failure (jugular venous distension, peripheral edema, and/or ascites) may follow.

4.2. General Approach

When pulmonary hypertension is suspected based on symptoms, signs, and risk factors, further evaluation is initiated. The findings of right-axis deviation and right ventricular hypertrophy on an electrocardiogram and right ventricular enlargement and/or prominence of pulmonary arteries on a chest radiograph are specific but not sensitive indicators of pulmonary hypertension. As with idiopathic PAH, echocardiography is the most useful screening tool, and repeated echocardiography in high-risk CTD patients, such as those with limited disease, has been suggested on an annual basis, as discussed below, to detect early manifestations of pulmonary hypertension. Right heart catheterization (RHC) remains necessary to confirm the diagnosis, though, and to exclude other causes of pulmonary hypertension such as

Table 1
**World Health Organization (WHO) Classification of Functional Status
of Patients with Pulmonary Hypertension (PH) (from Reference _76_)**

Functional Class	Description
I	Patients with PH in whom there is no limitation of usual physical activity; ordinary physical activity does not cause increased dyspnea, fatigue, chest pain, or presyncope.
II	Patients with PH who have mild limitation of physical activity. There is no discomfort at rest, but normal physical activity causes increased dyspnea, fatigue, chest pain, or presyncope.
III	Patients with PH who have a marked limitation of physical activity. There is no discomfort at rest, but less than ordinary activity causes increased dyspnea, fatigue, chest pain, or presyncope.
IV	Patients with PH who are unable to perform any physical activity at rest and who may have signs of right ventricular failure. Dyspnea and/or fatigue may be present at rest, and symptoms are increased by almost any physical activity.

left-sided heart disease or congenital shunts. A functional status should also be assessed, based on the modified NYHA/WHO functional classification and a six-minute walk test (Table 1), to serve as a baseline. The latter may have limited value, however, when CTD patients have significant musculoskeletal pain or arthropathy.

4.3. Pulmonary Function Testing

Although restriction is a common finding on pulmonary function testing in patients with SSc, perhaps related to stiffening of the chest wall and/or interstitial disease, it is usually mild unless there is advanced fibrosis. An isolated reduction in DLCO occurs in 20% of patients with limited SSc and is the most common abnormality found on pulmonary function testing in SSc (77,78). Although a reduction in DLCO is a nonspecific finding in SSc and only a minority (an estimated 11%) of such patients go on to develop pulmonary hypertension (78), most patients with pulmonary hypertension have a severely reduced DLCO, which is lower than similar SSc patients without pulmonary hypertension (17). In one study, 88% of SSc patients with pulmonary hypertension had a DLCO < 43% predicted, as opposed to only 12%

of those without pulmonary hypertension *(8)*. Thus, a DLCO < 43%
has been suggested as an indicator of pulmonary hypertension in CTD
patients, and a progressive decline of DLCO over time correlates with
the development of pulmonary hypertension. In fact, a decreasing
DLCO has been identified as the strongest predictor of pulmonary
hypertension *(16)* and inversely correlates ($r = 0.60$) with invasively
measured PA systolic pressure *(79)*.

However, some findings on the utility of DLCO in predicting
the presence of pulmonary hypertension in CTD patients have been
conflicting; in one study, 23 of 54 (43%) patients with SSc-PH had
a DLCO > 55%, demonstrating that a relatively preserved DLCO
is not sufficient to exclude the diagnosis of pulmonary hypertension
in patients with SSc. The correlation between DLCO and mean PA
pressure (mPAP) determined by right heart catheterization was also
quite weak in this study ($r^2 = 0.0908$) *(80)*. Differences in the patient
populations (limited SSc vs. diffuse SSc and the proportion of patients
with concomitant interstitial lung disease) as well as differences in the
definitions and severity for pulmonary hypertension probably explain
the inconsistencies between the studies. One approach to improving
the predictability of DLCO for pulmonary hypertension has been to
use an FVC (% predicted)/DLCO(% predicted) ratio > 1.6 to detect
those who have a disproportionate reduction in DLCO, although the
sensitivity and specificity of this approach are still under investigation
(Steen VD, personal communication). Despite the inconsistencies, the
American College of Chest Physicians' 2004 evidence-based clinical
practice guidelines for pulmonary arterial hypertension recommended
pulmonary function testing with diffusing capacity (DLCO) every 6 to
12 months in patients with SSc to improve the detection of pulmonary
vascular disease *(81)*.

4.4. Doppler Echocardiography

Doppler echocardiographic estimates of PA systolic pressure
correlate well with catheter-measured pressures in general, but they
are often inaccurate in individual patients *(81)*. Several studies have
specifically examined the performance of Doppler echocardiography
in detecting pulmonary hypertension in patients with SSc. In one
study of 33 SSc patients suspected of having pulmonary hypertension,
Doppler echocardiography had a sensitivity of 90% and a specificity of 75%, correctly identifying 19 of 21 patients with right heart
catheterization-proven pulmonary hypertension. Doppler echocardiography was also fairly accurate in this study, with a mean absolute

difference for PA systolic pressure between it and right heart catheter-ization of 11.4 mm Hg *(79)*. In a similar study of 54 patients with isolated SSc-PH, Doppler echocardiography had a sensitivity of 85% when a triscuspid gradient >30 was used as the threshold for defining pulmonary hypertension, but the specificity was only 42% *(80)*. In summary, Doppler echocardiography has good sensitivity (85–90%) but limited specificity in identifying SSc-PH. For this reason, it is an acceptable screening test, and the World Health Organization has recommended annual echocardiography to screen SSc patients for pulmonary hypertension. Presently, there are no studies assessing the utility of Doppler echocardiography as a screening test for pulmonary hypertension in other connective tissue diseases.

4.5. Brain Natriuretic Peptide

Brain natriuretic peptide (BNP) performs similar roles in patients with SSc-PH and idiopathic PAH, increasing in proportion to the degree of right ventricular hypertrophy and dysfunction, and serving as a prognostic indicator *(82)*. In a prospective study of 40 patients with SSc, a precursor of BNP, N-terminal proBNP (NT-proBNP), was measured at baseline, acutely following three doses of a calcium channel blocker, then six to nine months later. The 10 patients in this study with SSc-PH (based on estimated PA systolic pressure > 40 by Doppler echocardiography) had a higher mean NT-proBNP than patients without evidence of pulmonary hypertension. Short-term calcium channel blockade significantly decreased the NT-proBNP concentration (from 146 to 82) and decreased the number of patients with an elevated NT-proBNP from 13 to 3. At the later assessment six to nine months later, the significant differences were no longer apparent, although the number of patients available for long-term follow-up was small *(83)*. Thus, although this small study suggests that BNP may have a role in detecting patients with SSc who have underlying pulmonary hypertension, serving as a prognostic indicator and guiding therapy, this role remains to be established.

5. THERAPY OF SSC-PH

5.1. General Approach

The general approach to therapy of CTD-PH is similar to that for idiopathic PAH. In fact, virtually all of the recent randomized controlled trials assessing newer therapies for PAH have included patients with CTD, amounting to roughly 30% of patients in most of the trials. Thus, progress in treatment of CTD-PH and idiopathic PAH has paralleled one another and the main therapies for both include anticoagulation, oxygen, diuretics, and pulmonary vasodilator/antiproliferative agents. Currently FDA-approved agents for CTD-PH include prostanoids (treprostinil, eproprostenol, iloprost), endothelin-receptor antagonists (bosentan, with sitaxsentan and ambrisentan undergoing review), and phosphodiesterase-5 inhibitors (sildenafil, with tadalafil being investigated). These agents are discussed in detail in later chapters, and only evidence directly relevant to CTD-PH is discussed here. Table 2 summarizes the results of randomized controlled clinical trials that included patients with CTD-PH.

5.2. Anticoagulation, Oxygen, and Diuretics

A consensus of experts recommends that patients with PAH, including those with CTD-PH, be anticoagulated with warfarin, adjusting the dose to achieve an international normalized ratio (INR) of 1.5 to 2.5 (81). This is based mainly on two retrospective, uncontrolled studies demonstrating improved survival in patients with IPAH treated with anticoagulation (84,85). The consensus document noted that the indication for CTD-PH is controversial, that such patients may be at increased risk for gastrointestinal bleeding—presumably those with limited SSc and multiple telangiectasias, and that the risk/benefit ratio should be carefully considered for each patient before initiating therapy (81).

Again, in the absence of any controlled data, oxygen therapy is recommended to maintain an O_2 saturation >90% with the hope of ameliorating hypoxic vasoconstriction and remodeling and improving exercise capacity. Also, diuretic therapy should be instituted in patients with right heart failure and volume overload; however, this should be done carefully, as patients with right heart failure may be preload-dependent. These therapies are discussed in more detail in Chapter 11.

5.3. Immunosuppressives

Because many CTDs are considered to have an autoimmune/inflammatory component that contributes to pathogenesis, therapy with immunosuppressive agents, plasma exchange, and autologous stem cell transplantation have been attempted (20,23,86–96). Studies have been small, poorly controlled, and confounded by factors like vasodilator and other therapies; not surprisingly, results have been conflicting. Anti-inflammatory and immunosuppressive therapy has

Table 2
Summary of Randomized, Placebo-Controlled trials Including Patients with Connective Tissue Disease-Associated Pulmonary Hypertension

Study	Patients	NYHA	Outcome
Epoprostenol Badesch et al. (2000)	n = 111 SSc MCTD	II (4.5%) III (78.5%) IV (17%)	Statistically significant improvement in median distance walked, hemodynamics, NYHA class, and Borg dyspnea scores;no survival benefit (not sufficiently powered to detect).
Iloprost (inh) Olschewski et al. (2002)	n = 35/203*	III (58.6%) IV (41.4%)	Statistically significant benefit in combined endpoint of 10% improvement in 6MWT and functional class improvement in absence of clinical deterioration; no hemodynamic deterioration in iloprost group compared with placebo group.
Treprostinil (SQ) Oudiz et al. (2004)	n = 90 SLE SSc MCTD	II (10%) III (74.5%) IV (15.5%)	Improved exercise capacity, dyspnea-fatigue symptoms, pulmonary hemodynamics and trend toward improved quality of life.
Bosentan Rubin et al. (2002)	n = 63/213* SSc, SLE	III (91.5%) IV (8.5%)	Statistically significant improvement in 6MWT, functional class, Borg dyspnea score, time to clinical worsening; effects greater in IPAH than CTD-PH.
Sildenafil Galie et al. (2005)	n = 84/278* SSc, SLE, "other"	I (1 pt) II (38%) III (58%) IV (3%)	Improvement in exercise capacity, NYHA/WHO functional class, hemodynamics; no slowing of time to clinical worsening; not designed to assess mortality.

*n = number of patients with connective tissue disease/total number of patients in study; inh = inhaled.

been disappointing for SSc, but some case series show favorable responses in patients with SLE (87,91–93). On the other hand, another series of patients with SLE reported that five of six patients developed pulmonary hypertension while being treated with steroids (37). Thus, the role of immunomodulatory therapy in CTD-PH remains unclear.

5.4. Oral Antihypertensives

Early reports of treating patients with SSc-PH and MCTD-related PAH with oral vasodilators, including angiotensin converting enzyme inhibitors, calcium channel blockers, and alpha-adrenergic blockers, were mostly promising (97–101). An early small case series using calcium channel blockers in patients with SSc-PH and MCTD-related PAH demonstrated acute and longer-term (three to six months) hemodynamic improvement (98). Later, a case-control study found more and longer-duration calcium channel blocker use among SSc patients without pulmonary hypertension (61% and 2.7 years, respectively) as compared to SSc patients with pulmonary hypertension (37% and 0.9 years), suggesting a possible protective effect in this population (16). On the other hand, a hemodynamic study of 16 patients with SSc and severe PAH found no acute responses among 8 patients treated with calcium channel blockers (102). The ACCP consensus statement recommends that calcium channel blockers be considered in patients with CTD-PH whose mean PA pressure decreases at least 10 mm Hg to ≤40 mm Hg, with a concomitant increase or unchanged cardiac output (103). However, such a response among patients with CTD-PH is very unusual, and oral antihypertensives, including calcium channel blockers as well as ACE inhibitors and hydralazine, are considered to have a very limited role in pharmacotherapy. Of course, many patients with connective tissue disease take calcium channel blockers for Raynaud's phenomenon, and whether these have a protective effect against pulmonary hypertension, as suggested by the case-control study (16), remains to be proven.

5.5. Prostacyclins

Single-center, open-label trials of intravenous epoprostenol in patients with SSc-PH suggested that this patient population responds similarly to idiopathic PAH (102,104,105). In a subsequent multi-center, randomized controlled study, 111 patients with moderate to severe (78.5% NYHA class III, mean PVR 1016) SSc-PH and MCTD-PAH were treated with intravenous epoprostenol (mean dose: 11.2 ng/kg/min) for 12 weeks. Statistically significant improvements in median distance walked in six minutes, hemodynamics, NYHA class, and Borg dyspnea scores were similar to those observed for idiopathic PAH in an earlier pivotal trial *(106)*. In contrast to the idiopathic PAH trial, however, there was no survival benefit, perhaps because the study was underpowered for this outcome. In a small case series of six patients with severe (NYHA class III/IV, mean PVR 1120) SLE-related PAH, intravenous epoprostenol use was associated with improved NYHA class and improved hemodynamics in four patients after 9 to 16 months of therapy, with the longest reported follow-up of 2.5 years *(37)*. A note of caution derived from another small series that reported life-threatening thrombocytopenia in SLE patients on long-term intravenous epoprostenol treatment, despite evidence that the SLE was quiescent *(107)*. In sum, these results support the use of intravenous epoprostenol to treat severe (NYHA class III/IV) PAH associated with connective tissue disease as long as patients are closely monitored for possible complications.

Iloprost, a more stable analogue of epoprostenol, can be administered in intravenous, oral, and inhaled forms. Its use in CTD-PH patients has been less studied than epoprostenol, but one small trial of three patients with SSc-PH observed improvements in functional class, exercise tolerance, and pulmonary hemodynamics after 30 weeks of a continuous intravenous iloprost infusion *(108)*. In another small series, 12 patients with SSc but no pulmonary hypertension received iloprost intravenously for five days and had decreased levels of multiple serum proteins (sICAM, sE-selectin, sVCAM, VEGF, ET-1) along with a clinical improvement in Raynaud's phenomenon, suggesting reduced endothelial cell activation *(109)*.

Inhaled iloprost has also been studied. In one small, uncontrolled study of five patients with limited SSc and severe SSc-PH, treatment with inhaled iloprost for one year resulted in improved quality of life, functional class, and hemodynamics, a response that was maintained at two years in three of the five patients *(110)*. A subsequent, large, randomized, placebo-controlled pivotal trial of inhaled iloprost in pulmonary hypertension included 35 patients with CTD-PH, 13 of whom received treatment. Among all patients in the trial, a statistically significant benefit was demonstrated at 12 weeks in the combined primary endpoint of survival, a 10% improvement in six-minute walk distance, and functional class improvement. Numbers were too small for statistical analysis, but the CTD-PH subgroup tended to respond less to therapy than the idiopathic PAH subgroup *(111)*. Therefore, inhaled iloprost, which is an FDA-approved therapy for PAH in the United States, is a promising therapy for individuals who are reluctant or unable to manage a continuous intravenous infusion. The oral and intravenous forms of iloprost are not presently available in the United States.

An even more stable prostacyclin analogue (with a half-life of three to four hours and stable at room temperature), treprostinil has similar short-term hemodynamic effects as epoprostenol *(112)*. Subcutaneously administered treprostinil improved exercise capacity, dyspnea-fatigue index, and pulmonary hemodynamics in a large, multi-center, randomized, placebo-controlled, 12-week trial that included 90 patients with CTD-PH (SLE, SSc, MCTD). However, infusion site pain occurred in 83% of patients, limiting the uptitration of doses. Accordingly, the average dose of treprostinil was low (<9 ng/kg/min), and the overall improvement in six-minute walk distance was meager (median placebo-subtracted improvement of 25 m). However, patients on the highest doses of treprostinil tended to show the greatest improvement in the six-minute walk distance. Thus, subcutaneous treprostinil is an effective treatment for CTD-PH if adequate doses are used, but it may be limited by infusion site pain *(113)*.

Intravenous treprostinil was introduced more recently in response to the limitations of the subcutaneous route. In a prospective, multicenter, 12-week, open-label trial of intravenous treprostinil in 16 patients with PAH, including 6 with CTD-PH, patients treated with intra-venous treprostinil had statistically significant improvements in the six-minute walk test, Naughton–Balke treadmill test, Borg dyspnea score, and pulmonary hemodynamic parameters. In addition, six patients improved one to two NYHA/WHO functional classes, and there was no functional class deterioration. Side effects (extremity pain, jaw pain, nausea, headache, flushing, and diarrhea) were similar to those of intravenous epoprostenol *(114)*. Although no head-to-head comparisons have been done, and some evidence suggests that intra-venous treprostinil may be less potent than intravenous epoprostenol given in equivalent doses, it appears to be equally potent if the dose is aggressively uptitrated. It offers an attractive alternative to epoprostenol since the long half-life gives a safety margin and it does not require continuous refrigeration or daily mixing. These benefits may be especially important in patients with CTD-PH whose manual dexterity may be severely limited by the underlying disease process. Caution should be exercised, however, because the long-term efficacy and durability of response to intravenous treprostinil have not yet been established.

5.6. Endothelin-Receptor Antagonists

As discussed above, increased expression and release of the vasoconstrictor and mitogenic peptide endothelin-1 (ET-1) has been implicated in the pathogenesis of pulmonary hypertension and some connective tissue diseases. Thus, endothelin-receptor antagonists (ERAs) have been used to treat CTD-PH. In the pivotal BREATHE-1 trial, 213 patients with PAH, including 47 patients with SSc-PH and 16 with SLE-related PAH, were randomized to treatment with either bosentan or placebo. Compared to placebo, bosentan improved functional class, Borg dyspnea score, time to clinical worsening, and six-minute walk distance by approximately 40 m *(115)*, and these benefits were maintained for approximately one year *(116)*. The improvement was substantially less in the CTD-PH subgroup than in idiopathic PAH patients, however, with only a 3-m increase in six-minute walk distance over baseline. Bosentan's main effect was to prevent the nearly 40-m deterioration in six-minute walk distance that occurred in the placebo group. Studies evaluating the endothelin-receptor A selective antagonists sitaxsentan and ambrisentan have reported similar findings *(117,118)*. Preliminary one-year results of the STRIDE 2X open-label extension trial that compares sitaxsentan and bosentan suggest that sitaxsentan may be more effective than bosentan at preventing clinical worsening of CTD-PH, but this observation needs to be confirmed in a properly designed double-blind, randomized trial. Thus, ERAs appear to bring about more improvement in patients with idiopathic PAH than CTD-PH, but clinical stabilization and prevention of deterioration may be important benefits in the CTD-PH patients. In addition, some experimental evidence suggests that ERAs may offer benefit in patients with idiopathic pulmonary fibrosis, which could be important in selected CTD patients.

5.7. Phosphodiesterase-5 Inhibitors

Phosphodiesterase-5 (PDE5) degrades cyclic guanosine 3'-5' monophosphate (cGMP), the intracellular second messenger responsible for mediating the vasodilatory effects of nitric oxide (NO) and natriuretic peptides. Sildenafil is a selective PDE5 inhibitor that slows the degradation of cGMP, potentiates NO-mediated pulmonary vasodilation, and has antiproliferative effects on pulmonary vascular smooth muscle cells *(103,119)*. An early case report of a patient with SSc-PH who had improvements in pulmonary hemodynamics, brain natriuretic peptide level, and Raynaud's phenomenon after four months of sildenafil suggested a possible therapeutic role for sildenafil in SSc-PH and other forms of CTD-PH *(120)*. Subsequently, the pivotal double-blind, placebo-controlled trial of sildenafil for PAH, SUPER-1, enrolled 84 patients with CTD (of 278 patients enrolled), 38 with SSc-PH, 19 with SLE-related PAH, and 27 with "other" forms of CTD-PH. Responses in the CTD subgroup were similar to those of the larger PAH group: significant improvements in the six-minute walk distance (42 and 15 m from baseline for the 20- and 80-mg tid doses, respectively), pulmonary hemodynamics (20-mg dose), and NYHA/WHO functional class. The rate of clinical worsening was not slowed by any of the sildenafil doses compared to placebo, but the study was not powered to examine this outcome or mortality *(119)*. A randomized controlled trial on tadalafil that included patients with CTD-PH has recently been completed, but no results have yet been announced. In summary, the results on PDE5 inhibitors suggest that they are effective in CTD-PH and comparable in efficacy to ERAs, but no head-to-head trials have been or are likely to be performed.

6. SURGICAL TREATMENTS

The availability of effective medications to treat pulmonary hypertension has diminished the role of surgical treatments for CTD-PH. Lung transplantation remains an option for patients who fail to improve on optimal medical therapy. Complications of connective tissue diseases such as chronic aspiration due to esophageal dysmotility are of special concern in the lung transplant setting and have caused some centers to exclude CTD patients from consideration for lung transplantation. However, survival in CTD-PH following lung or heart-lung transplantation has not been different from that of idiopathic PAH *(121)*. Atrial septostomy is a consideration in patients not responding to medical therapy but has been used mainly in countries where the availability of effective pharmacotherapies is limited. Performed using graded balloon dilation during a cardiac catheterization, atrial septostomy unloads the failing right ventricle and may enhance right ventricular function. In one report, a patient with SSc-PH treated with atrial septostomy experienced improvements in exercise capacity and exertional syncope was abolished *(122)*. This procedure should be performed only at experienced centers and is best reserved for severe and refractory cases that are hemodynamically stable.

7. SUMMARY

Many connective tissue diseases, particularly limited systemic sclerosis, are associated with pulmonary arterial hypertension. The development of pulmonary hypertension in patients with connective tissue disease reduces functional capacity and imparts a worse prognosis. The pathophysiology and pathology of idiopathic PAH and CTD-PH are similar, but autoantibodies are more often seen with the latter, suggesting an autoimmune component. Numerous therapeutic options are now available to treat CTD-PH, including prostacyclins, endothelin-receptor antagonists, and phosphodiesterase-5 inhibitors. Most of the recent randomized controlled trials on these agents have enrolled patients with patients with connective tissue disease. On average, these agents are effective in patients with CTD-PH but seem to manifest less robust or sustained responses than in those with idiopathic PAH. Ongoing studies on combination therapy, simpler delivery systems, and agents that target different signaling pathways hold promise for continued advances in the treatment of CTD-PH.

REFERENCES

1. Simonneau G, Galie N, Rubin LJ, Langleben D, et al. Clinical classification of pulmonary hypertension. J Am Coll Cardiol 2004; 43:5S–12S.
2. Young RH, Mark GJ. Pulmonary vascular changes in scleroderma. Am J Med 1978; 64(6):998–1004.
3. Cool CD, Kennedy D, Voelkel NF, Tuder RM. Pathogenesis and evolution of plexiform lesions in pulmonary hypertension associated with scleroderma and human immunodeficiency virus infection. Hum Pathol 1997; 28(4):434–42.
4. Saito A, Takizawa H, Ito K, Yamamoto K, et al. A case of pulmonary veno-occlusive disease associated with systemic sclerosis. Respirology 2003; 8(3):383–5.
5. Gugnani MK, Pierson C, Vanderheide R, Girgis RE. Pulmonary edema complicating prostacyclin therapy in pulmonary hypertension associated with scleroderma: A case of pulmonary capillary hemangiomatosis. Arthritis Rheum 2000; 43(3):699–703.
6. Morassut PA, Walley VM, Smith CD. Pulmonary veno-occlusive disease and the CREST variant of scleroderma. Can J Cardiol 1992; 8(10):1055–8.
7. Fagan KA, Badesch DB. Pulmonary hypertension associated with connective tissue disease. Prog Cardiovasc Dis 2002; 45(3):225–34.
8. Ungerer RG, Tashkin DP, Furst D, Clements PJ, et al. Prevalence and clinical correlates of pulmonary arterial hypertension in progressive systemic sclerosis. Am J Med 1983; 75(1):65–74.
9. Mukerjee D, St George D, Coleiro B, Knight C, et al. Prevalence and outcome in systemic sclerosis associated pulmonary arterial hypertension: Application of a registry approach. Ann Rheum Dis 2003; 62(11): 1088–93.
10. Battle RW, Davitt MA, Cooper SM, Buckley LM, et al. Prevalence of pulmonary hypertension in limited and diffuse scleroderma. Chest 1996; 110(6):1515–9.

11. Pope JE, Lee P, Baron M, Dunne J, et al. Prevalence of elevated pulmonary arterial pressures measured by echocardiography in a multi-center study of patients with systemic sclerosis. J Rheumatol 2005; 32(7):1273–8.

12. Koh ET, Lee P, Gladman DD, Abu-Shakra M. Pulmonary hypertension in systemic sclerosis: An analysis of 17 patients. Br J Rheumatol 1996; 35(10): 989–93.

13. Schachna L, Wigley FM, Chang B, White B, et al. Age and risk of pulmonary arterial hypertension in scleroderma. Chest 2003; 124(6): 2098–104.

14. Yousem SA. The pulmonary pathologic manifestations of the CREST syndrome. Hum Pathol 1990; 21(5):467–74.

15. al Sabbagh MR, Steen VD, Zee BC, Nalesnik M, et al. Pulmonary arterial histology and morphometry in systemic sclerosis: A case-control autopsy study. J Rheumatol 1989; 16(8):1038–42.

16. Steen V, Medsger TA, Jr. Predictors of isolated pulmonary hypertension in patients with systemic sclerosis and limited cutaneous involvement. Arthritis Rheum 2003; 48(2):516–22.

17. Stupi AM, Steen VD, Owens GR, Barnes EL, et al. Pulmonary hypertension in the CREST syndrome variant of systemic sclerosis. Arthritis Rheum 1986; 29(4):515–24.

18. Lee P, Langevitz P, Alderdice CA, Aubrey M, et al. Mortality in systemic sclerosis (scleroderma). Quar J Med 1992; 82(298):139–48.

19. Kawut SM, Taichman DB, Archer-Chicko CL, Palevsky HI. et al. Hemodynamics and survival in patients with pulmonary arterial hypertension related to systemic sclerosis. Chest 2003; 123(2):344–50.

20. Bull TM, Fagan KA, Badesch DB. Pulmonary vascular manifestations of mixed connective tissue disease. Rheum Dis Clin North Am 2005; 31(3):451–64, vi.

21. Hosoda Y, Suzuki Y, Takano M, Tojo T, et al. Mixed connective tissue disease with pulmonary hypertension: A clinical and pathological study. J Rheum 1987; 14(4):826–30.

22. Esther JH, Sharp GC, Agia GA. Pulmonary hypertension in patients with connective tissue disease and anti-nuclear ribonucleoprotein. Arthritis Rheum 1981; 24:S105.

23. Sullivan WD, Hurst DJ, Harmon CE, Esther JH, et al. A prospective evaluation emphasizing pulmonary involvement in patients with mixed connective tissue disease. Medicine (Baltimore) 1984; 63(2):92–107.

24. Burdt MA, Hoffman RW, Deutscher SL, Wang GS, et al. Long-term outcome in mixed connective tissue disease: Longitudinal clinical and serologic findings. Arthritis Rheum 1999; 42(5):899–909.

25. Asherson RA, Morgan SH, Hackett D, Montanes P, et al. Rheumatoid arthritis and pulmonary hypertension. A report of three cases. J Rheum 1985; 12(1):154–9.

26. Balagopal VP, da Costa P, Greenstone MA. Fatal pulmonary hypertension and rheumatoid vasculitis. Eur Respir J 1995; 8(2):331–3.

27. Morikawa J, Kitamura K, Habuchi Y, Tsujimura Y, et al. Pulmonary hypertension in a patient with rheumatoid arthritis. Chest 1988; 93(4):876–8.
28. Young ID, Ford SE, Ford PM. The association of pulmonary hypertension with rheumatoid arthritis. J Rheum 1989; 16(9):1266–9.
29. Kay JM, Banik S. Unexplained pulmonary hypertension with pulmonary arteritis in rheumatoid disease. Br J Dis Chest 1977; 71(1):53–9.
30. Dawson JK, Goodson NG, Graham DR, Lynch MP. Raised pulmonary artery pressures measured with Doppler echocardiography in rheumatoid arthritis patients. Rheumatology (Oxford) 2000; 39(12):1320–5.
31. Baydur A, Mongan ES, Slager UT. Acute respiratory failure and pulmonary arteritis without parenchymal involvement: Demonstration in a patient with rheumatoid arthritis. Chest 1979; 75(4):518–20.
32. Pan TL, Thumboo J, Boey ML. Primary and secondary pulmonary hypertension in systemic lupus erythematosus. Lupus 2000; 9(5):338–42.
33. Shen JY, Chen SL, Wu YX, Tao RQ, et al. Pulmonary hypertension in systemic lupus erythematosus. Rheum Int 1999; 18(4):147–51.
34. Li EK, Tam LS. Pulmonary hypertension in systemic lupus erythematosus: Clinical association and survival in 18 patients. J Rheum 1999; 26(9):1923–9.
35. Simonson JS, Schiller NB, Petri M, Hellmann DB. Pulmonary hypertension in systemic lupus erythematosus. J Rheum 1989; 16(7): 918–25.
36. Falcao CA, Alves IC, Chahade WH, Duarte AL, et al. Echocardiographic abnormalities and antiphospholipid antibodies in patients with systemic lupus erythematosus. Arq Bras Cardiol 2002; 79(3):285–91.
37. Robbins IM, Gaine SP, Schilz R, Tapson VF, et al. Epoprostenol for treatment of pulmonary hypertension in patients with systemic lupus erythematosus. Chest 2000; 117(1):14–8.
38. Fayemi AO. Pulmonary vascular disease in systemic lupus erythematosus. Am J Clin Pathol 1976; 65(3):284–90.
39. Schwartzberg M, Lieberman DH, Getzoff B, Ehrlich GE. Systemic lupus erythematosus and pulmonary vascular hypertension. Arch Intern Med 1984; 144(3):605–7.
40. Sack KE, Bekheit S, Fadem SZ, Bedrossian CW. Severe pulmonary vascular disease in systemic lupus erythematosus. South Med J 1979; 72(8):1016–8.
41. Nair SS, Askari AD, Popelka CG, Kleinerman JF. Pulmonary hypertension and systemic lupus erythematosus. Arch Intern Med 1980; 140(1):109–11.
42. Hoeper MM. Pulmonary hypertension in collagen vascular disease. Eur Respir J 2002; 19(3):571–6.
43. Du L, Sullivan CC, Chu D, Cho AJ, et al. Signaling molecules in nonfamilial pulmonary hypertension. N Engl J Med 2003; 348(6): 500–9.

44. Kharitonov SA, Cailes JB, Black CM, Du Bois RM, et al. Decreased nitric oxide in the exhaled air of patients with systemic sclerosis with pulmonary hypertension. Thorax 1997; 52(12):1051–5.

45. Rolla G, Colagrande P, Scappaticci E, Chiavassa G, et al. Exhaled nitric oxide in systemic sclerosis: Relationships with lung involvement and pulmonary hypertension. J Rheum 2000; 27(7):1693–8.

46. Kawaguchi Y, Tochimoto A, Hara M, Kawamoto M, et al. NOS2 polymorphisms associated with the susceptibility to pulmonary arterial hypertension with systemic sclerosis: Contribution to the transcriptional activity. Arthritis Res Ther 2006; 8(4):R104.

47. Morse J, Barst R, Horn E, Cuervo N, et al. Pulmonary hypertension in scleroderma spectrum of disease: Lack of bone morphogenetic protein receptor 2 mutations. J Rheum 2002; 29(11):2379–81.

48. Yamane K, Miyauchi T, Suzuki N, Yuhara T, et al. Significance of plasma endothelin-1 levels in patients with systemic sclerosis. J Rheum 1992; 19(10):1566–71.

49. Vancheeswaran R, Magoulas T, Efrat G, Wheeler-Jones C, et al. Circulating endothelin-1 levels in systemic sclerosis subsets—A marker of fibrosis or vascular dysfunction? J Rheum 1994; 21(10):1838–44.

50. Morelli S, Ferri C, Polettini E, Bellini C, et al. Plasma endothelin-1 levels, pulmonary hypertension, and lung fibrosis in patients with systemic sclerosis. Am J Med 1995; 99(3):255–60.

51. Julkunen H, Saijonmaa O, Gronhagen-Riska C, Teppo AM, et al. Raised plasma concentrations of endothelin-1 in systemic lupus erythematosus. Ann Rheum Dis 1991; 50(7):526–7.

52. Kawaguchi Y, Suzuki K, Hara M, Hidaka T, et al. Increased endothelin-1 production in fibroblasts derived from patients with systemic sclerosis. Ann Rheum Dis 1994; 53(8):506–10.

53. Odoux C, Crestani B, Lebrun G, Rolland C, et al. Endothelin-1 secretion by alveolar macrophages in systemic sclerosis. Am J Respir Crit Care Med 1997; 156(5):1429–35.

54. Abraham DJ, Vancheeswaran R, Dashwood MR, Rajkumar VS, et al. Increased levels of endothelin-1 and differential endothelin type A and B receptor expression in scleroderma-associated fibrotic lung disease. Am J Pathol 1997; 151(3):831–41.

55. Hachulla E, Coghlan JG. A new era in the management of pulmonary arterial hypertension related to scleroderma: Endothelin receptor antagonism. Ann Rheum Dis 2004; 63(9):1009–14.

56. Ho KT, Reveille JD. The clinical relevance of autoantibodies in scleroderma. Arthritis Res Ther 2003; 5(2):80–93.

57. Cepeda EJ, Reveille JD. Autoantibodies in systemic sclerosis and fibrosing syndromes: Clinical indications and relevance. Curr Opin Rheum 2004; 16(6):723–32.

58. Steen VD, Powell DL, Medsger TA, Jr. Clinical correlations and prognosis based on serum autoantibodies in patients with systemic sclerosis. Arthritis Rheum 1988; 31(2):196–203.

59. Steen VD, Ziegler GL, Rodnan GP, Medsger TA, Jr. Clinical and laboratory associations of anticentromere antibody in patients with progressive systemic sclerosis. Arthritis Rheum 1984; 27(2):125–31.

60. Sacks DG, Okano Y, Steen VD, Curtiss E, et al. Isolated pulmonary hypertension in systemic sclerosis with diffuse cutaneous involvement: Association with serum anti-U3RNP antibody. J Rheum 1996; 23(4): 639–42.

61. Ulanet DB, Wigley FM, Gelber AC, Rosen A. Autoantibodies against B23, a nucleolar phosphoprotein, occur in scleroderma and are associated with pulmonary hypertension. Arthritis Rheum 2003; 49(1):85–92.

62. Yoshio T, Masuyama J, Sumiya M, Minota S, et al. Antiendothelial cell antibodies and their relation to pulmonary hypertension in systemic lupus erythematosus. J Rheum 1994; 21(11):2058–63.

63. Negi VS, Tripathy NK, Misra R, Nityanand S. Antiendothelial cell antibodies in scleroderma correlate with severe digital ischemia and pulmonary arterial hypertension. J Rheum 1998; 25(3):462–6.

64. Kuwana M, Kaburaki J, Okano Y, Tojo T, et al. Clinical and prognostic associations based on serum antinuclear antibodies in Japanese patients with systemic sclerosis. Arthritis Rheum 1994; 37(1):75–83.

65. Okawa-Takatsuji M, Aotsuka S, Fujinami M, Uwatoko S, et al. Up-regulation of intercellular adhesion molecule-1 (ICAM-1), endothelial leucocyte adhesion molecule-1 (ELAM-1) and class II MHC molecules on pulmonary artery endothelial cells by antibodies against U1-ribonucleoprotein. Clin Exp Immunol 1999; 116(1):174–80.

66. Bordron A, Dueymes M, Levy Y, Jamin C, et al. The binding of some human antiendothelial cell antibodies induces endothelial cell apoptosis. J Clin Invest 1998; 101(10):2029–35.

67. Sgonc R, Gruschwitz MS, Dietrich H, Recheis H, et al. Endothelial cell apoptosis is a primary pathogenetic event underlying skin lesions in avian and human scleroderma. J Clin Invest 1996; 98(3):785–92.

68. Sakao S, Taraseviciene-Stewart L, Wood K, Cool CD, et al. Apoptosis of pulmonary microvascular endothelial cells stimulates vascular smooth muscle cell growth. Am J Physiol Lung Cell Mol Physiol 2006; 291(3):L362–L368.

69. Filep JG, Bodolay E, Sipka S, Gyimesi E, et al. Plasma endothelin correlates with antiendothelial antibodies in patients with mixed connective tissue disease. Circulation 1995; 92(10):2969–74.

70. Balasubramaniam V, Le Cras TD, Ivy DD, Grover TR, et al. Role of platelet-derived growth factor in vascular remodeling during pulmonary hypertension in the ovine fetus. Am J Physiol Lung Cell Mol Physiol 2003; 284(5):L826–L833.

71. Humbert M, Monti G, Fartoukh M, Magnan A, et al. Platelet-derived growth factor expression in primary pulmonary hypertension: Comparison of HIV seropositive and HIV seronegative patients. Eur Respir J 1998; 11(3):554–9.

72. Schermuly RT, Dony E, Ghofrani HA, Pullamsetti S, et al. Reversal of experimental pulmonary hypertension by PDGF inhibition. J Clin Invest 2005; 115(10):2811–21.

73. Patterson KC, Weissmann A, Ahmadi T, Farber HW. Imatinib mesylate in the treatment of refractory idiopathic pulmonary arterial hypertension. Ann Intern Med 2006; 145(2):152–3.

74. Ghofrani HA, Seeger W, Grimminger F. Imatinib for the treatment of pulmonary arterial hypertension. N Engl J Med 2005; 353(13):1412–3.

75. Baroni SS, Santillo M, Bevilacqua F, Luchetti M, et al. Stimulatory autoantibodies to the PDGF receptor in systemic sclerosis. N Engl J Med 2006; 354(25):2667–76.

76. Barst RJ, McGoon M, Torbicki A, Sitbon O, et al. Diagnosis and Differential Assessment of Pulmonary Arterial Hypertension. J Am Coll Cardiol 2004; 43:40S–47S.

77. Owens GR, Fino GJ, Herbert DL, Steen VD, et al. Pulmonary function in progressive systemic sclerosis. Comparison of CREST syndrome variant with diffuse scleroderma. Chest 1983; 84(5):546–50.

78. Steen VD, Graham G, Conte C, Owens G, et al. Isolated diffusing capacity reduction in systemic sclerosis. Arthritis Rheum 1992; 35(7):765–70.

79. Denton CP, Cailes JB, Phillips GD, Wells AU, et al. Comparison of Doppler echocardiography and right heart catheterization to assess pulmonary hypertension in systemic sclerosis. Br J Rheum 1997; 36(2): 239–43.

80. Mukerjee D, St George D, Knight C, Davar J, et al. Echocardiography and pulmonary function as screening tests for pulmonary arterial hypertension in systemic sclerosis. Rheumatology (Oxford) 2004; 43(4):461–6.

81. McGoon M, Gutterman D, Steen V, Barst R, et al. Screening, early detection, and diagnosis of pulmonary arterial hypertension: ACCP evidence-based clinical practice guidelines. Chest 2004; 126(1 Suppl):14S–34S.

82. Nagaya N, Nishikimi T, Uematsu M, Satoh T, et al. Plasma brain natriuretic peptide as a prognostic indicator in patients with primary pulmonary hypertension. Circulation 2000; 102(8):865–70.

83. Allanore Y, Borderie D, Meune C, Cabanes L, et al. N-terminal pro-brain natriuretic peptide as a diagnostic marker of early pulmonary artery hypertension in patients with systemic sclerosis and effects of calcium-channel blockers. Arthritis Rheum 2003; 48(12):3503–8.

84. Rich S, Kaufmann E, Levy PS. The effect of high doses of calcium-channel blockers on survival in primary pulmonary hypertension. N Engl J Med 1992; 327(2):76–81.

85. Fuster V, Steele PM, Edwards WD, Gersh BJ, et al. Primary pulmonary hypertension: Natural history and the importance of thrombosis. Circulation 1984; 70(4):580–7.

86. Mariette X, Brenot F, Brouet JC. Recovery from pulmonary hypertension with steroid therapy in a patient with Sjogren's syndrome and polymyositis. J Rheum 1994; 21(4):772–3.

114. Tapson VF, Gomberg-Maitland M, McLaughlin VV, Benza RL, et al. Safety and efficacy of IV treprostinil for pulmonary arterial hypertension: A prospective, multicenter, open-label, 12-week trial. Chest 2006; 129(3):683–8.

115. Rubin LJ, Badesch DB, Barst RJ, Galie N, et al. Bosentan therapy for pulmonary arterial hypertension. *N Engl J Med* 2002; 346(12):896–903.

116. Sitbon O, Badesch DB, Channick RN, Frost A, et al. Effects of the dual endothelin receptor antagonist bosentan in patients with pulmonary arterial hypertension: A 1-year follow-up study. Chest 2003; 124(1):247–54.

117. Barst RJ, Langleben D, Frost A, Horn EM, et al. Sitaxsentan therapy for pulmonary arterial hypertension. Am J Respir Crit Care Med 2004; 169(4):441–7.

118. Galie N, Badesch D, Oudiz R, Simonneau G, et al. Ambrisentan therapy for pulmonary arterial hypertension. J Am Coll Cardiol 2005; 46(3): 529–35.

119. Galie N, Ghofrani HA, Torbicki A, Barst RJ, et al. Sildenafil citrate therapy for pulmonary arterial hypertension. N Engl J Med 2005; 353(20):2148–57.

120. Rosenkranz S, Diet F, Karasch T, Weihrauch J, et al. Sildenafil improved pulmonary hypertension and peripheral blood flow in a patient with scleroderma-associated lung fibrosis and the Raynaud phenomenon. Ann Intern Med 2003; 139(10):871–3.

121. Rosas V, Conte JV, Yang SC, Gaine SP, et al. Lung transplantation and systemic sclerosis. Ann Transplant 2000; 5(3):38–43.

122. Allcock RJ, O'Sullivan JJ, Corris PA. Palliation of systemic sclerosis-associated pulmonary hypertension by atrial septostomy. Arthritis Rheum 2001; 44(7):1660–2.

9

Pulmonary Hypertension Associated with HIV, Liver Disease, Sarcoidosis, and Sickle Cell Disease

Kimberly A. Fisher
and Elizabeth S. Klings

CONTENTS

INTRODUCTION
HIV-ASSOCIATED PULMONARY HYPERTENSION
PORTOPULMONARY HYPERTENSION
SARCOIDOSIS
SICKLE CELL DISEASE
CONCLUSIONS
REFERENCES

Abstract

HIV, portopulmonary hypertension, sarcoidosis, and sickle cell disease (SCD) are all associated with PH. Although specific histological features of the pulmonary vasculature may differ among the various entities, they share a number of similarities. The PH manifests itself in a minority of these patients, consistent with the idea that gene mutations may predispose certain individuals to developing PH, probably in combination with other factors. Multiple factors seem to contribute, including endothelial dysfunction, vasodilator/vasoconstrictor mediator imbalance, immunological and oxidant mechanisms, and structural abnormalities of the vasculature related to injected foreign material (mainly in HIV and some SCD patients) and to parenchymal destruction (particularly in sarcoidosis and SCD). In addition, some entities,

From: *Contemporary Cardiology: Pulmonary Hypertension*
Edited by: N. S. Hill and H. W. Farber © Humana Press, Totowa, NJ

such as portopulmonary hypertension and SCD, are characterized by relatively high cardiac outputs that may predispose to PH by means of increased shear stress. Patients with SCD not uncommonly have a component of pulmonary venous hypertension related to LV diastolic dysfunction, underscoring the need to perform right heart catheterizations to properly diagnose patients. The PAH in these entities is also often responsive to a variety of medical therapies, although this inference is based mainly on case reports and small cohort studies and not on properly designed randomized trials.

Key Words: sarcoidosis; HIV-associated pulmonary hypertension; portopulmonary hypertension; sickle cell disease; pulmonary hypertension pathogenesis.

1. INTRODUCTION

Pulmonary hypertension (PH) is a term that encompasses a spectrum of diseases in which there is elevation of the mean pulmonary artery (PA) pressure (≥ 25 mm Hg at rest or ≥ 30 mm Hg with exercise). In pulmonary arterial hypertension (PAH), evidence of left-sided cardiac dysfunction is lacking (typically a pulmonary artery occlusion pressure <15 mm Hg) *(1)*. Idiopathic or primary PAH (IPAH, formerly known as PPH), represents a small fraction of these patients and is limited to those cases in which all other causes of PH have been excluded *(2)*. The World Health Organization in 1998 sought to classify PH according to histopathology and response to vasodilator treatment. IPAH and disorders with similar histopathology were now described as pulmonary arterial hypertension (PAH) *(2)*. This chapter describes four different systemic diseases associated with PH: human immunodeficiency virus (HIV) disease, portal hypertension, sarcoidosis, and sickle cell disease (SCD). Although each of these systemic diseases is associated with PH, their disease manifestations differ. PH related to HIV disease or portal hypertension is similar to IPAH in both histopathology and response to treatment, but each is more aggressive and lethal than IPAH. PH related to sarcoidosis or SCD may have differing histological features than IPAH; however, each of these diseases does appear to respond to vasodilator therapy.

2. HIV-ASSOCIATED PULMONARY HYPERTENSION

Improved prophylaxis and treatment of the infectious complications of human immunodeficiency virus (HIV) infection have resulted in increased patient survival. This has been accompanied by a greater incidence of noninfectious complications of the virus such as HIV-associated pulmonary hypertension (HIV-PH). HIV-PH was first reported in 1987 by Kim and Factor *(3)*. Overall, the incidence has been estimated at 0.5%, a rate higher than the estimated incidence of IPAH in the general population (0.02%), suggesting a causal relationship between HIV infection and PH *(4,5)*. Pathologically, this disorder is characterized by a primary pulmonary arteriopathy similar to that observed in IPAH *(6)*. Recent data suggest an indirect role for the HIV virus in the development of this pathology. However, the etiology of HIV-PH remains largely unknown and is likely multifactorial.

The average age of patients with HIV-PH is 33 years, although it can be seen both in infancy and in the elderly *(5,7–9)*. Unlike IPAH in which females predominate, HIV-PH occurs more commonly in males, with a ratio of 1.5:1 *(8)*. HIV-PH was first described exclusively in hemophiliacs *(7)*, but, subsequently, intravenous drug use (IVDU) became the primary HIV risk factor associated with the development of PH (approximately 50% of cases) *(8)*. Approximately 20% of cases are associated with homosexuality and 15% of cases with transfusion *(8)*. No correlation has been observed between the occurrence of HIV-PH and the degree of immunosuppression or the presence of opportunistic infections *(7)*. Similarly, no correlation has been observed between pulmonary artery (PA) pressure and CD4 cell counts, although those who met CDC criteria for diagnosis of AIDS tended to have higher pressures. On average, PH was diagnosed approximately three years after the diagnosis of HIV infection, although in 6%, the diagnosis of PH occurred first *(7)*. It appears that HIV-PH is more aggressive and lethal than IPAH, with a one-year survival rate of 51% compared to 68% *(1,10,11)*.

2.1. Pathogenesis

2.1.1. HISTOPATHOLOGY

The histopathology of HIV-PH is similar to that observed in other forms of PAH such as IPAH, and PH associated with connective tissue disease, anorexigen use, or portal hypertension *(2)*. Plexogenic lesions, characterized by medial hypertrophy with concentric intimal proliferation, are the most common abnormalities in HIV-PH, occurring in up to 70% of patients *(5–7)*. Later in the course of disease, there is severe intimal proliferation resulting in near-complete obstruction of the vascular lumen with formation of channels *(5)* (Fig. 1). The vessels in patients with HIV-PH possess a greater amount of endothelial cell proliferation and less concentric/obliterative fibrosis than vessels from patients with other forms of PAH. In addition to the plexogenic arteriopathy, other observed vascular lesions include

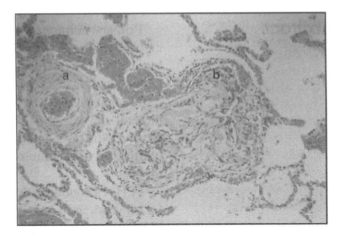

Fig. 1. Histologic section of the lungs of a patient with HIV-PH. This section demonstrates the characteristic vascular lesions observed. (**a**) Hypertrophy of the vascular media and (**b**) plexiform lesion. (Hematoxylin-eosin X63.)

thrombotic pulmonary arteriopathy and, in rare instances, pulmonary veno-occlusive disease *(5)*.

2.1.2. EFFECTS OF THE HIV VIRUS

The pathogenesis of HIV-PH, as in other forms of PH, remains largely unknown. Initially, it was thought to be, at least in part, due to coexisting conditions related to HIV infection. HIV-PH was first described in patients with classic hemophilia; based on these early cases, researchers theorized that the etiology of the pulmonary hypertension in HIV-infected patients was the hemophilia itself or perhaps the lyophilized factor VIII. Also of concern was the fact that many HIV-infected patients have confounding factors that have been independently associated with the development of pulmonary hypertension, such as intravenous drug abuse or hepatitis B and/or C infection. With time, however, most cases of pulmonary hypertension in HIV-infected individuals were identified in patients without coexisting risk factors. Thus, it seemed possible that development of pulmonary hypertension was related to the HIV infection itself.

Several investigators have postulated that PH is a disorder of dysregulated endothelial cell (EC) function characterized by uncontrolled proliferation and a vasoconstrictive phenotype *(12,13)*. This has led to an evaluation of the pulmonary vessels, and particularly the endothelium, for the presence of HIV expression. Studies evaluating the lungs of patients with HIV-PH failed to demonstrate the presence of HIV nucleic acid or HIV gag RNA by *in situ* hybridization or HIV-1 p24 antigen by immunohistochemistry *(9,14,15)*. Similarly, electron microscopy of the vascular endothelium did not demonstrate evidence of HIV viral particles *(5)*. Since direct infection of the endothelium by HIV does not occur, more recent studies have focused on an indirect role of the virus in the pathogenesis of HIV-PH.

HIV infection may play an indirect role in the development of HIV-PH via the production of cytokines (Fig. 2). In IPAH, inflammatory infiltrates containing B and T lymphocytes and macrophages have been noted within plexiform lesions *(5)*. Increased serum concentrations of the cytokines interleukin 1β (IL-1β) and IL-6 have been found in patients with IPAH; similar changes have been observed in the plasma cell dyscrasia associated with PH, POEMS (polyneuropathy, organomegaly, endocrinopathy, monoclonal gammopathy, and skin

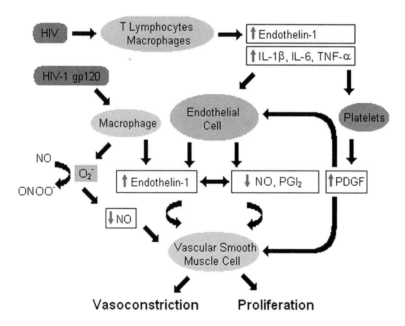

Fig. 2. Proposed pathogenesis of HIV-PH. The HIV virus stimulates endothelin-1, IL-1β, IL-6, and TNF-α from T lymphocytes and macrophages. These molecules decrease NO and PGI$_2$ production from the endothelium, which lead to increased smooth muscle contraction and proliferation. NO bioavailability is also affected by the production of O$_2^-$ by the macrophages and the preferential formation of ONOO$^-$. IL = interleukin; TNF = tumor necrosis factor; PDGF = platelet-derived growth factor; NO = nitric oxide; PGI$_2$ = prostacyclin; O$_2^-$ = superoxide; ONOO$^-$ = peroxynitrite.

changes) syndrome, suggesting a role for these cytokines in the development of pulmonary vascular disease *(16,17)*. Postulated mechanisms for cytokine action in the pathogenesis of PH include the induction of EC and smooth muscle cell proliferation, and the promotion of inflammatory cell migration via increased adhesion molecule expression *(18,19)*. The endothelium may also become pro-coagulant, potentially explaining the development of microthrombi observed histologically in patients with severe PH *(5)*. The effects of cytokines on the endothelium may be direct or indirectly mediated by platelet-derived growth factor (PDGF). PDGF is induced by IL-1β, and increased expression of this molecule has been demonstrated in the lungs of patients with IPAH and in those with HIV-PH *(16)*.

HIV tat protein may play a role in the pathogenesis of HIV-PH by several different mechanisms. First, the addition of the tat protein to cultured human umbilical vein EC (HUVEC) results in EC growth suggesting that tat may function as a proliferative agent *(20)*. Second, transfection of tat into human macrophages resulted in a dose-dependent repression of the bone morphogenetic protein receptor 2 gene *(BMPR2) (21)*. Mutations in *BMPR2* and its subsequent decreased effectiveness are associated with the familial form of IPAH *(22)*. Although the actual genetic alteration may differ in IPAH and HIV-PH, the target gene similarity is quite provocative and suggests a possible explanation for the similar histologies observed in both forms of the disease.

2.1.3. Vasoconstrictors and Vasodilators

Physiologically, PH represents a disease of pulmonary vasoconstriction and smooth muscle cell proliferation. Vascular tone is maintained via the interplay of vasoactive mediators such as the vasconstrictor endothelin-1 (ET-1) and the vasodilators nitric oxide (NO) and prostacyclin (PGI$_2$). This section describes the potential role of HIV infection in modulating the metabolism of these molecules (Fig. 2).

2.1.3.1. Endothelin-1. Interest in the role of ET-1, a vasoconstrictor and smooth muscle mitogen, in the development of PH arose from studies demonstrating increased plasma ET-1 levels in both IPAH and secondary forms of PH that correlated with the severity of disease *(23–26)*. ET-1 expression is increased in the vascular endothelium of the small muscular pulmonary arteries in IPAH patients; this has been correlated with pulmonary vascular resistance, linking the biology of this molecule with the pathophysiology of PH *(27)*. HIV-1 gp120 appears to stimulate the production of large quantities of ET-1 from macrophages, suggesting that the virus may play a primary role in the production of this vasoconstrictor within the lungs *(28)*. However, it is unclear if macrophage production of ET-1 correlates with plasma levels of ET-1 or the severity of PH in the HIV population.

2.1.3.2. Nitric Oxide.   NO is a molecule produced from L-arginine by endothelial nitric oxide synthase (eNOS) within the vascular endothelium *(29)*. It diffuses into the vascular smooth muscle, where it causes cellular relaxation through potentiation of cGMP *(30)*. Although NO is a potent vasodilator in its free form, it is preferentially converted to the powerful oxidants nitrite (NO_2), nitrate (NO_3), and peroxynitrite ($ONOO^-$) in the presence of oxygen and oxygen-related molecules *(29)*. Relative NO deficiency appears to play a role in the development of PH *(31–37)*. Although there is no direct evidence linking HIV infection to decreased NO bioactivity, there are several possible mechanisms by which this may occur. First, HIV infection of macrophages results in superoxide (O_2^-) generation, which converts NO to $ONOO^-$ *(28)*. Additionally, HIV infection may affect NO metabolism via ET-1. HIV can produce O_2^- through its interaction with the endothelin-receptor A (ET_A) receptor on the endothelium, thereby reducing NO bioavailability *(38)*. Additionally, ET-1 and NO appear to be involved in the regulation of each other via an autocrine feedback loop *(39)*, suggesting that when ET-1 production increases, NO is decreased.

2.1.3.3. Prostacyclin. PGI_2 is a powerful vasodilator and inhibitor of platelet adhesion produced by vascular endothelial and smooth muscle cells from arachidonic acid *(40–43)*. Therapeutically, a synthetic form of this molecule [epoprostenol (Flolan®)] improves symptoms, hemodynamics, and mortality in patients with IPAH *(44–46)*. In patients with HIV-PH, improvements in symptoms, NYHA class, and hemodynamics were noted in six patients on long-term epoprostenol *(47)*. These data suggest that PH is characterized by relative PGI_2 deficiency. Supporting this theory is the finding that mRNA and protein expression of PGI_2 synthase is decreased in the small and medium-sized pulmonary arteries of patients with both IPAH and HIV-PH *(12)*.

2.2. Autoimmunity and HLA Expression

Patients with HIV disease with and without PH have low titers of autoantibodies against cardiolipin IgG and IgM, glomerular basement membrane, and nuclear antibodies *(48)* likely resulting from nonspecific stimulation of B lymphocytes by HIV *(5)*. Patients with HIV-PH have a greater incidence of anti-cardiolipin IgM and anti-SS-B than control subjects *(5)*; the significance of this finding remains unclear.

A study of human leukocyte antigen (HLA) Class II alleles in 10 patients with HIV-PH demonstrated an increased frequency of HLA-DR6 and HLA-DR52 and of the linked alleles HLA-DRB1 1301/2, DRB3 0301, and DQBI 0603/4 compared to patients with IPAH and normal Caucasian controls. Additionally, HLA-DR6 and its DRB1 1301/2 subtypes were significantly increased in patients with HIV-PH compared with those having HIV infection alone *(49)*.

2.3. Toxic Substances

Chronic use of intravenous drugs is an independent risk factor for the development of PH; it occurs predominantly as a result of microthrombi of talc or methylcellulose of the injected material into the pulmonary vasculature *(50,51)*. Since injection drug users are at an increased risk for both HIV infection and PH, it is possible that foreign-body emboli contribute to the pathogenesis of HIV-PH. Thus, patients with HIV-PH related to IVDU may have higher PA pressures because of the two coexisting conditions; however, studies thus far have not supported this theory. Evaluation of patients with HIV-PH demonstrated no difference in mean systolic PAP in patients with a history of IVDU and those with other HIV risk factors *(9)*, suggesting that IVDU does not have an independent role in this process.

Another potential mechanism by which toxic substances can contribute to the development of PH is via chronic α-adrenergic stimulation; cocaine is the principal illicit agent in which this mechanism may be of importance. Stimulation of α-adrenergic receptors on vascular smooth muscle results in increased mRNA and protein synthesis of ET-1, PDGF, and vascular endothelial growth factor (VEGF) *(52)*, thereby leading to increased vasoconstriction and cellular proliferation *(53–56)*.

Chronic hypoxia also causes upregulation of the α-adrenergic receptor on the pulmonary vascular endothelium via activation of the transcription factor, hypoxia-inducible factor-1 (HIF-1). HIF-1 is a key mediator of hypoxia-induced VEGF gene expression, thereby inducing endothelial proliferation *(57)*. HIV patients may have an increased propensity for the development of chronic alveolar hypoxia because of recurrent pulmonary infections. Additionally, they appear to have an accelerated onset of chronic obstructive pulmonary disease (COPD) related to cigarette smoking *(58)*. Regardless of the inciting agent, the end result of α-adrenergic stimulation could produce vascular changes consistent with PH, suggesting a potential etiologic role for this mechanism in the development of HIV-PH.

2.4. Treatment

Significant therapeutic advances have been made in the treatment of HIV-PH since its original description in 1987. HIV infection is now more effectively treated with the advent of highly active anti-retroviral therapy (HAART). Pulmonary hypertension treatment has expanded to include numerous novel vasodilators. Several studies have examined the effects of these new treatments on the course of HIV-PH.

2.4.1. HAART THERAPY

The potential benefits of HAART therapy in treating HIV-PH were first noted in a case report describing a patient with progressive HIV-PH who was found to have decreased estimated right ventricular systolic pressure (RVSP) and normalization of right-sided dimensions by echocardiography after addition of HAART to the medical regimen *(59)*. In a retrospective study of 47 patients with HIV-PH, a decrease in the incidence of HIV-PH was noted (0.24% to 0.06–0.09%), which correlated with the introduction of HAART therapy. In patients stratified according to HIV treatment, serial echocardiograms revealed that patients treated with HAART had a median decrease in the RVSP-right atrial pressure (RAP) gradient of 21 mm Hg between the first and final echocardiograms. Additionally, there were stabilization of WHO/NYHA functional class and a decrease in mortality. No improvement in RVP-RAP, WHO/NYHA class, or mortality was noted in those patients receiving nucleoside reverse transcriptase inhibitors (NRTIs) alone *(60)*. In summary, HAART therapy appears to have a beneficial effect on the incidence, course, and outcome of HIV-PH, making HIV-PH an indication for the initiation of HAART.

2.4.2. VASODILATORS

The acute and long-term effects of epoprostenol infusion in HIV-PH have now been well described. Aguilar and Farber described six patients with HIV-PH (WHO/NYHA III or IV) who underwent treatment with epoprostenol *(47)*. Acutely, a decrease of 32.7% and 16.4% in pulmonary vascular resistance (PVR) and mean pulmonary artery pressure (PAP) and an increase of 51.4% in cardiac output (CO) were noted. Five of these six patients underwent repeat hemodynamic measurement after one year of treatment with epoprostenol; additional decreases in PVR (35.2%) and mean PAP (3.7%) and increases in CO (1.7%) were noted. These hemodynamic benefits were accompanied by an improvement in functional class (from WHO /NYHA class III-IV to I-II) *(47)*.

These findings have been confirmed and extended in a retrospective study examining 82 patients with HIV-PH, 20 of whom were treated with epoprostenol and followed for 6 to 47 months. Treatment with epoprostenol resulted in improved hemodynamics and functional status as measured by the six-minute walk test and WHO/NYHA class. Of note, the survival of NYHA class III–IV patients treated with epoprostenol and HAART was significantly better than in patients receiving HAART and conventional therapy (Fig. 3), suggesting an additive effect for epoprostenol in this population *(61)*.

The difficulty and risk of infection associated with the long-term use of epoprotenol to treat HIV-PH have led to exploration of other treatment regimens. Two small case series described the use of aerosolized iloprost or prostacyclin in HIV-PH. In one study, eight patients with severe HIV-PH underwent vasodilator trial with O_2, inhaled NO (iNO), and aerosolized iloprost. Only aerosolized iloprost produced a 30.6% decrease in PVR. Four of these patients

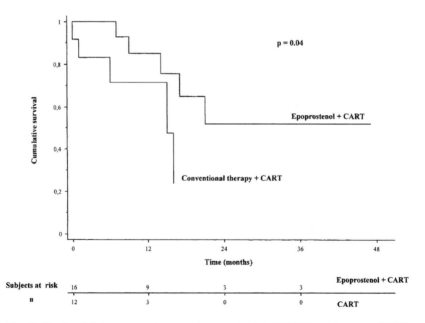

Fig. 3. Kaplan–Meier curves documenting survival in HIV-PH patients on CART and epoprostenol. Treatment with CART (combination antiretroviral therapy) and epoprostenol improves survival, compared with patients treated with CART alone. [From reference *(61)*, with permission]

received long-term aerosolized iloprost with nonsignificant trends toward improved six-minute walk test, decreased PVR, and improved WHO/NYHA class *(62)*. A smaller study of two patients with WHO/NYHA class IV HIV-PH treated with inhaled prostacyclin for seven months demonstrated a persistent decrease in mean PAP and PVR, but no change in CO. Both of these patients had a sustained improvement in echocardiographic findings and WHO/NYHA class *(63)*. Treprostinil, the subcutaneous form of prostacyclin, has been examined in a small study of three patients with HIV-PH who were treated with treprostinil for one year. All patients had improvement in their clinical status, measured by WHO/NYHA class and six-minute walk test. A decrease in systolic PAP by echocardiography was noted in two patients *(64)*. Based on these results, both inhaled and subcutaneous prostacyclins have potential as alternatives to intravenous epoprostenol in patients for which this therapy is unsuitable.

Other agents studied in the treatment of HIV-PH include the endothelin-receptor antagonist bosentan and the phosphodiesterase inhibitor sildenafil. Bosentan has been evaluated in a nonrandomized trial (BREATHE-4), in which 16 patients with HIV-PH (NYHA III-IV) were treated with bosentan for 16 weeks *(65)*. Clinically, this resulted in improved WHO/NYHA class, six-minute walk test, and score on the Borg dyspnea index. Hemodynamically, a 39% increase in cardiac index and a decrease in mPAP and PVR of 21% and 43%, respectively, occurred. Long-term follow-up (median: 556 days) data on 11 of these patients demonstrated maintained clinical and hemodynamic improvement. Two of the 16 developed an asymptomatic increase in transaminases, similar to that observed in other patient populations treated with bosentan. Treatment with bosentan produced no detectable changes in antiretroviral blood levels, CD4 count, or HIV viral load. Sildenafil has been shown in two case reports to produce clinical and echocardiographic improvement in patients with HIV-PH *(66,67)*. In summary, existing data suggest that HIV-PH resembles IPAH not just in terms of histopathology, but also in the response to traditional treatments for pulmonary hypertension, including epoprostenol, inhaled prostacyclin, sildenafil, and bosentan.

3. PORTOPULMONARY HYPERTENSION

The association of portal hypertension and pulmonary hypertension was first described in 1951 by Mantz and Craige *(68)*. A large autopsy study revealing histopathological changes of pulmonary hypertension in 0.73% of patients with cirrhosis, significantly greater than the prevalence of pulmonary hypertension (0.13%) found in the noncirrhotics, confirmed that this was a distinct clinical entity (69). Portopulmonary hypertension (PPHTN) is defined as pulmonary hypertension (mPAP ≥25 mm Hg at rest;≥30 mm Hg during exercise) in patients with portal hypertension (portal pressure >10 mm Hg). Clinical studies estimate the prevalence of PPHTN to be between 2% and 5% (70,71). Its presence appears to be indicative of more severe liver disease, as the prevalence is approximately 12% in patients being evaluated for orthotopic liver transplantation (OLT) (72) and 16.1% in patients with refractory ascites (73). The likelihood of developing PPHTN increases with the duration of portal hypertension, but studies are conflicting as to whether there is a direct correlation between PPHTN and the degree of portal hypertension (70,74,75).

In contrast to IPAH, which occurs primarily in women, PPHTN occurs with equal frequency in both genders. The mean age of presentation is in the fifth decade, whereas it is in the fourth decade for IPAH. Typically, PPHTN is diagnosed four to seven years following the diagnosis of portal hypertension (70), although, rarely, symptoms of PH can precede those of portal hypertension (76,77). PPHTN carries a worse prognosis than IPAH, with a mean survival of 15 months after diagnosis (78).

3.1. Pathogenesis

Histologically, the pulmonary vasculature in patients with PPHTN exhibits plexiform lesions, medial hypertrophy, intimal fibrosis, adventitial proliferation, and evidence of microthrombi, similar to IPAH. Reports of patients with portal hypertension in the absence of cirrhosis or liver disease developing PPHTN suggest a link between these two vascular processes (75,79–83). However, the low coincidence of PPHTN and portal hypertension and the finding in rats that portal vein ligation does not consistently lead to PPHTN (84,85) suggest an interplay of other mechanisms. Postulated mechanisms for the development of PPHTN include (1) increased pulmonary blood flow and altered vascular compliance leading to increased shear stress and (2) an imbalance between pulmonary vasodilators and vasoconstrictors.

One potential mechanism by which portal hypertension results in PPHTN is via increased shear stress. It has been theorized that portal hypertension results in increased pulmonary blood flow, thereby increasing shear stress, a known mechanism of endothelial injury. In support of this theory, Kuo et al. found that 41% of patients awaiting OLT without preexisting pulmonary hypertension developed pulmonary hypertension following volume infusion, suggesting that patients with cirrhosis may have an underlying defect in pulmonary vascular compliance, even in the absence of overt pulmonary hypertension *(86)*. However, the fact that the amount of blood shunted from the portal system has not been found to be an independent risk factor for pulmonary hypertension raises the possibility that increased shear stress is not the sole factor responsible for the development of pulmonary arteriopathy *(87)*.

As in IPAH, an imbalance between pulmonary vasodilators and vasoconstrictors likely plays a role in the pathogenesis of PPHTN. Decreased expression of the vasodilator PGI_2 synthase in small and medium-sized pulmonary arteries has been found in patients with PPHTN *(12)*. In addition, cirrhotic rats have been found to have decreased eNOS activity in the liver, potentially mediated through increased caveolin-1 binding *(88)*. However, in a rat model of PPHTN, increased inducible NOS expression was found in the pulmonary vascular endothelium *(89)*, suggesting an unclear role for NO in this process. Cirrhotics have increased ET-1 levels, compared with controls, with the highest levels being observed in those with PPHTN *(73)*.

The balance of vascular mediators may be altered in PPHTN by direct passage into the inferior vena cava (IVC) and pulmonary circulation, thereby avoiding hepatic metabolism. In support of this theory, elevated levels of the vasoconstrictors prostaglandin $F_2\alpha$, thromboxane B_2, and angiotensin 1 have been observed in the IVC in PPHTN patients *(80)*. Serotonin, another potent vasoconstrictor normally metabolized in the liver, has been implicated in the pathogenesis of IPAH. Changes in platelet serotonin concentration have been found in PH patients and cirrhotics, suggesting a role for serotonin in PPHTN *(90)*. Overall, there appears to be an increased propensity toward vasoconstriction in PPHTN. A number of these mediators have a dual function as smooth muscle mitogens, leading to induction of smooth muscle hyperplasia.

3.2. Diagnosis and Treatment

Patients with PPHTN often present insidiously with progressive dyspnea on exertion. In advanced disease, lightheadedness, syncope, and exertional chest pain can be observed. The presence of ascites and lower extremity edema is more difficult to interpret in the setting of portal hypertension, as they can both reflect right ventricular failure or portal hypertension. If PPHTN is suspected, transthoracic echocardiography is the mainstay of initial evaluation. Colle et al. *(91)*

prospectively compared echocardiography and right heart catheterization (RHC), performed within one week of each other, in a group of 165 patients being evaluated for OLT. Of the 148 patients without findings of pulmonary hypertension on echocardiography, none was found to have PPHTN by RHC, giving echocardiography a 100% negative predictive value (Fig. 4). Seventeen patients had echocardiographic findings of PPHTN (systolic pulmonary artery pressure calculated ≥30 mm Hg), 10 of whom had PPHTN confirmed by RHC. Thus, echocardiography had a sensitivity of 100%, a specificity of 96%, and a positive predictive value of 59%. Based on these data, echocardiography is sufficient to exclude the diagnosis of PPHTN in suspected cases or as screening for evaluation for OLT. However, if echocardiography suggests PPHTN, RHC is necessary to demonstrate (or exclude) elevated PVR.

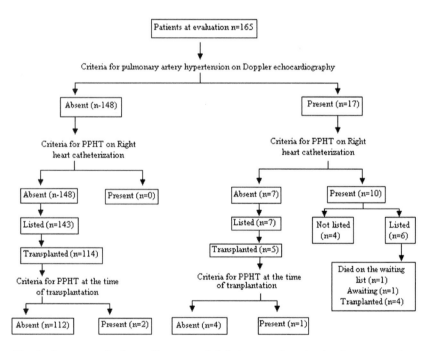

Fig. 4. Accuracy of echocardiogram and right heart catheterization in preoperative assessment of patients with portopulmonary hypertension. In those with normal echocardiograms, 112 of 114 patients had no evidence of pulmonary hypertension on right heart catheterization or at the time of surgery. Right heart catheterization is most helpful in preoperative assessment of those with PH on echocardiogram. [From reference *(91)*, with permission]

Pharmacological agents demonstrated to decrease PAP and PVR in patients with PPHTN include inhaled NO (iNO) *(92)*, beta blockers *(93,94)*, nitrates *(95)*, bosentan *(96)*, sildenafil *(97)*, and epoprostenol *(87,98)*. Inhaled NO has limited clinical utility in the long-term treatment of patients because of difficulty with administration. Traditional vasodilators such as beta blockers and nitrates have been ineffective in the treatment of pulmonary hypertension as a result of systemic hypotension. Of the newer pulmonary vasodilators, epoprostenol, the synthetic form of PGI_2, has been the best studied in this patient group. Krowka et al. *(87)* reported their experience with both acute and long-term epoprostenol administration in 15 patients with PPHTN. They found an acute improvement in both mean PAP (mPAP) and PVR. Notably, there was a somewhat larger decrease in mPAP and PVR noted than observed in patients with IPAH. However, at baseline, the PPHTN patients had lower mPAP and PVR and higher CO than their IPAH counterparts, suggesting less severe, and possibly more vasoresponsive, disease. Confirming previous findings by Kuo et al. *(98)*, there were significant further improvements in PVR, MPAP, and CO with the long-term administration of epoprostenol in patients with PPHTN. Reports of worsening splenomegaly and thrombocytopenia during use of epoprostenol for PPHTN *(99)* suggest the need for caution in treating these patients. The nonspecific endothelin-receptor antagonist bosentan, although beneficial in the treatment of IPAH, carries an 8% to 10% risk of transaminitis, making its use less than ideal in patients with hepatic dysfunction *(100)*. However, two case reports document both safe and effective use of bosentan in treating PPHTN, one in a patient with progressive PPHTN after OLT, and one in a patient not considered for OLT due to advanced age *(96,101)*. In addition, a case report of the successful use of the phosphodiesterase-5 inhibitor sildenafil in the treatment of PPHTN suggests that further studies using this agent are warranted *(97)*.

Historically, PPHTN has been considered a contraindication to liver transplantation, due to excessive mortality. Subsequent studies have demonstrated minimal increased risk with mPAP < 35 mm Hg, making this a hemodynamic goal of vasodilator therapy *(102)*. Furthermore, there are reports documenting the resolution of pulmonary hypertension after OLT. Case reports of successful OLT after long-term use of epoprostenol *(103–105)* are the basis for the increasingly standard practice of using long-term epoprostenol to normalize pulmonary hemodynamics, as a bridge to OLT.

4. SARCOIDOSIS

Pulmonary hypertension (PH) occurs in up to 28% of patients with pulmonary sarcoidosis *(106)*. It appears to be more common in those with advanced disease; 50% of patients with stage III sarcoid have evidence of PH at rest, and all have elevated PAP with exercise *(106)*.

4.1. Pathogenesis

The etiology of PH associated with sarcoidosis is unclear and likely multifactorial. Initially, it was thought to result from fibrosis of the pulmonary vasculature occurring in the setting of extensive parenchymal disease; however, a growing body of literature supports a role for direct invasion of the intima and media of the pulmonary arteries with noncaseating granulomas, thereby resulting in encroachment of the vascular flow *(106,107)*. In addition to the histopathology, the favorable clinical response observed to vasodilators suggests that vasoconstriction is an important contributor to the disease process. This correlates with the observation, in some patients, that the severity of PH is worse than the extent of parenchymal disease *(106)*.

4.2. Treatment

In a number of small clinical studies, PH secondary to sarcoidosis has been responsive to vasodilators. Two studies demonstrated an acute hemodynamic response to epoprostenol in a small number of patients with PH related to sarcoidosis *(106,108)*. Preston and colleagues demonstrated an acute hemodynamic response in seven of eight patients to inhaled NO, four of six patients to epoprostenol, and two of five patients to calcium channel blockers. Long-term inhaled NO resulted in improved symptoms and hemodynamics in three patients after one year of treatment *(106)*.

5. SICKLE CELL DISEASE

Pulmonary hypertension is becoming an increasingly recognized complication of sickle cell disease (SCD), occurring in 30% to 40% of patients *(109,110)*. PH in SCD has emerged as an important cause of morbidity and mortality over the past decade with the development of life-prolonging treatments such as transfusion therapy, antibiotic prophylaxis, and hydroxyurea. The PAP observed in this population is frequently lower than that observed in patients with IPAH; often PA systolic pressures (PASP) are less than 50 mm Hg *(109)*. However, the presence of PH in SCD appears to be an independent risk factor for mortality in these patients, with two-year mortality rates approaching 50%, even with a PASP of as low as $\geq$30 mm Hg *(110)*. Additionally, evidence of pulmonary arteriopathy is found in a high percentage of autopsy studies performed on SCD patients who experience sudden cardiac death *(111)*.

5.1. Pathogenesis

The etiology of PH related to SCD is likely multifactorial. Although PH was traditionally thought to occur as a result of multiple episodes of acute chest syndrome, recent evidence supports the notion that patients with SCD experience a spectrum of vaso-occlusive processes over their lifetime and that subclinical pulmonary vaso-occlusion may play a role in the development of sickle cell chronic lung disease *(109)*. Placing these patients at particular risk for the development of PH is the occurrence of increased cytokine production, shear stress, and localized hypoxia during pulmonary vaso-occlusion, each of which has been implicated in the pathogenesis of IPAH. Additionally, the presence of PH in other hemolytic disorders, such as thalassemia, hereditary spherocytosis, and paroxysmal nocturnal hemoglobinuria, suggests a role for cell-free hemoglobin in this process *(112–114)*. One potential mechanism by which free hemoglobin can play a role in the development of PH is via its role as an NO scavenger *(115)*. Additionally, the sickle red blood cell (RBC) is a source of reactive oxygen species (ROS), such as O_2^- and hydrogen peroxide (H_2O_2) *(116)*. Upon lysis, ROS can be released into the bloodstream and react with NO to form nitrosative metabolites, thereby decreasing NO bioavailability *(116,117)* and promoting pulmonary vasoconstriction.

Autopsy studies of SCD patients have demonstrated that evidence of pulmonary arteriopathy is much more widespread than expected by clinical presentation. Of 20 SCD patients who underwent autopsies after dying from various causes in one study, all had evidence of pulmonary vascular disease. Approximately 50% of patients had evidence of the irreversible plexiform lesions within their lungs, although many had more reversible lesions of PH, such as medial hypertrophy, intimal fibroelastosis, and cellular intimal hyperplasia, present *(111)*. These data suggest that the incidence of PH in the SCD population is grossly underestimated by current antemortem clinical testing and that this represents an important area of future investigative work.

5.2. Diagnosis and Treatment

Very limited data are available regarding the diagnosis and treatment of PH secondary to SCD. Although patients with end-stage disease present similarly to those with other forms of PH with progressive dyspnea, screening echocardiograms and autopsy studies suggest that many with PH related to SCD are asymptomatic. In general, these patients are older than SCD patients without PH, with a mean age of approximately 37 years *(110)*. Although patients with hemoglobin SS disease generally have more symptomatic vaso-occlusive events and more evidence of end-organ disease, interestingly, this may not be the case for PH related to SCD, which in some studies occurs in equal frequency in those without SS disease *(108)*. A recent large-scale study evaluating 175 patients with SCD found PH by echocardiogram in approximately 33% *(109)*, confirming the results observed in the older, smaller studies. PH in this study was defined as a tricuspid regurgitant jet velocity > 2.5 m/s, corresponding to a PASP $\geq$30 mm Hg. In this study, right heart catheterization of 20 patients with PH related to SCD demonstrated mean PA pressures that are moderately elevated (approximately 36 mm Hg), but, in contrast to other forms of PH, there was a persistently high CO observed (approximately 8.6 l/min) *(109)*. It is likely that this high-output cardiac failure relates to the anemic state of these patients and possible that this accounts for the frequent lack of symptoms in these patients. Studies evaluating the treatment of PH related to SCD have been quite limited. In two small studies, containing four and eight patients, respectively, intravenous epoprostenol had acute therapeutic hemodynamic effects in approximately 75% of cases *(109)*. Treatment strategies devised to increase NO bioavailability have begun to be studied. Supplementation of L-arginine, the NO precursor, acutely reversed PH in 12 SCD patients studied by echocardiography *(118)*. A trial evaluating the use of sildenafil for treatment of PH in SCD is underway. As the median survival of patients who have RHC evidence of PH was 25.6 months, it appears to be essential that larger-scale trials of vasodilators, such as epoprostenol and sildenafil, be conducted in this population.

6. CONCLUSIONS

HIV, portopulmonary hypertension, sarcoidosis, and sickle cell disease (SCD) are all associated with PH. Although specific histological features of the pulmonary vasculature may differ among the various entities, they share a number of similarities. The PH manifests itself in a minority of these patients, consistent with the idea that gene mutations may predispose certain individuals to developing PH, probably in combination with other factors. Multiple factors seem to contribute, including endothelial dysfunction, vasodilator/vasoconstrictor mediator imbalance, immunologic and oxidant mechanisms, and structural abnormalities of the vasculature related to injected foreign material (mainly in HIV and some SCD patients) and to parenchymal destruction (particularly in sarcoidosis and SCD). In addition, some entities, such as portopulmonary hypertension and SCD, are characterized by relatively high cardiac outputs that may predispose to PH by means of increased shear stress. Patients with SCD not uncommonly have a component of pulmonary venous hypertension related to LV diastolic dysfunction, underscoring the need to perform right heart catheterizations to properly diagnose patients. The PAH in these entities is also often responsive to a variety of medical therapies, although this inference is based mainly on case reports and small cohort studies and not on properly designed randomized trials.

REFERENCES

1. Rubin LJ. Primary pulmonary hypertension. N Engl J Med 1997; 336: 111–7.
2. Rich S. Primary pulmonary hypertension. Executive summary from the world symposium World Health Organization 1998.
3. Kim KK, Factor SM. Membranoproliferative glomerulonephritis and plexogenic pulmonary arteriopathy in a homosexual man with acquired immunodeficiency syndrome. Hum Pathol 1987; 18:1293–6.
4. Speich R, Jenni R, Opravil M, Pfab M, Russi EW. Primary pulmonary hypertension in HIV infection. Chest 1991; 100(1268):1271.
5. Pellicelli AM, Palmieri F, Cicalini S, Petrosillo N. Pathogenesis of HIV-related pulmonary hypertension. Ann NY Acad Sci 2001; 946:82–94.
6. Cool CD, Kennedy D, Voelkel NF, Tuder RM. Pathogenesis and evolution of plexiform lesions in pulmonary hypertension associated with scleroderma and human immunodeficiency virus infection. Hum Pathol 1997; 28:434–42.
7. Mehta NJ, Khan IA, Mehta RN, Sepkowitz DA. HIV-related pulmonary hypertension: Analytic review of 131 cases. Chest 2000; 118:1133–41.
8. Petrosillo N, Pellicelli AM, Boumis E, Ippolito G. Clinical manifestations of HIV-related pulmonary hypertension. Ann NY Acad Sci 2001; 946:223–35.
9. Pellicelli AM, Palmieri F, D'Ambrosio CD, Riando A, et al. Role of human immunodeficiency virus in primary pulmonary hypertension. Angiology 1998; 49:1005–11.

10. Mesa RA, Edell ES, Dunn WF, Edwards WD. Human immunodeficiency virus infection and pulmonary hypertension: Two new cases and a review of 86 reported cases. Mayo Clin Proc 1998; 73:37–45.

11. D'Alonzo GE, Barst RJ, Ayres SM, Bergofsky EH, et al. Survival in patients with primary pulmonary hypertension. Ann Intern Med 1991; 115:343–9.

12. Tuder RM, Cool CD, Geraci MW, Wang J, et al. Prostacyclin synthase expression is decreased in lungs from patients with severe pulmonary hypertension. Am J Respir Crit Care Med 1999; 159:1925–32.

13. Tuder RM, Broves BM, Badesch DB, Voelkel NF. Exuberant endothelial cell growth and elements of inflammation are present in plexiform lesions of pulmonary hypertension. Am J Pathol 1994; 144:275–85.

14. Chalifoux LV, Simon MA, Pauley DR, Mackey JJ, et.al. Arteriopathy in macaques infected with simian immunodeficiency virus. Lab Invest 1992; 67:338–49.

15. Mette SA, Palevsky HI, Pietra GG, et.al. Primary pulmonary hypertension in association with human immunodeficiency virus infection. Am Rev Respir Dis 1992; 145:1196–2000.

16. Humbert M, Monit G, Brenot F, et al. Increased interleukin-1 and interleukin-6 serum concentrations in severe primary pulmonary hypertension. Am J Respir Crit Care Med 1995; 151:1629–31.

17. Lesprit P, Godeau B, Authier FJ, Soubrier M, et al. Pulmonary hypertension in POEMS syndrome: A new feature mediated by cytokines. Am J Respir Crit Care Med 1998; 157:907–11.

18. Carlos TM, Schwartz BR, Kovach NL, Yee E, et al. Vascular cell adhesion molecule-1 mediates lymphocyte adherence to cytokine-activated cultured human endothelial cells. Blood 1990; 76:965–70.

19. Chen YH, Lin SJ, Ku HH, Shiao MS, et al. Salvianolic acid B attenuates VCAM-1 and ICAM-1 expression in TNF-α treated human aortic endothelial cells. J Cell Biochem 2001; 82:512–21.

20. Caldwell RL, Egan BS, Shepherd VL. HIV-1 Tat represses transcription from the mannose receptor promoter. J Immunol 2000; 165:7035–41.

21. Caldwell RL, Gaddipadi R, Shepherd V, Lane K. Pulmonary hypertension in HIV-infected individuals may involve transcriptional regulation of BMPRII. Am J Respir Crit Care Med 2002; 165:A636.

22. Deng Z, Morse JH, Slager SL, et al. Familial primary pulmonary hypertension (gene PPH1) is caused by mutations in the bone morphogenetic protein receptor-II gene. Am J Hum Genet 2000; 67:737–44.

23. MacLean MR. Endothelin-1 and serotonin: Mediators of primary and secondary pulmonary hypertension? J Lab Clin Med 1999; 134:105–14.

24. Stewart DJ, Levy RD, Cernacek P, Langleben D. Increased plasma endothelin-1 in pulmonary hypertension: Marker or mediator of disease. Ann Intern Med 1991; 114:464–9.

25. Yoshibayashi M, Nishioka K, Nakao K, Saito Y, et al. Plasma endothelin concentrations in patients with primary pulmonary hypertension associated with congenital heart defects: Evidence for increased

production of endothelin in pulmonary circulation. Circulation 1991; 84:2280–5.

26. Cody RJ, Haas GJ, Binkley PF, Capers Q, Kelley R. Plasma endothelin correlates with the extent of pulmonary hypertension in patients with chronic congestive heart failure. Circulation 1992; 85:504–9.

27. Giaid A, Yanagisawa M, Langleben D, Michel RP, et al. Expression of endothelin-1 in the lungs of patients with pulmonary hypertension. N Engl J Med 1993; 328:1732–9.

28. Ehrenreich H, Rieckmann P, Sinowatz F, et al. Potent stimulation of monocytic endothelin-1 production by HIV-1 glycoprotein 120. J Immunol 1993; 150:4601–9.

29. Stamler JS, Singel DJ, Loscalzo J. Biochemistry of nitric oxide and its redox-activated forms. Science 1992; 258:1898–902.

30. Arnal JF, Dinh-Xuan AT, Pueyo M, et al. Endothelium-derived nitric oxide and vascular physiology and pathology. Cell Mol Life Sci 1999; 55:1078–87.

31. Wanstall JC, Hughes IE, O'Donnell SR. Evidence that nitric oxide from the endothelium attenuates inherent tone in isolated pulmonary arteries from rats with hypoxic pulmonary hypertension. Br J Pharm 1995; 114:109–14.

32. Adnot S, Raffestin B, Eddahibi S, et al. Loss of endothelial-dependent relaxant activity in the pulmonary circulation of rats exposed to chronic hypoxia. J Clin Invest 1991; 87:155–62.

33. Warren JB, Maltby NH, McCormack D, Parnes PJ. Pulmonary endothelium-derived relaxing factor is impaired in hypoxia. Clin Sci 1989; 77:671–6.

34. Fagan KA, Tyler RC, Sato K, et al. Relative contributions of endothelial, inducible and neuronal NOS to tone in the murine pulmonary circulation. Am J Physiol 1999; 277:L472–L478.

35. Fagan KA, Fouty BW, Tyler RC, et al. The pulmonary circulation of homozygous or heterozygous eNOS-null mice is hyperresponsive to mild hypoxia. J Clin Invest 1999; 103:291–9.

36. Voelkel NF, Tuder RM. Cellular and molecular mechanisms in the pathogenesis of severe pulmonary hypertension. Eur Respir J 1995; 8: 2129–38.

37. Sitbon O, Brenot F, Denjean A, et al. Inhaled nitric oxide as a screening agent in primary pulmonary hypertension. Am J Respir Crit Care Med 1995; 151:384–9.

38. Wedgwood S, McMullen DM, Bekker JM, Fineman JR, Black SM. Role for endothelin-1-induced superoxide and peroxynitrite production in rebound pulmonary hypertension associated with inhaled nitric oxide therapy. Circ Res 2001; 89:357–64.

39. Lal H, Woodward B, Williams KI. Investigations of the contributions of nitric oxide and prostaglandins to the actions of endothelins and sarafotoxin 6c in rat isolated perfused lungs. Br J Pharmacol 1996; 118: 1931–8.

40. Alhenc-Gelas F, Tsai SJ, Callahan KS, Campbell WB, Johnson AR. Stimulation of prostaglandin formation by vasoactive mediators in cultured human endothelial cells. Prostaglandins 1982; 24:723–42.
41. Smith DL, Dewitt DL, Allen ML. Bimodal distribution of the prostaglandin I2 synthase antigen in smooth muscle cells. J Biol Chem 1993; 258:5922–6.
42. Gerber JG, Voelkel NF, Nies AS, McMurtry IF, Reeves JT. Moderation of hypoxic vasoconstriction by infused arachidonic acid: Role of PGI_2. J Appl Physiol 1980; 49:107–12.
43. Owen NE. Prostacyclin can inhibit DNA synthesis in vascular smooth muscle cells. In JM Bailey, ed. Prostaglandins, Leukotrienes and Lipoxins. New York: Plenum Press, 2004.
44. Rubin LJ, Mendoza J, Hood M, et al. Treatment of primary pulmonary hypertension with continuous intravenous prostacyclin (epoprostenol): Results of a randomized trial. Ann Intern Med 1990; 112:485–91.
45. Barst RJ, Rubin LJ, McGoon MD, Caldwell EJ, Long WA, Levy PS. Survival in primary pulmonary hypertension with long-term continuous intravenous prostacyclin. Ann Intern Med 1994; 121:409–15.
46. McLaughlin VV, Genthner DE, Panella MM, Rich S. Reduction in pulmonary vascular resistance with long-term epoprostenol (prostacylin) therapy in primary pulmonary hypertension. N Engl J Med 1998; 338:273–7.
47. Aguilar RV, Farber HW. Long-term epoprostenol (prostacyclin) therapy in HIV-associated pulmonary hypertension. Am J Respir Crit Care Med 2000; 162:1846–50.
48. Opravil M, Pechere M, Speich R, et al. HIV-associated primary pulmonary hypertension: A case control study. Am J Respir Crit Care Med 1997; 155:990–5.
49. Morse JH, Barst RJ, Itescu S, Flaster ER, et al. Primary pulmonary hypertension in HIV infection: An outcome determined by particular HLA Class II alleles. Am J Respir Crit Care Med 1996; 153:1299–301.
50. Tomashefski JF, Hirsch CS. The pulmonary vascular lesions of intravenous drug abuse. Hum Pathol 1980; 11:133–45.
51. Kendra KP, Farber HW. Foreign body granulomatosis. In S Weinberger, ed. UPTODATE, Pulmonary and Critical Care Medicine, 2004.
52. Guillemin K, Krasnow MA. The hypoxic response: Huffing or HIFing. Cell 1997; 89:9–12.
53. Escamilla R, et al. Pulmonary veno-occlusive disease in an HIV-infected intravenous drug abuser. Eur Respir J 1995; 8:1982–4.
54. Yu SM, et al. Mechanism of catecholamine-induced proliferation of smooth muscle cells. Circulation 1996; 94:547–54.
55. Chen LQ, et al. Regulation of vascular smooth muscle growth by α-1-adrenoreceptor subtypes *in vitro* and *in situ*. J Biol Chem 1995; 270:30980–8.
56. deBlois D, et al. Chronic α-1-adrenoreceptor stimulation increases DNA synthesis in rat arterial wall: Modulation of responsiveness after vascular injury. Arterioscler Thromb Vasc Biol 1996; 16:1122–9.

57. Kimura H, Esumi H. Reciprocal regulation between nitric oxide and vascular endothelial growth factor in angiogenesis. Acta Biochimica Polonica 2003; 50(1):49–59.
58. Diaz PT, et al. Increased susceptibility to pulmonary emphysema among HIV-seropositive smokers. Ann Intern Med 2000; 132:369–72.
59. Speich R, Jenni R, Opravil M, Jaccard R. Regression of HIV-associated pulmonary arterial hypertension and long-term survival during antiretroviral therapy. Swiss Med Wkly 2001; 131:663–5.
60. Zuber JP, Calmy A, Evison JM, Hasse B, Schiffer V, Wagels T, et al. Pulmonary arterial hypertension related to HIV infection: Improved hemodynamics and survival associated with antiretroviral therapy. Clin Infect Dis 4 A.D. 2004; 38:1178–85.
61. Nunes H, Humber M, Sitbon O, Morse JH, Deng Z, Knowles JA, et al. Prognostic factors for survival in human immuodeficiency virus-associated pulmonary arterial hypertension. Am J Respir Crit Care Med 2003; 167:1433–9.
62. Ghofrani HA, Friese G, Discher T, Olschewski H, Schermuly RT, Weissmann N, et al. Inhaled iloprost is a potent acute pulmonary vasodilator in HIV-related severe pulmonary hypertension. Eur Respir J 2004; 23(2):321–6.
63. Stricker H, Domenighetti G, Mombelli G. Prostacyclin for HIV-associated pulmonary hypertension. Ann Intern Med 1997; 127(11):1043.
64. Cea-Calvo L. Treatment of HIV-associated pulmonary hypertension with trepostinil. Rev Esp Cardiol 2003; 56(4):421–5.
65. Sitbon O, Gressin V, Speich R, Macdonald PS, Opravil M, Cooper DA, et al. Bosentan for human immunodeficiency virus-associated pulmonary arterial hypertension. Am J Respir Crit Care Med 2004; 170(11): 1212–1217.
66. Carlsen J, Kjeldsen K, Gerstoft J. Sildenafil as a successful treatment of otherwise fatal HIV-related pulmonary hypertension. AIDS 2002; 16(11):1568–9.
67. Schumacher YO, Zdebik A, Huonker M, Kreisel W. Sildenafil in HIV-related pulmonary hypertension. AIDS 2001; 15(13):1747–8.
68. Mantz FA, Craige E. Portal axis thrombosis with spontaneous portacaval shun and resultant cor pulmonale. Arch Pathol 1951; 52:91–7.
69. McDonnell PJ, Toye PA, Hutchins GM. Primary pulmonary hypertension and cirrhosis: Are they related? Am Rev Respir Dis 1983; 127:437–41.
70. Hadengue A, Benhayoun MK, Lebrec D. Pulmonary hypertension complicating portal hypertension: Prevalence and relation to splanchnic hemodynamics. Gastroenterology 1991; 100:520–8.
71. Yang YY, Lin HC, Lee WC. Portopulmonary hypertension: Distinctive hemodynamic and clinical manifestations. J Gastroenterol 2001; 36: 181–6.
72. Donovan CL, Marcovitz PA, Punch JD. Two-dimensional, and dobutamine stress echocardiography in the pre-operative assessment of

patients with end-stage liver disease prior to orthotopic liver transplantation. Transplantation 1996; 61:1180–8.

73. Benjaminov FS, Prentice M, Sniderman KW, Siu S, Liu P, Wong F. Portopulmonary hypertension in decompensated cirrhosis with refractory ascites. Gut 2003; 52:1355–62.

74. Auletta M, Oliviero U, Iasiuolo L. Pulmonary hypertension associated with liver cirrhosis: An echocardiographic study. Angiology 2000; 51:1013–20.

75. Budhiraja R, Hassoun PM. Portopulmonary hypertension. A tale of two circulations. Chest 2003; 123(2):562–76.

76. Molden D, Abraham JL. Pulmonary hypertension: Its association with hepatic cirrhosis and iron accumulation. Arch Pathol Lab Med 1982; 106:328–31.

77. Tasaka S, Kanazawa M, Nakamura H, et al. An autopsied case of primary pulmonary hypertension complicated by hepatopulmonary syndrome [in Japanese]. Nihon Kyobu Shikkan Gakkai Zasshi 1995; 33:90–4.

78. Robalino BD, Moodie DS. Association between primary pulmonary hypertension and portal hypertension: Analysis of its pathophysiology and clinical, laboratory and hemodynamic manifestations. J Am Coll Cardiol 1991; 17(2):492–8.

79. Goenka MK, Mehta SK, Malik AK, et al. Fatal pulmonary arterial hypertension complicating noncirrhotic portal fibrosis. Am J Gastroenterol 1992; 87:1203–5.

80. Tokiwa K, Iwai N, Nakamura K, et al. Pulmonary hypertension as a fatal complication of extrahepatic portal hypertension. Eur J Pediatr Surg 1993; 3:373–5.

81. Woolf D, Voigt MD, Jaskiewickz K, et al. Pulmonary hypertension associated with non-cirrhotic portal hypertension in systemic lupus erythematosus. Postgrad Med J 1994; 70:41–3.

82. Cohen MD, Rubin LJ, Taylor WE, et al. Primary pulmonary hypertension: An unusual case associated with extrahepatic portal hypertension. Hepatology 1993; 3:588–92.

83. Bernthal AC, Eybel Ce, Payne JA. Primary pulmonary hypertension after portocaval shunt. J Clin Gastroenterol 1997; 5:353–6.

84. Kibria G, Smith P, Heath D, et al. Observations on the rare association between portal and pulmonary hypertension. Thorax 1980; 35:945–9.

85. Hiyama E. Pulmonary vascular changes after portasystemic shunt operation in rats [in Japanese]. Nippon Geka Gakkai Zasshi 1989; 90: 874–85.

86. Kuo PC, Schroeder RA, Vagelos RH, Valantine H, Garcia G, Alfrey EJ, et al. Volume-mediated pulmonary responses in liver transplant candidates. Clin Transplant 1996; 10(1):521–7.

87. Krowka MJ, Frantz RP, McGoon MD, Severson C, Plevak DJ, Wiesner RH. Improvement in pulmonary hemodynamics during intravenous epoprostenol (prostacyclin): A study of 15 patients with moderate to severe portopulmonary hypertension. Hepatology 1999; 30:641–8.

88. Shah V, Toruner M, Haddad F, Cadelina G, Papapetropoulos A, Choo K, et al. Imparied endothelial nitric oxide synthase activity associated with enhanced caveolin binding in experimental cirrhosis in the rat. Gastroenterology 1999; 117(5):1222–8.

89. Schroeder RA, Ewing CA, Sitzmann JV, Kuo PC. Pulmonary expression of iNOS and HO-1 protein is upregulated in a rat model of prehepatic portal hypertension. Dig Dis Sci 2000; 45(12):2405–10.

90. Laffi G, Marra F, Gresele P, Romagnoli P, Palermo A, Bartolini O, et al. Evidence for a storage pool defect in platelets from cirrhotic patients with defective aggregation. Gastroenterology 1992; 103(2):641–6.

91. Colle IO, Moreau R, Godinho E, Belghiti J, Ettori F, Cohen-Solal A, et al. Diagnosis of portopulmonary hypertension in candidates for liver transplantation: A prospective study. Hepatology 2003; 37(2):401–9.

92. Findlay JY, Harrison BA, Plevak DJ, et al. Inhaled nitric oxide reduces pulmonary artery pressures in portopulmonary hypertension. Liver Transpl Surg 1999; 5:381–7.

93. Buchhorn R, Hulpke-Wette M, Wessel A, et al. β-Blocker therapy in an infant with pulmonary hypertension. Eur J Pediatr 1999; 158:1007–8.

94. Boot H, Visser FC, Thijs JC, et al. Pulmonary hypertension complicating portal hypertension: A case report with suggestions for a different therapeutic approach. Eur Heart J 1987; 8:656–60.

95. Ribas J, Angrill J, Barbera JA, et al. Isosorbide-5-mononitrate in the treatment of pulmonary hypertension associated with portal hypertension. Eur Respir J 1999; 13:210–2.

96. Clift PF, Bramhall S, Isaac JL. Successful treatment of severe portopulmonary hypertension after liver transplantation by bosentan. Transplantation 2004; 77(11):1774–5.

97. Makisalo H, Koivusalo A, Vakkuri A, Hockerstedt K. Sildenafil for portopulmonary hypertension in a patient undergoing liver transplantation. Liver Transpl 2004; 10(7):945–50.

98. Kuo PC, Johnson LB, Plotkin JS, et al. Continuous intravenous infusion of epoprostenol for the treatment of portopulmonary hypertension. Transplantation 1997; 63:604–6.

99. Findlay JY, Plevak DJ, Krowka MJ, et al. Progressive splenomegaly after epoprostenol therapy in portopulmonary hypertension. Liver Transpl Surg 1999; 5:362–5.

100. Rubin LJ, Badesch DB, Barst RJ, Nazzareno G, Black CM, Keogh A, et al. Bosentan therapy for pulmonary arterial hypertension. N Engl J Med 2002; 346(12):896–903.

101. Halank M, Miehlke S, Hoeffken G, Schmeisser A, Schulze M, Strasser RH. Use of oral endothelin-receptor antagonist bosentan in the treatment of portopulmonary hypertension. Transplantation 2004; 77(11):1775–6.

102. Krowka MJ, Plevak DJ, Findlay JY, Rosen CB, Wiesner RH, Krom RA. Pulmonary hemodynamics and perioperative cardiopulmonary-related mortality in patients with portopulmonary hypertension undergoing liver transplantation. Liver Transpl 2000; 6(4):443–50.

103. Krowka MJ. Hepatopulmonary syndrome versus portopulmonary hypertension: Distinctions and dilemmas. Hepatology 1997; 25(5):1282–4.

104. Plotkin JS, Kuo PC, Rubin LJ, Gaine S, Howell CD, Laurin J, et al. Successful use of chronic epoprostenol as a bridge to liver transplantation in severe portopulmonary hypertension. Transplantation 1998; 65(4): 457–9.

105. Kuo PC, Plotkin JS, Gaine S, Schroeder RA, Rustgi VK, Rubin LJ, et al. Portopulmonary hypertension and the liver transplant candidate. Transplantation 1999; 67(8):1087–93.

106. Preston IR, Klinger JR, Landzberg MJ, Houtchens J, Nelson D, Hill NS. Vasoresponsiveness of sarcoidosis-associated pulmonary hypertension. Chest 2001; 120:866–72.

107. Smith LJ, Lawrence JB, Katzenstein AA. Vascular sarcoidosis: A rare cause of pulmonary hypertension. Am J Med Sci 1983; 285:38–44.

108. Jones K, Higenbottam T, Wallwork J. Pulmonary vasodilation with prostacyclin in primary and secondary pulmonary hypertension. Chest 1989; 96:784–9.

109. Gladwin MT, Sachdev V, Jison ML, et al. Pulmonary hypertension as a risk factor for death in patients with sickle cell disease. N Engl J Med 2004; 350:880–6.

110. Castro O, Hoque M, Brown BD. Pulmonary hypertension in sickle cell disease: Cardiac catheterization results and survival. Blood 2003; 101:1257–61.

111. Haque AK, Gokhale S, Rampy BA, Adegboyega P, Duarte A, Saldana MJ. Pulmonary hypertension in sickle cell hemoglobinopathy: A clinicopathologic study of 20 cases. Hum Pathol 2002; 33:1037–43.

112. Aessopos A, Farmakis D, Karagiorga M, et al. Cardiac involvement in thalassemia intermedia: A multicenter study. Blood 2001; 97:3411–6.

113. Hayag-Barin JE, Smith RE, Tucker FC. Hereditary spherocytosis, thrombocytosis, and chronic pulmonary emboli: A case report and review of the literature. Am J Hematol 1998; 57:82–4.

114. Heller PG, Grinberg AR, Lencioni M, Molina MM, Roncoroni AJ. Pulmonary hypertension in paroxysmal nocturnal hemoglobinuria. Chest 1992; 102:642–3.

115. Reiter CD, Wang X, Tanus-Santos JE, Hogg N, Cannon RO, Schechter AN, et al. Cell-free hemoglobin limits nitric oxide bioavailability in sickle cell disease. Nat Med 2002; 8:1383–9.

116. Hebbel RP, Eaton JW, Balasingam M, Steinberg MH. Spontaneous oxygen radical generation by sickle erythrocytes. J Clin Invest 1982; 70:1253–9.

117. Schachter L, Warth JA, Gordon EM, et al. Altered amount and activity of superoxide dismutase in sickle cell disease. FASEB J 1988; 2:237–43.

118. Claudia-Morris CR, Morris SM, Hagar W, van Warmerdam J, Claster S, et al. Arginine therapy: A new treatment for pulmonary hypertension in sickle cell disease. Am J Respir Crit Care Med 2003; 168:63–9.

10 Chronic Thromboembolic Pulmonary Hypertension

Victor J. Test, William R. Auger, and Peter F. Fedullo

Contents

Introduction
Pathogenesis
Clinical Presentation and History
Physical Examination
Diagnostic Evaluation
Surgical Selection
Surgical Approach
Postoperative Course
Surgical Outcome
Long-Term Outcome
Medical Therapy
Lung Transplantation
Summary
References

Abstract

Chronic thromboembolic pulmonary hypertension (CTEPH) is an important form of pulmonary hypertension to detect because prompt treatment can lead to a surgical cure. The true incidence is unknown, but it is estimated to occur in 1% to 3% of patients following acute thromboembolism. Detection may be difficult, because symptoms are nonspecific and other diagnoses are often made before that of CTEPH is entertained. Routinely screening all pulmonary hypertension

From: *Contemporary Cardiology: Pulmonary Hypertension*
Edited by: N. S. Hill and H. W. Farber © Humana Press, Totowa, NJ

patients with a ventilation–perfusion scan will detect most, however. Candidates for thromboendarterectomy are evaluated using right heart catheterization, computerized tomographic angiography, and pulmonary angiography, seeking those with proximal obstructions that can be removed surgically. Patients who are not candidates for thromboendarterectomy because of comorbidities, very high pulmonary vascular resistances. or mainly distal disease may still receive medical therapy or be considered for lung transplantation.

Key Words: chronic thromboembolic pulmonary hypertension; thromboendarterectomy; lung transplantation; thromboembolism; pulmonary angiography; pulmonary angioscopy.

1. INTRODUCTION

Chronic thromboembolic pulmonary hypertension (CTEPH) represents a unique cause of secondary pulmonary hypertension by virtue of its potentially remedial nature. Therefore, it is imperative to identify patients with this disorder. Unlike most other variants of pulmonary hypertension in which modest improvements in functional status and clinical stability are the usual achievable therapeutic endpoints, thromboembolic pulmonary hypertension is potentially curable.

The first surgical procedure for CTEPH was performed in 1958 *(1,2)*. Over the next 26 years, only 85 patients who had undergone thromboendarterectomy were reported in the medical literature, with a mortality of 22% *(3)*. Since 1985, the number of pulmonary thromboendarterectomies has increased dramatically, the majority (over 2,000) having been performed at the University of California at San Diego. Other centers have begun to perform the procedure, including those in Canada, Great Britain, France, Austria, Germany, Italy, Australia, and the Netherlands. The overall surgical mortality has declined to the range of 4% to 8% as established programs have enhanced their skills with the preoperative assessment, surgical management, and perioperative care of patients suffering from this disease *(4–6)*. As is the case with other highly complex surgical procedures requiring a multidisciplinary approach, mortality seems to be related to the surgical volume *(7–9)*.

Our understanding of the epidemiology of CTEPH is evolving. Based on the number of patients referred for thromboendarterectomy, it was originally thought that 0.1% to 1% of patients who suffered from pulmonary embolism would subsequently develop pulmonary hypertension *(7)*. However, more recent data suggest that 0.8% to as many as 3.1% of patients may develop CTEPH after an initial episode of pulmonary embolism *(10,91)*, with an even higher occurrence after recurrent thromboembolic events *(10)*. Considering that an estimated 300,000 to 400,000 acute pulmonary embolic events occur annually in the United States and that the number of annual pulmonary thromboendarterectomies approximates only 300 *(11)*, the disease is either less common than the estimated figures or is underrecognized and thereby not treated.

2. PATHOGENESIS

Although the mechanisms by which patients develop CTEPH are not fully understood, incomplete resolution of pulmonary emboli rather than *in situ* thrombosis of the pulmonary arteries appears to be the major contributor *(12,13)*. Acute pulmonary embolism in patients without preexisting cardiopulmonary disease results in pulmonary hypertension when at least 30% of the pulmonary vascular bed is obstructed *(14)*. In the setting of preexisting cardiopulmonary disease, the degree of obstruction necessary to cause pulmonary hypertension is less *(14)*. In patients without preexisting cardiopulmonary disease, the relationship between pulmonary artery systolic pressure and the degree of pulmonary vascular obstruction is relatively linear to a maximal pulmonary artery systolic pressure of approximately 60 to 70 mm Hg. Beyond 70% obstruction of the pulmonary vascular bed, the normal right ventricle is incapable of compensation and right ventricular failure ensues.

Approximately 50% of patients presenting with acute symptomatic pulmonary embolism have echocardiographic evidence of right ventricular dysfunction *(26)*. Afterwards, echocardiographic and pulmonary perfusion scan abnormalities typically stabilize over four to six weeks *(15,16)*. However, normalization of perfusion scan defects occurs in less than 50% of patients when evaluated six months after the acute event *(23)*. Persistence of echocardiographic abnormalities at four to six weeks predicts persistent echocardiographic abnormalities at one year and identifies those at risk of developing chronic thomboembolic pulmonary hypertension *(16)*. In one prospective study of 78 patients with an estimated systolic pulmonary artery pressure by echocardiogram of greater than 56 mm Hg at the initial diagnosis of pulmonary embolism, echocardiogram abnormalities persisted at one year in 5.1% (4 of 78 patients) *(17,94)*.

2.1. Pathophysiology

The explanation for failure of clot lysis in patients with CTEPH and subsequent incorporation of thromboembolic material into the arterial wall remains elusive. No abnormalities of the fibrinolytic system of such patients have been reported, although some patients with the disease may have fibrinogen that resists thrombolysis *(18)*. A patient with CTEPH was reported in whom the fibrinogen gamma chains were abnormally sialylated *(28)*.

In addition to proximal vessel obstruction, patients with CTEPH often have distal vascular changes suggestive of those that occur in idiopathic pulmonary hypertension *(22)*. This has been hypothesized to represent a secondary pulmonary vasculopathy caused by the high pulmonary arterial pressures and sheer stress *(22)*. Other etiologies for these secondary changes have also been sought. Mutations of the bone morphogenetic protein receptor type 2 (*BMPR2*) gene have been associated with the development of idiopathic and familial pulmonary arterial hypertension but have not been found in patients with chronic thromboembolic pulmonary hypertension *(19–21)*. As has been reported with other forms of pulmonary hypertension though, angiopoetin-1 and endothelin-1 are upregulated in CTEPH *(22,23)*.

The concept of dual compartment pulmonary vascular involvement by CTEPH, with one compartment consisting of proximal large vessel obstruction and the other of distal small vessel obliteration, was suggested by Moser and Braunwald in 1973 based on the finding of microvascular obliteration in lung biopsies from pulmonary thromboendarterectomy patients *(22,25,26)*. Progressive small vessel disease may explain the worsening of hemodynamics and symptoms that is seen occasionally despite a lack of radiologically discernable progression in large vessels *(26)*. The proportion of large vessel obstruction versus small vessel obliteration is crucial to the hemodynamic consequences of the disease and the response to surgical therapy *(4)*. The greater the contribution of small vessel arteriopathy to the increased pulmonary vascular resistance, the higher the potential morbidity and mortality of surgical intervention and the lower the possibility of hemodynamic benefit *(4)*. The utility of partitioning of the pulmonary vascular resistance to predict response to pulmonary thromboendarterectomy has reinforced the concept *(27)*. Occasionally, *in situ* thrombosis of dilated central pulmonary arteries has been described in idiopathic pulmonary hypertension. These can be difficult to differentiate from the central thromboemboli of CTEPH, but in contrast to those of CTEPH, they are generally of little hemodynamic significance, so partitioning techniques can be helpful in making the distinction.

2.2. Risk Factors

The incidence of CTEPH in patients with a prior history of pulmonary embolism has been reported to be in the range of 0.1% to 3.1% *(7,10)*. The incidence in patients with a history of multiple thromboembolic events may be as high as 13.4% *(10)*. In the study by Pengo et al. *(17)*, risk factors for the development of CTEPH included younger age, larger perfusion defects, idiopathic pulmonary embolism, and multiple embolic episodes. In addition, patients with anatomically massive pulmonary embolism may be at higher risk for the development of CTEPH. In a study where massive pulmonary embolism was defined as a greater than 50% obstruction of the pulmonary vascular bed, the incidence of CTEPH was 20.2% despite the use of thrombolytic agents *(29)*.

The antiphospholipid antibody syndrome is the most common hypercoagulable state associated with CTEPH, occurring in up to 20% of patients *(30–32)*. The frequencies of factor V Leiden, protein S or C deficiency, and prothrombin 20210 mutation have not been found to be more common in CTEPH than in the general population *(30,31)*. Increased levels (41% of 122 patients with CTEPH) of factor VIII have been reported in one small study, while hyperhomocysteinemia (50% of 14 patients with CTEPH) was reported in another *(31,32)*. These findings will need to be confirmed in a larger series. Lastly, CTEPH has been associated with myeloproliferative syndromes as well as chronic inflammatory states, chronic ventriculoatrial shunts, splenectomy, and chronic indwelling central venous lines *(24)*.

3. CLINICAL PRESENTATION AND HISTORY

The symptoms of CTEPH are very similar to those of idiopathic pulmonary arterial hypertension and are often present for months to years prior to diagnosis. The most common initial symptom is dyspnea on exertion that typically worsens over time. Often, patients and physicians attribute the symptoms to other common problems such as deconditioning, asthma, obesity, underlying lung disease, or cigarette smoking before the true diagnosis is established. Delay in diagnosis also occurs because the symptoms are often insidious in onset and the physical examination findings are subtle. Patients with a more active lifestyle usually recognize the symptoms earlier in the course of the disease than do more sedentary patients. As the symptoms progress, the patients may complain of exertional presyncope, palpitations, cough, hemoptysis, or dyspnea with bending over. Chest pain may be a harbinger of right ventricular ischemia. Syncope is an alarming symptom that raises concern for advanced heart failure and should prompt an urgent evaluation.

A history of previous deep venous thrombosis or pulmonary embolism may be elusive in these patients. In one series, 63% of patients had no specific history of acute venous thromboembolism *(33)*. On careful questioning though, many patients may recall a history of phlebitis, hemoptysis, pleurisy, or pneumonia that may have represented an undiagnosed thromboembolic event. In addition, CTEPH may present months or years after an acute episode of venous thromboembolism.

4. PHYSICAL EXAMINATION

Physical findings vary depending on the severity and duration of the pulmonary hypertension. Early in the course of the disease, narrowing of the aortic and pulmonic components of the second heart sound occurs with accentuation of the pulmonic component. These findings may be difficult to appreciate in obese patients or those with COPD. As the pulmonary hypertension worsens and the right heart compensates by enlarging and hypertrophying, the classic findings of pulmonary hypertension become more evident. These include widened or fixed splitting of the second heart sound, a left parasternal impulse or lift where the enlarged right heart taps against the chest wall, and the systolic murmur of tricuspid regurgitation along the left and right sternal borders. Evidence of right heart failure includes neck vein distention, a right-sided S3 or S4, jugular venous distention, hepatojugular reflux, ascites, hepatomegaly, or lower extremity edema. Approximately 30% of patients with CTEPH have a pulmonary flow murmur *(34)*, caused by turbulent flow across the partially obstructed pulmonary arteries that produces a bruit best heard over the posterior lung fields during an inspiratory hold maneuver. These bruits have been described in other conditions that result in focal narrowing of the pulmonary arteries such as arteritis and pulmonary artery sarcoma but are not typically heard in idiopathic PAH.

5. DIAGNOSTIC EVALUATION

5.1. Laboratory Studies

The complete blood count and blood chemistries are usually unrevealing in patients with CTEPH. The transaminases, alkaline phosphatase, and bilirubin may be elevated in the setting of passive liver congestion. Thrombocytopenia should raise the possibilities of heparin-induced thrombocytopenia or the antiphospholipid antibody syndrome. A prolonged activated partial thromboplastin time (aPTT) should suggest the possibility of a lupus anticoagulant or anticardiolipin antibody. Brain natriuretic peptide (BNP) may be elevated and correlates with the level of the right atrial pressure, pulmonary hypertension, and reduction in cardiac output *(35)*. Hyperuricemia is a marker of severe pulmonary hypertension and a worse prognosis *(36)*.

5.2. Pulmonary Function Testing

Pulmonary function should be tested to seek other confounding disorders such as emphysema or interstitial lung disease. Twenty percent of patients with CTEPH will have mild to moderate restrictive spirometric defects associated with parenchymal scarring thought to be the result of prior infarcts *(37)*. The diffusion capacity is usually decreased, but if it is severely reduced, additional diagnoses should be considered such as pulmonary veno-occlusive disease or parenchymal lung disease *(38)*. A normal diffusion capacity does not exclude the diagnosis of CTEPH, nor does the diffusion abnormality usually normalize after thromboendarterectomy *(40)*. Typically, the alveolar-arterial gradient and dead space ventilation are increased because of V/Q mismatching, and oxygen saturation drops with exercise because of diffusion limitation and a diminished ability to raise cardiac output, leading to a decrease in mixed venous oxygen saturation *(39)*.

5.3. Echocardiography

Echocardiographic findings that are common in CTEPH include right ventricular hypertrophy, right atrial and right ventricular enlargement, and increased tricuspid regurgitation *(41,42)*. The echocardiogram may also demonstrate a pericardial effusion, flattening of the ventricular septum, or a paradoxical shift of the ventricular septum that suggests more advanced right heart failure. Contrast echocardiography is useful in detecting the presence of an intracardiac shunt. Rarely, the echocardiogram may detect evidence of an intracardiac or intravascular clot, but this is more common in acute thromboembolic disease. A normal echocardiogram probably rules out severe but not mild pulmonary hypertension, and the inability to accurately measure the tricuspid regurgitation jet leads to an over- or underestimation of the pulmonary artery pressure. Thus, an abnormal echocardiogram or even a normal one in the presence of worrisome symptoms should be confirmed with cardiac catheterization.

5.4. Chest Radiography

Chest radiographic abnormalities encountered in CTEPH are nonspecific but may suggest the presence of the disease. Pulmonary arteries are often asymmetrically enlarged centrally and abruptly decrease in caliber distally, corresponding to the "pouch" defect seen angiographically, related to central vascular dilatation with a distal clot (Fig. 1). Patchy oligemia may be present along with areas of hyperemia. Pleural-based scars consistent with prior infarct may be present. The silhouette of the heart may demonstrate enlargement of the right atrium or the right ventricle. Atrial enlargement is best noted on the PA view, and right ventricular enlargement is best seen on the lateral view in the retrosternal space. The presence of Kerley B lines

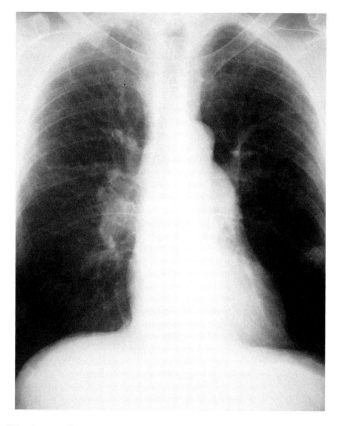

Fig. 1. PA chest radiograph showing asymmetry of the main pulmonary arteries with abrupt termination of the central pulmonary arteries and a peripheral scar. (Courtesy of P.F. Fedullo, MD)

suggests the possibility not only of left ventricular failure but also of pulmonary veno-occlusive disease.

5.5. Ventilation–Perfusion Lung Scanning

Once the diagnosis of CTEPH is considered, steps should be taken to determine whether the thromboembolic disease is surgically accessible. Ventilation–perfusion lung scanning is used to differentiate central versus peripheral obstruction of the pulmonary arteries. In CTEPH, the V/Q scan typically reveals multiple segmental or larger perfusion defects *(43,44)* (Figure 2). In idiopathic pulmonary arterial hypertension, small *in situ* thromboses may occur in distal vessels, but the perfusion scan either is normal or has a nonsegmental "moth-eaten" appearance with a basilar redistribution of flow (Figure 3).

The ventilation–perfusion lung scan is thought to be more sensitive for CTEPH than computerized tomographic angiography, which is why the American College of Chest Physicians' guidelines identify ventilation–perfusion scanning as the preferred initial screening test.

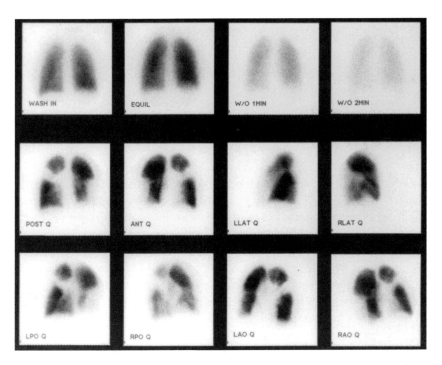

Fig. 2. Typical ventilation–perfusion lung scan for CTEPH showing multiple unmatched segmental defects. (Courtesy of P.F. Fedullo, MD)

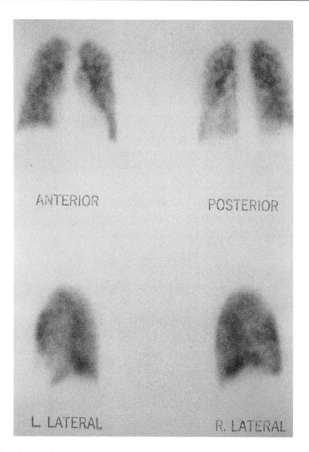

Fig. 3. Classic ventilation–perfusion lung scan for idiopathic pulmonary hypertension. (Courtesy of P.F. Fedullo, MD)

Worsley et al. demonstrated that 24 of 25 patients with CTEPH had "high-probability" scans and the remaining patient had an "intermediate–probability" scan *(52)*. Thus, the sensitivity for CTEPH was 100% for a high- or intermediate-probability ventilation–perfusion lung scan (and specificity was 86%) *(45)*. However, because partial occlusion of a vessel can still result in distal blood flow, ventilation–perfusion scanning may underestimate the degree of obstruction, and the size and the number of defects do not correlate well with the pulmonary hemodynamics determined at catheterization *(46)*.

The presence of even a single mismatched ventilation–perfusion defect in a patient with otherwise unexplained pulmonary hypertension or dyspnea should prompt consideration of CTEPH. However, the differential diagnosis of segmental or larger mismatched defects in a patient with pulmonary hypertension is quite broad and includes pulmonary artery sarcoma, large vessel vasculitides, mediastinal fibrosis, mediastinal lymphadenopathy with vascular compression, sickle cell anemia, and pulmonary veno-occlusive disease *(38)*.

5.6. Computerized Tomography and Magnetic Resonance Imaging

Findings on helical contrasted computed tomography scanning of the pulmonary arteries that can be helpful in diagnosing CTEPH include thrombus in and dilation of the central pulmonary arteries, right ventricular enlargement, and parenchymal abnormalities such as a mosaic attenuation pattern and peripheral scarring (suggesting old pulmonary infarcts) *(47,48)*. In addition, one can see an abrupt termination or decrease in caliber of the pulmonary arteries. Another advantage of CT angiography is that other pathologies can be detected, such as intravascular neoplasms (Fig. 3). Visualization of the smaller segmental pulmonary arteries may be inadequate, however, and thin-walled lining of the thrombus may not be detected. In addition, central *in situ* thrombosis cannot be separated from chronic thromboembolic disease.

Recently, a series of 60 patients undergoing thromboendarterectomy suggested that helical computed tomography is useful in predicting postoperative hemodynamic improvement. Predictors of postoperative pulmonary vascular resistance included the presence or absence of a central thrombus, the number of subpleural densities, dilation of the bronchial arteries, and (by ventilation–perfusion lung scanning) the number of lung segments with abnormal perfusion *(49)*.

Magnetic resonance angiography is also useful for defining anatomy and the extent of obstruction in CTEPH *(47)*. Presently, it is not used routinely in patients who can undergo conventional angiography, but in comparison with helical computed tomographic angiography, it appears to be equivalent for identifying the signs of CTEPH *(50)*. Of course, both computerized tomographic angiography and magnetic resonance angiography provide a wealth of additional anatomic information, permitting the detection of alternative diagnoses that may be associated with pulmonary hypertension such as central obstructing tumors, pulmonary venous stenoses, or fibrosing mediastinitis. Computerized tomographic angiography should be obtained when alternative diagnoses such as these are being entertained or the severity of parenchymal disease by chest X-ray indicates that ventilation–perfusion lung scan findings are likely to be unrevealing.

5.7. Right Heart Catheterization and Pulmonary Angiography and Angioscopy

Essential steps in the preoperative evaluation of patients with CTEPH are the right heart catheterization and pulmonary angiography. Right heart catheterization is imperative to confirm the diagnosis and severity of pulmonary hypertension and to provide prognostic information. Catheterization permits accurate measurement of the pulmonary artery pressure as well as of the right atrial pressure, pulmonary artery occlusion pressure, and cardiac output. Patients with borderline pulmonary artery pressures at rest undergo symptom-limited exercise during catheterization to detect abnormal elevations *(51)*. In patients with sufficient chronic thromboembolic obstruction to limit the usual recruitment of pulmonary vessels that occurs with increases in cardiac output, the pulmonary artery pressure will climb in an almost linear fashion and the normal decline in pulmonary vascular resistance will not occur *(51)*. In CTEPH patients with risk factors for coronary artery disease, left heart catheterization with coronary angiography is also performed prior to contemplated surgery.

Pulmonary angiography is essential in the preoperative evaluation of the patient with CTEPH to define the location and extent of anatomic obstruction. The angiographic appearance of CTEPH is distinct from that encountered in acute pulmonary embolism, although both processes can be seen simultaneously. Angiographic abnormalities associated with CTEPH include pouch defects, pulmonary artery webs or bands, intimal irregularities, abrupt angular narrowing of the pulmonary arteries, and complete obstruction of the main, lobar, or central pulmonary arteries (Figs. 4, 5, and 6a and 6b). Often, more than one pattern is seen. Also, other diseases can cause similar findings, including pulmonary artery sarcoma, which can completely obstruct the central pulmonary arteries, or vasculitis and extrinsic compression of the pulmonary arteries, which can cause band-like narrowing.

Pulmonary angiography requires considerable experience to perform properly and interpret accurately, and with the increasing reliance on computerized tomographic angiography, it is no longer widely available. In addition, pulmonary angiography has been thought to pose considerable risk in the setting of severe pulmonary hypertension. However, the procedure can be performed safely by experienced angiographers who use well-established safety techniques *(52,53)*. The biplane acquisition technique should be used when possible. Routine use of the lateral view is extremely helpful in determining the proximal

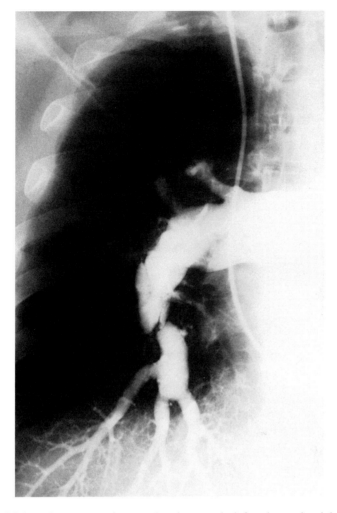

Fig. 4. Right pulmonary angiogram showing a web deformity to the right lower lobar artery and central pulmonary artery irregularity. (Courtesy of P.F. Fedullo, MD)

location and anatomical extent of the obstructing emboli and, therefore, the surgical accessibility.

Pulmonary angioscopy is used as an adjunct to pulmonary angiography. Approximately 10% of cases that are being evaluated for thromboendarterectomy at the University of California at San Diego undergo angioscopy to confirm operability when the extent of proximal disease is not certain from angiography. In the early years of pulmonary thromboendarterectomy, angioscopy was used more frequently but has been displaced by improved imaging techniques and interpretation *(54)*. The

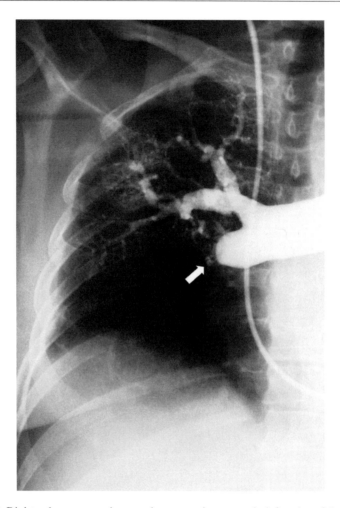

Fig. 5. Right pulmonary angiogram demonstrating a pouch deformity of the inter-lobar artery and irregularity of the right upper lobar artery. (Courtesy of P.F. Fedullo, MD)

angioscope is a fiber-optic flexible scope that is 120 cm in length and 3 mm in diameter. A transparent balloon is fastened onto the distal end of the scope. After the angioscope is passed through an introducer, preferably in the right internal jugular vein, it is passed through the right atrium and right ventricle and into the right and left pulmonary arteries, where it can be guided into each of the lobar arteries. The distal balloon is inflated with carbon dioxide, which transiently obstructs proximal blood flow and allows visualization of the vascular bed. The

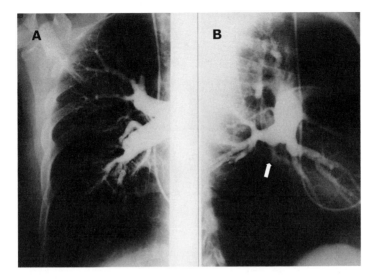

Fig. 6. (a) Right pulmonary angiogram demonstrating multiple abnormalities with abrupt tapering of multiple vessels and webs on the PA view. (b) The lateral view enhances the knowledge of the anatomy by clearly demonstrating absence of flow to the right lower lobe (arrow). (Courtesy of P.F. Fedullo, MD)

typical angioscopic findings of CTEPH include pitting of the vascular surface, bands, webs, and pitted masses of chronic embolic material *(54)* (Fig. 7).

6. SURGICAL SELECTION

Selection of good candidates for thromboendarterectomy can be quite challenging. The main criteria include the surgical accessibility of the thromboembolic material, the hemodynamic and symptomatic status of the patient, and the potential hemodynamic benefit from the procedure. As part of the decision-making process, the patient's comorbidities such as morbid obesity, severe underlying parenchymal lung disease, chronic renal insufficiency, diabetes mellitus, coronary artery disease, hepatic dysfunction, malnutrition, and advanced age are considered. Age is not a contraindication to surgical intervention, and octogenarians in otherwise good health have successfully undergone the procedure.

The untreated prognosis of advanced CTEPH is very poor, so high-risk patients are often considered. However, patients with advanced lung disease pose a special challenge. They are at high risk for prolonged mechanical ventilation in the postoperative period and

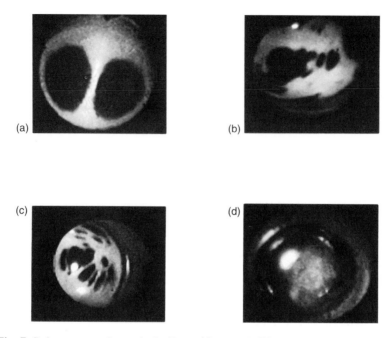

Fig. 7. Pulmonary angioscopic findings: (a) normal; (b) pitting of the intima seen in CTEPH; (c) web formation seen in CTEPH; (d) subacute thrombus or mass. (Courtesy of P.F. Fedullo, MD)

may have little symptomatic improvement even when the pulmonary hemodynamic result is favorable.

Special attention must be given to the pulmonary vascular resistance in selecting patients for surgery. In the majority of published series of patients undergoing pulmonary thromboendarterectomy, the typical range of pulmonary vascular resistance is 700 to 1100 dyne/s^{-1}/cm^{-5} *(4,55–60)*. In general, most patients have a pulmonary vascular resistance greater than 300 dyne/s^{-1}/cm^{-5}. Patients with pulmonary vascular resistances less than 300 dyne/s^{-1}/cm^{-5} occasionally undergo surgery to relieve dyspnea related to their high dead space ventilation. These patients typically have unilateral pulmonary arterial occlusion, have an active lifestyle, or live at a high altitude. On occasion, patients with no evidence of resting pulmonary hypertension may be offered surgery if they have an increase in pulmonary artery pressure with exercise associated with symptomatic impairment. Patients with extremely high pulmonary vascular resistances (greater than 1200 dyne/s^{-1}/cm^{-5}) may occasionally be offered surgery, but the risk of perioperative mortality is high and significant pulmonary hypertension is likely to persist after surgery *(4,94)*.

The most important aspects of the preoperative assessment are to determine whether the thromboembolic disease is surgically accessible and how much of the increased pulmonary vascular resistance is attributable to proximal obstruction. In experienced surgical hands, the central, lobar, and proximal segmental pulmonary arteries are accessible to thromboendarterectomy. Preoperative partitioning of the contributing elements of the increased pulmonary vascular resistance into operable and nonoperable components is important because failure to significantly lower pulmonary vascular resistance not only limits long-term outcome but also contributes to the persistence of severe pulmonary hypertension and right ventricular dysfunction postoperatively that may be associated with hemodynamic instability and death.

A technique that has been developed to objectively "partition" the vascular resistance into proximal and distal compartments uses a special pulmonary artery catheter and a computer-generated pulmonary capillary wedge tracing. The computer calculates the decay of the wedge tracing curve and generates a percentage of upstream resistance. Investigators have demonstrated that the upstream resistance percentage is higher in patients with CTEPH than in other forms of pulmonary hypertension *(61)*. In a study of 26 patients who underwent pulmonary thromboendarterectomy, the postoperative improvement in pulmonary hemodynamics correlated with the preoperative upstream resistance percentage and the four patients with high upstream resistance percentages had an increased mortality *(62)*. This technique holds promise for assisting in the preoperative selection of patients with CTEPH.

7. SURGICAL APPROACH

Details of the thromboendarterectomy procedure have been described extensively elsewhere *(101)*. However, several features of the procedure should be emphasized here. Although a thoracotomy approach has been used in the past, the standard approach now is a median sternotomy with cardiopulmonary bypass and hypothermic circulatory arrest. A sternotomy provides better access to the central pulmonary vessels of both lungs and reduces the risk of hemorrhage caused by disruption of the extensive bronchial collateral circulation and pulmonary adhesions that may develop following pulmonary artery obstruction. A sternotomy approach also provides adequate exposure for additional procedures that might need to be performed. In a review of 1,190 patients undergoing thromboendarterectomy at the UCSD Medical Center, 90 patients (7.6%) required additional procedures exclusive of closure of a patent foramen ovale (which is performed in approximately 30% of thromboendarterectomy procedures) *(63)*. Of the 90 patients, 83 underwent coronary artery bypass surgery, 3 tricuspid valve repair, 2 mitral valve repair, and 2 aortic valve replacement *(64)*. The thromboendarterectomy procedure also involves periods of complete hypothermic circulatory arrest to assure a bloodless operative field and optimal exposure of the pulmonary vascular intima. Circulatory arrest periods are limited to 20 minutes, with resumption of blood flow and restoration of mixed venous O_2 saturation between each interruption *(63)*.

The procedure is a true thromboendarterectomy, not an embolectomy. The chronic thromboembolic material is fibrotic and incorporated into the native vascular lumen. The neo-intima must be meticulously dissected away from the native intima, and considerable surgical experience is required to identify the correct operative plane. The removal of nonadherent, partially organized thrombus within the lumen of the central pulmonary arteries is ineffective in reducing

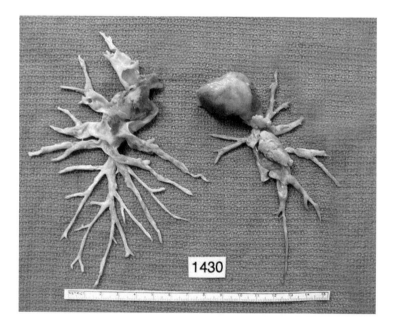

Fig. 8. Typical surgical specimen from a pulmonary thromboendarterectomy for CTEPH. Note the involvement of the segmental arterial branches. (Courtesy of P.F. Fedullo, MD)

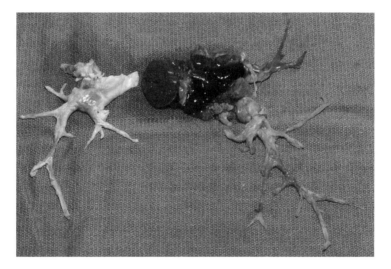

Fig. 9. Typical surgical specimen from a pulmonary thromboendarterectomy for CTEPH. Note the involvement of the segmental arterial branches and the subacute thrombus on the right (left pulmonary artery). (Courtesy of P.F. Fedullo, MD)

right ventricular afterload, whereas creation of too deep a plane poses the risk of pulmonary artery perforation and massive pulmonary hemorrhage when perfusion is restored. The surgical specimen often resembles a cast of the pulmonary arteries (Fig. 8), sometimes containing a mixture of fresh and old clots (Fig. 9).

Modifications of the surgical approach continue to be explored, aiming to decrease surgical risks and improve long-term hemodynamic outcomes. These include the use of intraoperative video-assisted angioscopy to enhance visibility in the distal pulmonary arteries, thereby allowing surgical intervention in patients with previously inaccessible disease; division rather than retraction of the superior vena cava to improve visualization of the right pulmonary artery; selective antegrade cerebral perfusion and moderate rather than deep hypothermia to decrease the risk of neurologic sequelae; and bronchial artery occlusion to minimize retrograde bronchial artery flow *(65,66,73,74,84,94,95,97).*

8. POSTOPERATIVE COURSE

Careful postoperative management is essential for a successful outcome following pulmonary thromboendarterectomy. Although pulmonary hemodynamics improves immediately after surgery in the majority of patients, the postoperative course can be complicated. In addition to those common to other forms of cardiac surgery (arrhythmias, atelectasis, wound infection, pericardial effusions, delirium), patients undergoing pulmonary thromboendarterectomy often experience three unique postoperative complications capable of significantly impairing gas exchange and hemodynamic stability: pulmonary artery "steal," reperfusion pulmonary edema, and persistent pulmonary hypertension *(68,69)*.

Pulmonary artery "steal" represents a postoperative redistribution of pulmonary arterial blood flow away from previously well-perfused segments and into the newly endarterectomized segments *(69)*. Although the basis for this phenomenon remains speculative, it is likely related to the sudden reduction of resistance in the endarterectomized vessels and temporary loss of normal vasoregulation in the pulmonary vascular bed following thromboendarterectomy. Long-term follow-up has demonstrated that pulmonary vascular steal resolves in the majority of patients *(71)*.

Reperfusion pulmonary edema appears to represent a form of high-permeability lung injury that occurs in those areas of the lung from which proximal thromboembolic obstructions have been removed *(67,68)*. Appearing up to 72 hours after surgery, it is highly variable in severity, ranging from a mild form that causes transient postoperative hypoxemia to an acute, hemorrhagic, and fatal complication. Management of gas exchange in the patient with significant reperfusion injury can be extremely challenging and is worsened when there is a component of the "steal" phenomenon. In this circumstance, the blood flow is redistributed to the edematous, injured lung, which has low compliance and is thus relatively poorly ventilated (Fig. 10).

Management of acute lung injury post-thromboendarterectomy is supportive; although the preferred ventilator strategy is unproven, a low tidal volume approach (less than 8 ml/kg) and avoidance of inotropic agents appear to lower mortality compared to a high tidal volume strategy (10–15 ml/kg) *(70)*. The lower tidal volume strategy may worsen hypoxemia and should be used cautiously pending further studies. Other unproven therapies include inhaled nitric oxide, which may improve gas exchange transiently, and high-dose corticosteroids. A small, randomized trial compared the intraoperative and early postoperative use of Cylexin, a selectin-mediated neutrophil adhesion-blocking agent. This drug decreased the incidence of lung injury after thromboendarterectomy by 50% (60% in the control group vs. 31% in the treatment group) but had no impact on mortality, ventilator days, or length of intensive care unit stay *(71)*. The prostacyclin analogue

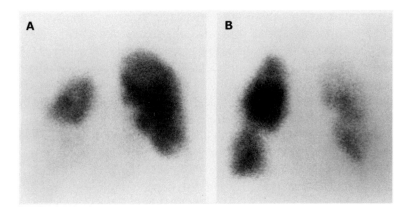

ANTERIOR   ANTERIOR

Fig. 10. (a) Preoperative and (b) postoperative ventilation–perfusion lung scan demonstrating reperfusion of the right upper lobe and right lower lobe with "steal phenomena." Note the reperfusion of the right lower lobe and the relative nonsegmental decrease in perfusion of the left lung. (Courtesy of P.F. Fedullo, MD)

iloprost has been reported to decrease reperfusion lung injury in lung transplant patients but has not yet been studied after pulmonary thromboendarterectomy *(72)*. Lastly, extracorporeal support (ECCO2) has been used successfully in patients in whom aggressive support is failing in patients with a good hemodynamic result from the endarterectomy.

The most difficult problem in the perioperative period is management of patients with persistent pulmonary hypertension. The initial step in management of these patients occurs in the operating room. Although it is routine when pulmonary vascular resistance can be lowered adequately, closure of a patent foramen ovale should not be undertaken in patients with severe pulmonary hypertension whose thromboendarterectomies were inadequate. In fact, patients unable to discontinue cardiopulmonary bypass due to right ventricular failure may benefit from the enlargement of an existing patent foramen ovale or the creation of a new atrial septal communication to unload the right ventricle. Of course, such an intervention may be associated with severe postoperative hypoxemia and should be attempted only when weaning from cardiopulmonary bypass cannot be achieved by any other means.

The early intensive care management goals for the patient with persistent pulmonary hypertension and right ventricular failure following attempted thromboendarterectomy are to minimize systemic oxygen consumption and right ventricular afterload, optimize right ventricular preload, and provide aggressive inotropic support. However, afterload reduction in this patient population is fraught with difficulty. Pulmonary vascular resistance is often fixed, and attempts at pharmacological manipulation of right ventricular afterload may simply decrease the systemic blood pressure and right coronary artery perfusion pressure. Inhaled nitric oxide at a concentration of 20 to 40 ppm seems ideal for this circumstance because it has negligible systemic effects *(92,93)*. Unfortunately, our experience with it in the setting of persistent postoperative pulmonary hypertension has been disappointing. More recently, inhaled iloprost has been utilized in patients with residual pulmonary hypertension following thromboendarterectomy *(98)*. In a small cohort of patients, inhaled iloprost achieved a significant improvement in pulmonary artery pressure and cardiac output without adverse effects on systemic hemodynamics when compared to placebo.

9. SURGICAL OUTCOME

Despite the potential for life-threatening complications, the perioperative mortality of patients undergoing pulmonary thromboendarterectomy has improved in recent years. Perioperative mortality for patients undergoing pulmonary thromboendarterectomy at the University of California at San Diego was 17% for the first 200 patients who underwent the operation from 1970 to 1990 *(4)*. In a series from UCSD from 1998 until 2002, 500 patients underwent pulmonary thromboendarterectomy, with a hospital mortality rate of 4.4% *(4)*. Preoperative factors that may adversely affect surgical outcome include age greater than 70 years, the presence of multiple comorbid conditions, preoperative pulmonary vascular resistance, severe right heart failure with high right atrial pressures, and the duration of pulmonary hypertension prior to surgery *(4,59,74,96)*. The preoperative pulmonary vascular resistance seems to be particularly important in predicting the surgical outcome. In one series, the mortality was 1.3% if the preoperative pulmonary vascular resistance was less than 1000 dyne/s^{-1}/cm^{-5} and 10.1% if the preoperative pulmonary vascular resistance was greater than 1000 dyne/s^{-1}/cm^{-5} *(4)*. The postoperative pulmonary vascular resistance also predicts outcome. Perioperative mortality is 30.6% if the postoperative pulmonary vascular resistance is greater than 500 dyne/s^{-1}/cm^{-5} and 0.9% if less *(4)*.

10. LONG-TERM OUTCOME

The majority of patients who receive pulmonary thromboen-darterectomy have favorable short-term and long-term functional and hemodynamic outcomes. Most patients initially in World Health Organization/New York Heart Association (WHO/NYHA) functional class III or IV preoperatively return to class I or II postoperatively and are able to resume normal activities. A significant reduction and at times normalization of pulmonary artery pressures and resistances can also be achieved. In the largest series to date, the mean pulmonary artery pressure decreased from 46 ± 11.0 mm Hg to 28 ± 10.1 mm Hg and the mean pulmonary vascular resistance from 893 ± 443.5 dyne/s^{-1}/cm^{-5} to 285 ± 214.7 dyne/s^{-1}/cm^{-5}, preoperatively to postoperatively, respectively *(4)*. Similar improvements have been observed in right ventricular function by echocardiography, exercise capacity, and quality of life *(75–81)*. These effects can be long-lasting, but the patient should be maintained on lifelong warfarin or other anticoagulant to prevent the recurrence of CTEPH.

Repeat thromboendarterectomy has been performed successfully in a number of patients who suffered a recurrent postoperative embolic event or who initially underwent an inadequate procedure, by way of either thoracotomy or sternotomy. A second procedure can be performed with morbidity and mortality comparable to the primary procedure, but the subsequent improvements in hemodynamics are less impressive *(81)*.

11. MEDICAL THERAPY

Traditionally, the medical therapy for patients who did not receive surgery for chronic thromboembolic disease was anticoagulation and supportive care. The five-year survival rate associated with this approach was 30% when the mean pulmonary artery pressure was greater than 40 mm Hg and was 10% when it was greater than 50 mm Hg *(81)*. Another similar study reported a survival of 20% or less at three years for patients with a mean pulmonary artery pressure greater than 30 mm Hg *(99)*.

In recent years, a number of the newer agents introduced to treat pulmonary hypertension have been tried for CTEPH. Widely accepted indications for the medical management of CTEPH include inoperable or distal chronic thromboembolic pulmonary hypertension, use preoperatively in patients with severe right heart failure or pulmonary vascular resistances greater than 1000 dyne/s^{-1}/cm^{-5}, and refusal of surgery. Medical therapy is also indicated for long-term use in patients with residual pulmonary hypertension after pulmonary thromboendarterectomy.

Although no sizable randomized, controlled trial has examined medical therapy in CTEPH patients per se, small numbers have been included in a number of the published series. A randomized study of 201 patients with pulmonary hypertension treated with iloprost or placebo for 12 weeks included 57 CTEPH patients *(82)*. Although both idiopathic and nonidiopathic PAH patients in this trial manifested improvements in hemodynamics, WHO/NYHA class, and quality of life compared to placebo, the CTEPH patients were not analyzed separately *(82)*. In a second small study, 10 patients with CTEPH received iloprost immediately before and after thromboendarterectomy *(83)*. Interestingly, there was no hemodynamic response to the medication prior to surgery, but the mean pulmonary artery pressure and pulmonary vascular resistance decreased and the cardiac output increased when the medication was administered postoperatively *(83)*.

Small numbers of patients with chronic thromboembolic pulmonary hypertension have been included in numerous clinical trials for various agents including prostacyclins, bosentan, and sildenafil *(83,85–87)*. Many of these studies suggest an improvement in clinical status, hemodynamics, and exercise capacity. Beraprost, an oral prostacyclin available in Japan but not in the United States, has demonstrated improvements in exercise capacity as well as in the overall clinical status in a number of small studies of three to six months' duration *(88–90)*. Epoprostenol has been used in patients as a bridge to thromboendarterectomy *(100)*. In one study, nine patients were placed on epoprostenol prior to pulmonary thromboendarterectomy *(100)*. In this cohort of patients, six patients demonstrated clinical stability or improvement *(100)*. All patients ultimately underwent surgical intervention with significant hemodynamic improvement *(100)*. A one-year study using bosentan in 47 patients with inoperable CTEPH also demonstrated improvements in exercise capacity and clinical status based upon six-minute walk test and hemodynamics *(101)*. Ghofrani et al. published a study of 12 patients with inoperable CTEPH that were treated with Sildenafil *(101)*. These patients demonstrated an improvement in hemodynamics and exercise capacity after six months *(100)*.

Considering the poor prognosis of patients with inoperable CTEPH or with residual pulmonary hypertension after surgery and the evidence suggesting beneficial effects, a trial of medical therapy should be offered to such patients. The threshold for elevation of mean pulmonary artery pressure or pulmonary vascular resistance above which medical therapy should be initiated has not yet been clearly defined, but our practice is to provide it when the postoperative pulmonary vascular resistance is greater than 400 or 500 dyne/s^{-1}/cm^{-5}. Patients with modest elevations in pulmonary vascular resistance (between 300 and 400 dyne/s^{-1}/cm^{-5}) are followed with annual echocardiograms and clinical evaluations and may be considered for treatment if symptoms progress or pulmonary hemodynamics deteriorates.

12. LUNG TRANSPLANTATION

Lung transplantation remains an option for patients not considered candidates for thromboendarterectomy or for those with an inadequate functional and pulmonary hemodynamic recovery following surgery. Candidates have usually failed medical therapy as well and satisfy the other standard guidelines for transplantation. There are currently no data on how CTEPH patients fare following lung transplantation compared to other categories of patients.

13. SUMMARY

CTEPH is an important form of pulmonary hypertension to detect because prompt treatment can lead to a surgical cure. The true incidence is unknown, but it is estimated to occur in 1% to 3% of patients following acute thromboembolism, which suggests that many cases are missed. Detection may be difficult, because symptoms are nonspecific and other diagnoses are often made before that of CTEPH is entertained. Routinely screening all pulmonary hypertension patients with a ventilation perfusion scan will detect most, however. Candidates for thromboendarterectomy are evaluated using right heart catheterization, computerized tomographic angiography, and pulmonary angiography seeking those with proximal obstructions that can be removed surgically. Patients who are not candidates for thromboendarterectomy because of comorbidities, very high pulmonary vascular resistances, or mainly distal disease may still receive medical therapy or be considered for lung transplantation.

REFERENCES

1. Carroll D. Chronic obstruction of major pulmonary arteries. Am J Med 1950; 9:175–85.

2. Jamieson SW, Auger WR, Fedullo PF, et al. Experience and results with 150 pulmonary thromboendarterectomy operations over a 29-month period. J Thorac Cardiovasc Surg 1993; 106:116–27.

3. Fedullo PF, Auger WR, Channick RN, et al. Chronic thromboembolic pulmonary hypertension. Clin Chest Med 1995; 16:353–74.

4. Daily PO, Auger WR. Historical perspective: Surgery for chronic thromboembolic disease. Sem Thorac Cardiovasc Surg 1999; 11:143–51.

5. Daily PO, Dembitsky WP, Jamieson SW. The evolution and the current state of the art of pulmonary thromboendarterectomy. Sem Thorac Cardiovasc Surg 1999; 11:152–63.

6. Jamieson SW, Kapelanski DP. Pulmonary endarterectomy. Curr Probl Surg 2000; 37:165–252.

7. Kapelanski DP, Macoviak JA, Jamieson SW. Surgical intervention in the treatment of pulmonary embolism and chronic thromboembolic pulmonary hypertension. In M Oudkerk, EJR van Beek, JW Ten Cate, eds. Pulmonary Embolism. Berlin: Blackwell Science, 1999, pp. 382–397.

8. Hollister LE, Cull VL. The syndrome of chronic thrombosis of major pulmonary arteries. Am J Med 1956; 21:312–20.

9. Houk VN, Hufnagel CA, McClenathan JE, et al. Chronic thrombotic obstruction of major pulmonary arteries: Report of a case successfully treated by thromboendarterectomy, and a review of the literature. Am J Med 1963; 35:269–82.

10. Chitwood WR, Lyerly HK, Sabiston DC. Surgical management of chronic pulmonary embolism. Ann Surg 1985; 201:11–26.

11. Jamieson SW, Kapelanski DP, Sakakibara N, et al. Pulmonary endarterectomy: Experience and lessons learned in 1500 cases. Ann Thorac Surg 2003; 76:1457–62.

12. Rubens F, Wells P, Bencze S, Bourke M. Surgical treatment of chronic thromboembolic pulmonary hypertension. Can Respir J 2000; 7:49–57.

13. D'Armini AM, Cattadori B, Monterosso C, et al. Pulmonary thromboendarterectomy in patients with chronic thromboembolic pulmonary hypertension: Hemodynamic characteristics and changes. Eur J Cardiothorac Surg 2000; 18:696–702.

14. Fedullo PF, Auger WR, Kerr KM, Rubin LJ. Chronic thromboembolic pulmonary hypertension. N Engl J Med 2001; 345:1465–72.

15. Ando M, Okita Y, Tagusari O, et al. Surgical treatment for chronic thromboembolic pulmonary hypertension under profound hypothermia and circulatory arrest in 24 patients. J Card Surg 1999; 14:377–85.

16. Masuda M, Nakajima N. Our experience of surgical treatment for chronic pulmonary thromboembolism. Ann Thorac Cardiovasc Surg 2001; 7: 261–5.

17. Pengo V, Lensing AW, Prins MH, et al. Incidence of chronic thromboembolic pulmonary hypertension after pulmonary embolism. N Engl J Med 2004; 350:2257–64.

18. Dalen JE, Alpert JS. Natural history of pulmonary embolism. Prog Cardiovasc Dis 1975; 17:259–70.

19. Egermayer P, Peacock AJ. Is pulmonary embolism a common cause of pulmonary hypertension? Limitations of the embolic hypothesis. Eur Respir J 2000; 15:440–8.
20. Fedullo PF, Rubin LJ, Kerr KM, et al. The natural history of acute and chronic thromboembolic disease: The search for the missing link. Eur Respir J 2000; 15:435–7 (ed).
21. McIntyre KM, Sasahara AA. The hemodynamic response to pulmonary embolism in patients without prior cardiopulmonary disease. Am J Cardiol 1971; 28:288–94.
22. Wolfe MW, Lee RT, Feldstein ML, et al. Prognostic significance of right ventricular hypokinesis and perfusion lung scan defects in pulmonary embolism. Am Heart J 1994; 127:1371–5.
23. Wartski M, Collignon MA. Incomplete recovery of lung perfusion after 3 months in patients with acute pulmonary embolism treated with antithrombotic agents. J Nucl Med 2000; 41:1043–8.
24. Ribeiro A, Lindmarker P, Johnsson H, et al. Pulmonary embolism: A follow-up study of the relation between the degree of right ventricular overload and the extent of perfusion defects. J Intern Med 1999; 245:601–10.
25. Moser KM, Auger WR, Fedullo PF. Chronic major-vessel thromboembolic pulmonary hypertension. Circulation 1990; 81:1735–43.
26. Ribeiro A, Lindmarker P, Johnsson H, et al. Pulmonary embolism: One-year follow-up with echocardiography Doppler and five-year survival analysis. Circulation 1999; 99:1325–30.
27. Liu P, Meneveau N, Schiele F, Bassand JP. Predictors of long-term clinical outcome of patients with acute massive pulmonary embolism after thrombolytic therapy. Chin Med J (Engl) 2003; 116:503–9.
28. Naudziunas A, Miliauskas S. Factor V Leiden and post thromboembolic pulmonary hypertension. Medicina (Kaunas) 2003; 39:1171–4.
29. Wolf M, Boyer-Neumann C, Parent F, et al. Thrombotic risk factors in pulmonary hypertension. Eur Respir J 2000; 15:395–9.
30. Auger WR, Permpikul P, Moser KM. Lupus anticoagulant, heparin use, and thrombocytopenia in patients with chronic thromboembolic pulmonary hypertension: A preliminary report. Am J Med 1995; 99:392–6.
31. Olman MA, Marsh JJ, Lang IM, et al. Endogenous fibrinolytic system in chronic large-vessel thromboembolic pulmonary hypertension. Circulation 1992; 86:1241–8.
32. Bonderman D, Turecek PL, Jakowitsch J, et al. High prevalence of elevated clotting factor VIII in chronic thromboembolic pulmonary hypertension. Thromb Haemost 2003; 90:372–6.
33. Colorio CC, Martinuzzo ME, Forastiero RR, et al. Thrombophilic tendencies in chronic thromboembolic pulmonary hypertension. Blood Coagul Fibrinolysis 2001; 12:427–32.
34. Meignan M, Rosso J, Gauthier H, et al. Systematic lung scans reveal a high frequency of silent pulmonary embolism in patients with proximal deep venous thrombosis. Arch Intern Med 2000; 160:159–64.

35. Karwinski B, Svendsen E. Comparison of clinical and postmortem diagnosis of pulmonary embolism. J Clin Pathol 1989; 42:135–9.
36. Moser KM, Bloor CM. Pulmonary vascular lesions occurring in patients with chronic major-vessel thromboembolic pulmonary hypertension. Chest 1993; 103:684–92.
37. Auger WR, Moser KM. Pulmonary flow murmurs; a distinctive physical sign found in chronic pulmonary thromboembolic disease. Clin Res 1989; 37:145A.
38. Nagaya N, Uematsu M, Satoh T, et al. Serum uric acid levels correlate with the severity and the mortality of primary pulmonary hypertension. Am J Respir Crit Care Med 1999; 160:487–92.
39. Voelkel MA, Wynne KM, Badesch DB, et al. Hyperuricemia in severe pulmonary hypertension. Chest 2000; 117:19–24.
40. Nagaya N, Ando M, Oya H, et al. Plasma brain natriuretic peptide as a noninvasive marker for efficacy of pulmonary thromboendarterectomy. Ann Thorac Surg 2002; 74:180–4.
41. Kapitan KS, Buchbinder M, Wagner PD, et al. Mechanisms of hypoxemia in chronic thromboembolic pulmonary hypertension. Am Rev Respir Dis 1989; 139:1149–54.
42. Morris TA, Auger WR, Ysrael MZ, et al. Parenchymal scarring is associated with restrictive spirometric defects in patients with chronic thromboembolic pulmonary hypertension. Chest 1996; 110:399–403.
43. D'Alonzo GE, Bower JS, Dantzker DR. Differentiation of patients with primary and thromboembolic pulmonary hypertension. Chest 1984; 85:457–61.
44. Currie PJ, Seward JB, Chan KL, et al. Continuous wave Doppler determination of right ventricular pressure: A simultaneous Doppler-catheterization study in 127 patients. J Am Coll Cardiol 1985; 6: 750–6.
45. Berger M, Haimowitz A, Van Tosh A, et al. Quantitative assessment of pulmonary hypertension in patients with tricuspid regurgitation using continuous wave Doppler ultrasound. J Am Coll Cardiol 1985; 6: 359–65.
46. Mahmud E, Raisinghani A, Hassankhani A, et al. Correlation of left ventricular diastolic filling characteristics with right ventricular overload and pulmonary artery pressure in chronic thromboembolic pulmonary hypertension. J Am Coll Cardiol 2002; 40:318–24.
47. Ghio S, Raineri C, Scelsi L, et al. Usefulness and limits of transthoracic echocardiography in the evaluation of patients with primary and chronic thromboembolic pulmonary hypertension. J Am Soc Echocardiogr 2002; 15:1374–80.
48. Sun XG, Hansen JE, Oudiz RJ, Wasserman K. Pulmonary function in primary pulmonary hypertension. J Am Coll Cardiol 2003; 41:1028–35.
49. Bernstein RJ, Ford RL, Clausen JL, Moser KM. Membrane diffusion and capillary blood volume in chronic thromboembolic pulmonary hypertension. Chest 1996; 110:1430–6.

50. Fishman AJ, Moser KM, Fedullo PF. Perfusion lung scans vs pulmonary angiography in evaluation of suspected primary pulmonary hypertension. Chest 1983; 84:679–83.

51. Lisbona R, Kreisman H, Novales-Diaz J, et al. Perfusion lung scanning: Differentiation of primary from thromboembolic pulmonary hypertension. Am J Roentgenol 1985; 144:27–30.

52. Worsley DF, Palevsky HI, Alavi A. Ventilation-perfusion lung scanning in the evaluation of pulmonary hypertension. J Nucl Med 1994; 35: 793–6.

53. Azarian R, Wartski M, Collignon MA, et al. Lung perfusion scans and hemodynamics in acute and chronic pulmonary embolism. J Nucl Med 1997; 38:980–3.

54. Ryan KL, Fedullo PF, Davis GB, et al. Perfusion scan findings understate the severity of angiographic and hemodynamic compromise in chronic thromboembolic pulmonary hypertension. Chest 1988; 93:1180–5.

55. Bergin CJ, Sirlin CB, Hauschildt JP, et al. Chronic thromboembolism: Diagnosis with helical CT and MR imaging with angiographic and surgical correlation. Radiology 1997; 204:695–702.

56. King MA, Ysrael M, Bergin CJ. Chronic thromboembolic pulmonary hypertension: CT findings. Am J Roentgenol 1998; 170:955–60.

57. Bergin CJ, Rios G, King MA, et al. Accuracy of high-resolution CT in identifying chronic pulmonary thromboembolic disease. Am J Roentgenol 1996; 166:1371–7.

58. Bergin CJ, Hauschildt JP, Brown MA, et al. Identifying the cause of unilateral hypoperfusion in patients suspected to have chronic pulmonary thromboembolism: Diagnostic accuracy of helical CT and conventional angiography. Radiology 1999; 213:743–9.

59. Kreitner KF, Ley S, Kauczor HU, et al. Chronic thromboembolic pulmonary hypertension: Pre- and postoperative assessment with breath-hold MR imaging techniques. Radiology 2004; 232:535–43.

60. Ley S, Kauczor HU, Heussel CP, et al. Value of contrast-enhanced MR angiography and helical CT angiography in chronic thromboembolic pulmonary hypertension. Eur Radiol 2003; 13:2365–71.

61. Fedullo PF, Auger WR, Moser KM, et al. Hemodynamic response to exercise in patients with chronic, major vessel thromboembolic pulmonary hypertension. Am Rev Respir Dis 1990; 141:A-890 (Abstract).

62. Auger WR, Fedullo PF, Moser KM, et al. Chronic major-vessel chronic thromboembolic pulmonary artery obstruction: Appearance of angiography. Radiology 1992; 182:393–8.

63. Pitton MB, Duber C, Mayer E, Thelen M. Hemodynamic effects of nonionic contrast bolus injection and oxygen inhalation during pulmonary angiography in patients with chronic major-vessel thromboembolic pulmonary hypertension. Circulation 1996; 94:2485–91.

64. Nicod P, Peterson K, Levine M, et al. Pulmonary angiography in severe chronic pulmonary hypertension. Ann Intern Med 1987; 107:565–8.

65. Shure D, Gregoratos G, Moser KM. Fiberoptic angioscopy: Role in the diagnosis of chronic pulmonary artery obstruction. Ann Intern Med 1985; 103:844–50.

66. Sompradeekul S, Fedullo PF, Kerr KM, et al. The role of pulmonary angioscopy in the preoperative assessment of patients with thromboembolic pulmonary hypertension (CTEPH). Am J Respir Crit Care Med 1999; 159:A-456 (Abstract).

67. Channick RN, Auger WR, Fedullo PF, et al. Angioscopy. in SH Feinsilver, AM Fein, eds. Textbook of Bronchoscopy. Philadelphia: Williams and Wilkins, 1995, pp. 477–485.

68. Fedullo PF, Auger WR, Channick RN, et al. Chronic thromboembolic pulmonary hypertension. Clin Chest Med 2001; 22:561–83.

69. Nakajima N, Masuda M, Mogi K. The surgical treatment for chronic pulmonary thromboembolism. Our experience and current review of the literature. Ann Thorac Cardiovasc Surg 1997; 3:15–21.

70. Mayer E, Kramm T, Dahm M, et al. Early results of pulmonary thromboendarterectomy in chronic thromboembolic pulmonary hypertension. Z Kardiol 1997; 86:920–7.

71. Gilbert TB, Gaine SP, Rubin LJ, Sequeira AJ. Short-term outcome and predictors of adverse events following pulmonary thromboendarterectomy. World J Surg 1998; 22:1029–32.

72. Miller WT, Osiason AW, Langlotz CP, Palevsky HI. Reperfusion edema after thromboendarterectomy: Radiographic patterns of disease. J Thorac Imag 1998; 13:178–83.

73. Dartevelle P, Fadel E, Chapelier A, et al. Angioscopic video-assisted pulmonary endarterectomy for post-embolic pulmonary hypertension. Eur J Cardiothorac Surg 1999; 16:38–43.

74. Mares P, Gilbert TB, Tschernko EM, et al. Pulmonary artery thromboendarterectomy: A comparison of two different postoperative treatment strategies. Anesth Analg 2000; 90:267–73.

75. Tscholl D, Langer F, Wendler O, et al. Pulmonary thromboendarterectomy—Risk factors for early survival and hemodynamic improvement. Eur J Cardiothorac Surg 2001; 19:771–6.

76. Hagl C, Khaladj N, Peters T, et al. Technical advances in pulmonary thromboendarterectomy for chronic thromboembolic pulmonary hypertension. Eur J Cardiothorac Surg 2003; 23:776–81.

77. Kafi SA, Mélot C, Vachiéry JL, Brimoulle S, Naeije R. Partitioning of the pulmonary vascular resistance in primary pulmonary hypertension. J Am Coll Cardiol 1998; 31:1372–6.

78. Fesler P, Pagnamenta A, Vachiery JL, et al. Single arterial occlusion to locate resistance in patients with pulmonary hypertension. Eur Respir J 2003; 21:31–6.

79. Kim NH, Fesler P, Channick RN, et al. Preoperative partitioning of pulmonary vascular resistance correlates with early outcome after thromboendarterectomy for chronic thromboembolic pulmonary hypertension. Circulation 2004; 109:18–22.

80. Hartz RS. Surgery for chronic thromboembolic pulmonary hypertension. World J Surg 1999; 23:1137–47.

81. Thistlethwaite PA, Auger WR, Madani MM, et al. Pulmonary thromboendarterectomy combined with other cardiac operations: Indications, surgical approach, and outcome. Ann Thorac Surg 2001; 72:13–9.

82. Zeebregts CJ, Dossche KM, Morshuis WJ, et al. Surgical thromboendarterectomy for chronic thrombembolic pulmonary hypertension using circulatory arrest with selective antegrade cerebral perfusion. Acta Chir Belg 1998; 98:95–7.

83. Zund G, Pretre R, Niederhauser U, et al. Improved exposure of the pulmonary arteries for thromboendarterectomy. Ann Thorac Surg 1998; 66:1821–3.

84. Dartevelle P, Fadel E, Mussot S, et al. Chronic thrombembolic pulmonary hypertension . Eur Respir J 2004; 23:637–48.

85. Kapelanski DP, Macoviak JA, Jamieson SW. Surgical interventions in the treatment of pulmonary embolism and chronic thromboembolic pulmonary hypertension. In M Oudkerk, EJR van Beels, JW Ten Cate, eds. Pulmonary Embolism. Berlin: Blackwell Science, 1999, pp. 382–397.

86. Fedullo PF, Auger WR, Dembitsky WP. Postoperative management of the patient undergoing pulmonary thromboendarterectomy. Sem Thorac Cardiovasc Surg 1999; 11:172–8.

87. Olman MA, Auger WR, Fedullo PF, et al. Pulmonary vascular steal in chronic thromboembolic pulmonary hypertension. Chest 1990; 98: 1430–4.

88. Moser KM, Metersky ML, Auger WR, et al. Resolution of vascular steal after pulmonary thromboendarterectomy. Chest 1993; 104:1441–4.

89. Levinson RM, Shure D, Moser KM. Reperfusion pulmonary edema after pulmonary artery thromboendarterectomy. Am Rev Respir Dis 1986; 134:1241–5.

90. Kerr KM, Auger WR, Marsh J, et al. The use of Cylexin (CY-1503) in prevention of reperfusion lung injury in patients undergoing pulmonary thromboendarterectomy. Am J Respir Crit Care Med 2000; 162:14–20.

91. *The Acute Respiratory Distress Syndrome Network.* Ventilation with lower tidal volumes as compared with traditional tidal volumes for acute lung injury and the acute respiratory distress syndrome. N Engl J Med 2000; 342:1301–8.

92. Dupont H, Le Corre F, Fierobe L, et al. Efficiency of inhaled nitric oxide as rescue therapy during severe ARDS: Survival and factors associated with the first response. J Crit Care 1999; 14:107–13.

93. Pinelli G, Mertes PM, Carteaux JP, et al. Inhaled nitric oxide as an adjunct to pulmonary thromboendarterectomy. Ann Thorac Surg 1996; 61:227–99.

94. Gardeback M, Larsen FF, Radegran K. Nitric oxide improves hypoxaemia following reperfusion oedema after pulmonary thromboendarterectomy. Br J Anaesth 1995; 75:798–800.

95. Troncy E, Collet JP, Shapiro S, et al. Inhaled nitric oxide in acute respiratory distress syndrome: A pilot randomized controlled study. Am J Respir Crit Care Med 1998; 157:1483–8.
96. Hartz RS, Byrne JG, Levitsky S, et al. Predictors of mortality in pulmonary thromboendarterectomy. Ann Thorac Surg 1996; 62:1255–9.
97. Birkmeyer JD, Siewers AE, Finlayson EV, et al. Hospital volume and surgical mortality in the United States. N Engl J Med 2002; 346:1128–37.
98. Birkmeyer JD, Stukel TA, Siewers AE, et al. Surgeon volume and operative mortality in the United States. N Engl J Med 2003; 349: 2117–27.
99. Lewczuk J, Piszko P, Jagas J, et al. Prognostic factors in medically treated patients with chronic pulmonary embolism. Chest 2001; 119:818–23.
100. Bresser P, Fedullo PF, Auger WR, et al. Continuous intravenous eporostenol for chronic thromboembolic pulmonary hypertension. Eur Respir J 2004; 23:595–600.
101. Ghofrani HA, Schermuly T, Rose F, et al. Sildenafil for long-term treatment of nonoperable chronic thromboembolic pulmonary hypertension. Am J Respir Crit Care Med 2003; 167:1139–41.

11 General Therapeutic Approach and Traditional Therapies

Nicholas S. Hill
and Elizabeth S. Klings

CONTENTS

INTRODUCTION
REVERSIBLE FACTORS CONTRIBUTING
  TO PULMONARY HYPERTENSION
SUMMARY
REFERENCES

Abstract

The availability of newer, effective agents to treat pulmonary hypertension should not cause clinicians to lose sight of the fact that many traditional therapies can still be useful. As part of the diagnostic evaluation, reversible contributing factors to pulmonary hypertension should be identified and treated as ways of palliating symptoms or even, in some cases, effectively treating the disease. Fluid overload, polycythemia, and hypoxemia are all factors that can be ameliorated, sometimes with dramatic symptomatic benefit. Treatment of presumed *in situ* thrombosis may slow progression of the disease. Sleep apnea and vasoconstriction can respond to appropriate therapy, sometimes with a near-curative effect. These factors should be sought with appropriate testing (sleep studies and vasoreactivity testing, respectively), because therapy can often bring substantial amelioration. Routinely seeking out and treating all potentially reversible factors should be considered one of the fundamental principles of managing pulmonary hypertension.

From: *Contemporary Cardiology: Pulmonary Hypertension*
Edited by: N. S. Hill and H. W. Farber © Humana Press, Totowa, NJ

Key Words: hypoxic vasoconstriction; calcium channel blocker therapy; diuretics; vasodilator therapy; polycythemia; pulmonary hypertension therapy; oxygen supplementation.

1. INTRODUCTION

Although the use of pulmonary vasodilators has revolutionized the treatment of pulmonary hypertension, the potential value of traditional therapies should not be overlooked. These therapies derive from the diagnostic evaluation, one purpose of which is to identify potentially reversible factors that might be contributing to the severity of pulmonary hypertension and symptoms. Factors such as volume overload, polycythemia, supraventricular arrythmias, hypoxemia, and vasoconstriction can be ameliorated, sometimes with dramatic effect. These therapies are often palliative, but they can achieve substantial symptomatic benefit. This chapter examines the use of traditional therapies to treat pulmonary hypertension, based on the findings of the diagnostic evaluation and guided by consensus recommendations or authors' opinion because little scientific evidence is available for guidance.

2. REVERSIBLE FACTORS CONTRIBUTING TO PULMONARY HYPERTENSION

2.1. Fluid Overload

Fluid overload is nearly universal in patients with advanced pulmonary hypertension, particularly if they have coexistent left ventricular disease. This occurs as compensation for diminishing cardiac output, in part via the increased release of aldosterone, promoting sodium retention by the kidney. Although the dilated heart secretes atrial and brain natriuretic hormones (ANP and BNP) that, in addition to their natriuretic actions, are pulmonary vasodilators and oppose the actions of aldosterone *(1)*, this is insufficient to maintain fluid homeostasis. As more fluid is retained, right-sided filling pressure increases, leading to the typical manifestations of lower extremity edema, ascites, and neck vein distention.

With further progression, the liver enlarges, more fluid accumulates in the legs and abdomen, and, eventually, anasarca ensues. When patients reach this stage, they become very symptomatic, feeling bloated because of the ascites and leg edema. Additionally, they become dyspneic with almost any exertion. Bowel edema may precipitate anorexia, malabsorption, and hypoproteinemia, which intensify the fluid overload. Patients may have accumulated 10 or more liters of excess fluid during this process, and diuretic administration can markedly ameliorate the symptoms and improve functional capacity.

To correct volume overload in patients with pulmonary hypertension, loop diuretics are the preferred initial agents because of their rapid onset of action and potency. Severely overloaded patients should be hospitalized and treated with intravenous diuretics, as bowel wall edema will prevent adequate intestinal absorption of these medications. Less severe cases can be treated on an outpatient basis with oral therapy. Patients with normal renal function can be started on 20 to 40 mg of furosemide, 1 mg of bumetanide, or 10 to 20 mg of torsemide daily (Table 1). Patients with renal insufficiency or who were previously taking diuretics may require higher initial doses. Patients should be asked to weigh themselves daily and return for frequent outpatient visits to assess the adequacy of fluid removal, symptomatic response, mobilization of edema and/or ascites, and reduced body weight. It is imperative to avoid overdiuresis, which can cause intravascular volume depletion and worsening renal function. As patients with pulmonary hypertension can be extremely preload-sensitive, systemic hypotension is another risk of reduced intravascular volume.

As patients are diuresed, renal function (BUN and creatinine) and electrolytes should be monitored, with attention to the development of prerenal azotemia, hypokalemia, and metabolic alkalosis. Also, at high doses of diuretics, magnesium may be depleted. Often, oral supplementation with potassium and less frequently, magnesium, is required to maintain electrolyte homeostasis. Adequate diuresis requires appropriate dose escalation of the chosen diuretic. The clinician should start with a dose at the lower end of the range and increase the dose until urine output is demonstrably increased. Giving a subtherapeutic diuretic dose twice a day is likely to be less successful than giving a dose that promotes adequate diuresis once daily. The choice among many possible dosage regimens depends mainly on the preference and experience of the clinician, but recommendations for furosemide, for example, set the maximal oral dosage in the range of 200 to 240 mg twice daily and for torsemide at approximately 200 mg daily (see Table 1).

If patients fail to respond adequately to a single loop diuretic, additional diuretics can be added to potentiate the diuretic effect. Hydrochlorothiazide at 25 to 50 mg daily or metolazone at 2.5 to 10 mg daily are popular choices, although metolazone appears to be more potent. Typically, metolazone will be administered 30 minutes prior to the dose of loop diuretic. Patients must be monitored closely for

intravascular volume and electrolyte depletion. Multiple consecutive days of such a combination are rarely needed and may be hazardous.

Potassium replacement is usually necessary with aggressive dosing of diuretics and should be guided by frequent testing of serum potassium levels. Rather than high doses of oral potassium, a potassium-sparing diuretic such as aldactone or triamterene can be added that might also potentiate the diuretic effect. Whether aldactone has any salutary effect on right ventricular function, as has been suggested for left ventricular function *(2)*, is unclear.

Several additional options are available for patients with recalcitrant fluid retention despite maximal outpatient therapy. In hospitalized patients, intravenous furosemide, either intermittently or by continuous infusion, may be used to induce diuresis (see Table 1). The continuous intravenous infusion is highly effective at inducing a diuresis, even in patients with renal insufficiency, and can avoid hypotension that may be a problem with intermittent high-dose therapy. If a low cardiac output state is suspected, inotropic therapy with dobutamine or milrinone may enhance diuresis. Patients with pulmonary hypertension secondary to congestive heart failure on maximal therapy may benefit from the addition of intravenous nesiritide (BNP), which can potentiate reductions in pulmonary arterial pressure and enhance cardiac output *(3)*. For patients with intractable ascites, intermittent paracentesis can be palliative, as can thoracenteses for refractory pleural effusions. Few studies have examined techniques for the optimal use of diuretics in patients with advanced pulmonary hypertension, but there is no question that adequate control of volume overload can greatly relieve symptoms for these patients.

2.2. Hypoxemia

Arterial hypoxemia commonly accompanies pulmonary hypertension. Sometimes the hypoxemia causes the pulmonary hypertension, such as when hypoventilation gives rise to sustained alveolar hypoxia, stimulating hypoxic pulmonary hypertension and the structural changes referred to as remodeling. These responses are thought to be the major ones predisposing to cor pulmonale (structural and/or functional changes of the right heart as a consequence of pulmonary hypertension due to respiratory abnormalities) (WHO Group 2). This form of pulmonary hypertension is usually relatively mild and responds at least partially to oxygen supplementation. In patients with reversible hypoventilation syndromes, such as those with chest-wall deformities or neuromuscular disease, augmentation of ventilation with nocturnal noninvasive ventilation can completely reverse the pulmonary hypertension, even without supplemental oxygen therapy *(4)*.

More often, though, the hypoxemia is secondary to shunts, ventilation–perfusion mismatch, diffusion limitation, low mixed venous O_2 saturation, or some combination of these mechanisms. The foramen ovale, an atrial aperture that is necessary for the fetal circulation but normally closes after birth, may remain patent in approximately 25% of normal individuals. A patent foramen ovale causes right-to-left shunting in pulmonary hypertension patients when the right atrial pressure exceeds the left atrial pressure. Hypoxemia caused by intracardiac shunting is not accompanied by alveolar hypoxia, however, and is a less potent stimulus for hypoxic vasoconstriction than alveolar hypoxia *(5)*. Accordingly, oxygen supplementation is less likely to ameliorate pulmonary hypertension in patients with intracardiac shunts than in patients with alveolar hypoxia, even though it is indicated in an attempt to minimize the adverse effects of hypoxemia on exercise capacity. Eisenmenger's syndrome denotes a congenital shunt such as an atrial or ventricular septal defect that gradually reverses direction from left to right to right to left as pulmonary pressures increase, sometimes causing profound hypoxemia that is recalcitrant to oxygen therapy.

Exercise-induced hypoxemia is common in pulmonary hypertension patients, even in those with normal oxygenation at rest, and has prognostic implications. The more severe the exercise-induced hypoxemia, the worse the prognosis *(7)*. Exercise-induced hypoxemia occurs in the setting of increased blood velocity that leads to a diffusion limitation and failure of oxygen tension to equilibrate across the alveolar capillary membrane. If cardiac output is low, the increased extraction of oxygen from the blood reduces the mixed venous oxygen saturation and widens the arteriovenous gradient. Nocturnal hypoxemia is also common, related to changes in breathing pattern or body position and possibly obstructive sleep apnea (see below).

Daytime oxygenation should be assessed in patients with pulmonary hypertension using rest and exercise oximetry. In some patients, exercise ability may be inadequate to induce hypoxemia. The addition of nocturnal oximetry to the diagnostic algorithm may be useful to detect patients with isolated nocturnal hypoxemia as well as those with underlying obstructive sleep apnea. Arterial blood gases should be measured if alveolar hypoventilation is suspected to determine the $PaCO_2$. Patients with suspected left-to-right shunts should undergo Doppler echocardiography. Transesophageal echography is more accurate in detecting such shunts than transthoracic. With intracardiac shunts, "bubbles" are seen in the left atrium within two or three heartbeats of saline injection, whereas with intrapulmonary shunts, such as arteriovenous malformations, bubbles are seen after four or five heartbeats.

Oxygen supplementation is recommended in hypoxemic patients with PAH "to maintain oxygen saturation >90% at all times" (6). Medicare guidelines permit coverage of supplemental oxygen if PaO_2 or O_2 saturation falls to or below 55 mm Hg or 88%, respectively, at rest, during exercise, or nocturnally (for more than 5 consecutive minutes), and to or below 60 mm Hg or 90% with evidence of dependent edema or other manifestations of cor pulmonale (most pulmonary hypertension patients qualify for this). Although oxygen therapy has not been shown to prolong survival in patients with pulmonary hypertension as it has in hypoxemic COPD patients, 100% oxygen has been shown to be a weak pulmonary vasodilator, lowering mean PA pressure from 56 to 53 mm Hg and pulmonary vascular resistance from 14 to 10.6 Wood units in a group of 23 patients with mixed forms of pulmonary hypertension (8). It also probably improves functional capacity, particularly in patients with exercise-induced hypoxemia.

Maintaining desirable levels of oxygenation in patients with pulmonary hypertension (i.e., >89%) can be very challenging, particularly in the presence of large shunts or during exercise in patients with exercise-induced hypoxemia. Although the typical supplementary O_2 rate is in the 2–4 L/min range, delivery of up to 20-L/min oxygen supplementation can be achieved in the home using multiple tank systems. Combining systems such as masks, nasal cannulae, and pendants can maximize FiO_2 in severely hypoxemic patients. In some patients, maintenance of O_2 saturations of >89% is impossible using noninvasive oxygen-supplementation systems, and exercise-induced oxygen desaturations to the low 80% range, or sometimes even lower, must be accepted if the patient is to be managed at home. These patients should receive continuous-flow oxygen supplementation because oxygen-conserving systems usually perform poorly in them.

Transtracheal oxygen is an alternative approach that supplies O_2 at rates as high as 12 L/min via a small-bore percutaneous intratracheal catheter and is more efficient than noninvasive O_2 delivery systems. However, many patients are reluctant to accept a percutaneous catheter, and no published data are available to guide its use in pulmonary hypertension patients. Furthermore, most patients with moderate to severe pulmonary hypertension take anticoagulants, which might exacerbate the bleeding problems that sometimes complicate transtracheal oxygen delivery.

In summary, although oxygen supplementation guidelines established for COPD patients are generally applied to patients with pulmonary hypertension, few data are available to establish the efficacy of this approach. Clinicians are encouraged to attempt to maintain O_2 saturations of at least 90% at all times to assure adequate saturation of hemoglobin. However, whether administration of O_2 supplementation to patients with hypoxemia limited to exercise or to sleep favorably alters prognosis or even exercise capacity is not known. Efforts to maintain O_2 saturations in the desired range in patients with severe shunting may be futile, so lower saturations may have to be accepted. Nevertheless, some of these patients, particularly those with congenital shunts, may tolerate the low saturations quite well for years.

2.3. Polycythemia

The viscosity of whole blood is a function of the hematocrit and, according to Poiseuille's law of fluid dynamics, is directly related to resistance (9). Physiological studies performed decades ago revealed that pulmonary vascular resistance rises markedly at high hematocrits. As demonstrated in isolated dog lungs (Fig. 1), pulmonary vascular

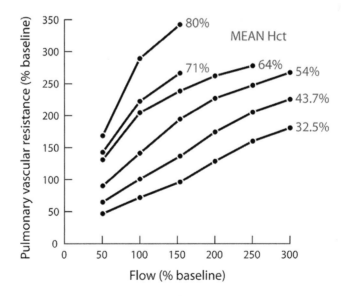

Fig. 1. Pulmonary vascular resistance (as percent of baseline) is shown as blood flow is increased (as percent of baseline) at different hematocrits in isolated dog lungs. Resistance is much higher at high hematocrits. [From reference (10), with permission.]

resistance virtually doubles when the hematocrit rises to 60% and triples at a hematocrit of 80% *(10)*.

These studies are based on acute manipulations of the hematocrit, but the effects of long-term alterations of the hematocrit may not parallel the acute effects. Erythropoietin given subcutaneously to rats for several weeks to increase the hematocrit failed to augment the effects of chronic hypoxia on pulmonary hemodynamics and right ventricular hypertrophy *(11)*. This was associated with a reduction in the severity of remodeling in peripheral pulmonary vessels compared to hypoxic controls, suggesting a compensatory release of an antiproliferative mediator, perhaps nitric oxide, in response to the high hematocrit *(12)*.

Clinicians have long recommended phlebotomy to lower the resistance if the hematocrit becomes too high *(13)*. This has been associated with improved cerebral blood flow and exercise capacity in patients with COPD *(14)*. The optimal hematocrit for patients with PAH has never been precisely determined and undoubtedly varies from individual to individual, but in the past, phlebotomy has been recommended at hematocrits exceeding 56%. Phlebotomy is rarely necessary today, however, because oxygen supplementation usually ameliorates hypoxemia sufficiently to avoid vigorous stimulation of erythropoietin release. In addition, repeated phlebotomy is now discouraged because it can lead to iron deficiency and microcytosis that can secondarily increase blood viscosity *(15)*.

2.4. In Situ *Thrombosis/Venous Thromboembolism*

Thromboses are found in the peripheral arteries of many patients with advanced PAH and are thought to be formed *in situ (16)*. These are hypothesized to result from a clotting disorder, either congenital or acquired, that underlies the pathogenesis of PAH. An alternative possible mechanism is a disruption of normal homeostatic mechanisms at the endothelial surface caused by endothelial cell injury. In the setting of increased pulmonary pressures and structural abnormalities, increased stasis within the pulmonary vasculature may further increase the propensity toward thrombus formation. Thromboses are thought to contribute to elevation of pulmonary vascular resistance and disease progression.

As right atrial pressure rises in the presence of moderate to severe pulmonary hypertension, stasis in the systemic venous circulation becomes a risk factor for venous thromboembolism. This raises the concern that even a small pulmonary embolism could be lethal when the pulmonary vascular resistance is already so elevated. A slight further increase could provoke hemodynamic collapse. Prevention of these potential complications—*in situ* thrombosis and pulmonary embolism—serves as the rationale for anticoagulation therapy for pulmonary hypertension.

Unfortunately, the appeal of the rationale to use anticoagulation in patients with PAH is not matched by the strength of the supporting evidence. Fuster et al. *(17)* performed a retrospective analysis of 120 patients with various forms of pulmonary hypertension and found that of those with available histopathology, 57% had evidence of thromboembolism. Furthermore, the use of anticoagulant therapy was associated with improved survival. Because of its retrospective design, however, the study was subject to selection bias. A prospective study by Rich et al. on patients with IPAH *(18)* also found that warfarin therapy was associated with improved survival during five years of follow-up, regardless of whether or not the response to concomitant calcium channel blocker therapy was favorable. In a third study *(19)*, 7 patients treated with warfarin combined with a vasodilator (isoproterenol or nifedipine) were compared with 13 untreated patients. The treated patients had significantly better survivals than the untreated ones. Although these studies support the idea that anticoagulation therapy is beneficial for patients with PAH, the lack of both randomization and a placebo group renders these data susceptible to a number of potential confounders and makes the drawing of definitive conclusions difficult. As of yet, no sufficiently powered randomized placebo controlled trial has demonstrated that anticoagulation therapy truly improves survival in PAH patients, and its benefit remains hypothetical.

Despite the limited evidence, warfarin anticoagulation is currently recommended for the therapy of idiopathic PAH (IPAH) and "should be considered" for other forms of PAH according to the ACCP consensus guidelines *(6)*. However, we would not recommend anticoagulation for patients with PAH related to sickle cell disease in light of the increased risk of intracerebral hemorrhage in this population. Of course, anticoagulation is clearly indicated for chronic thromboembolic pulmonary hypertension (WHO Group 4).

Despite the consensus supporting the use of anticoagulation for patients with PAH, many questions about specific applications are unanswered. For example, it is unclear whether patients with mild pulmonary hypertension should be treated, because the evidence of benefit was derived mainly from patients with more severe disease. It is also unknown whether patients with other forms of PAH besides IPAH, or those in other WHO diagnostic groups (excepting chronic thromboembolism), benefit. It is also unclear how much anticoagulation is sufficient, although slightly less than full anticoagulant doses—that is, international normalized ratios (INRs) ranging from 1.5 to 2.5— are commonly used. Pending the acquisition of more evidence, the authors' recommendations for the use of anticoagulation in patients with pulmonary hypertension are presented in Table 2.

2.5. Right Ventricular Dysfunction

Acute right heart dysfunction and its management are discussed in Chapter 17. The present discussion focuses on more gradual loss of right ventricular function in the face of chronic pulmonary hypertension. As pulmonary hypertension progresses, the right ventricle dilates and loses contractility, changes that are easily detectable with transthoracic echocardiography. Although higher PA pressures are associated with worse right ventricular function, there is marked variability among individuals related to the rapidity of progression of

Table 2
Recommendations on Use of Anticoagulation for PAH*

WHO Groups of Pulmonary Hypertension
  Group 1
    Idiopathic PAH (strongest recommendation)
    Familial PAH
    PAH related to connective tissue disease
      (caution if multiple telangiectasias or history of multiple epistaxes
      or gastrointestinal bleeding)
    Appetite-suppressant-related PAH
    HIV-related**
    Portopulmonary hypertension**
  Group 4
    Chronic thromboembolic pulmonary hypertension
Severity of Pulmonary Hypertension
  WHO functional class II or greater
  Moderate to severe pulmonary hypertension
    Mean PA pressure >30–35 mm Hg or
    Pulmonary vascular resistance >350–400 dyne/s^{-1}/cm^{-5}
Target International Normalized Ratio (INR)
  1.5 to 2.5

*Based on authors' opinion.
**Except in patients with bleeding diathesis.
Source: Adapted from N. Hill, Pulmonary Hypertension Therapy, Summit Publishers, New York, 2006.

the pulmonary hypertension and poorly understood factors governing the ability of the right ventricle to remodel in the setting of elevated end-diastolic pressures. Some patients present with severe right ventricular dilatation and dysfunction in the face of only modest elevations of pressures; others may sustain normal right ventricular size and function despite systemic-level pulmonary arterial pressures.

Although the most effective way to restore right ventricular function is to reduce the pressure overload by decreasing the pulmonary hypertension, this is not always achievable. If the pulmonary hypertension and right ventricular dysfunction remain severe, some clinicians use digoxin to enhance contractility and, for patients taking calcium channel blockers, to protect the ventricle against the negative inotropic effects (20). In experimental animals, digoxin has a weak pulmonary vasoconstrictor effect, and evidence demonstrating benefit in advanced pulmonary hypertension, in either animal models or clinical settings, is virtually nonexistent (21). In a study of 17 PAH patients with right ventricular failure, digoxin increased cardiac output (3.5 to 3.8 L/min) and ANP levels and lowered norepinephrine levels two hours after intravenous administration (19). The authors concluded that the use of digoxin "is warranted" in pulmonary hypertension patients with right heart failure.

However, the ACCP Clinical Practice Guidelines Committee chose not to discuss the use of digoxin for pulmonary hypertension (6). Thus, the use of digoxin to treat right ventricular dysfunction in the face of recalcitrant severe pulmonary hypertension must be considered optional, and a clearer indication in the face of pulmonary hypertension would be to use it for rate control in patients with atrial fibrillation. If digoxin is to be used, avoidance of toxicity is of paramount importance, particularly in patients with coexistent renal insufficiency. Doses exceeding 0.125 mg daily would be inadvisable in patients with low cardiac output states whose renal perfusion might be compromised.

2.6. Sleep-Disordered Breathing

Sleep-disordered breathing is very prevalent in the United States, with estimates ranging up to 24% of the older male population. Conservative estimates place the prevalence at 4% of adult males and 2% of adult females (22). Consisting of frank apneas, partially obstructing hypopneas, and respiratory event-related arousals, sleep-disordered breathing has been associated with an increased prevalence of comorbidities, including systemic hypertension, myocardial infarction, and strokes (23). An association between obstructive sleep apnea (OSA) and pulmonary hypertension has also been posited, presumably because the intermittent nocturnal hypoxia stimulates hypoxic vasoconstriction.

The prevalence of pulmonary hypertension among patients with OSA has been reported to range from 17% to 52%, but most of these studies have been limited by relatively small sample size and an excessively liberal criterion for defining pulmonary hypertension (i.e., a mean PA pressure $\geq$ 20 mm Hg) *(24)*. Some of the studies have included patients with obesity and underlying lung disease and have found an association between the presence of pulmonary hypertension and higher body mass index, higher $PaCO_2$, lower PaO_2, and worse FEV1 *(24)*. This has led to the speculation that the association between pulmonary hypertension and sleep-disordered breathing is mainly due to an "overlap" syndrome *(25)*. Furthermore, in some studies, the pulmonary hypertension of OSA patients has been associated primarily with left ventricular diastolic dysfunction *(26)*, thought to be related to endothelial dysfunction and systemic hypertension seen in many patients with obstructive sleep apnea.

Thus, unless patients have severe sleep apnea associated with sustained alveolar hypoventilation, or there are significant comorbidities such as severe chronic obstructive pulmonary disease, OSA is thought to lead mainly to mild pulmonary hypertension, occasionally moderate and only rarely severe. In one series of 100 consecutive OSA patients undergoing right heart catheterization, 42 had mean PA pressure greater than 20 mm Hg, but only approximately 10% had mean PA pressures higher than 40 mm Hg and only one patient's exceeded 50 mm Hg *(27)* (Fig. 2).

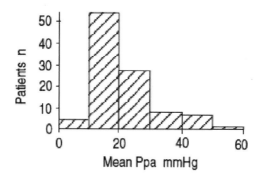

Fig. 2. Distribution of mean pulmonary artery pressures (P_{PA}) determined by pulmonary artery catheterization in 100 consecutive patients referred to a Sleep Disorders Center and found to have respiratory disturbance indices (RDI) > 20/hr. [From reference *(27)*, with permission.]

Conversely, patients with PAH are thought to have an increased incidence of associated OSA. However, one widely quoted study *(28)* observed a prevalence of 77% of patients having nocturnal oxygen desaturations, but actual apneas/hypopneas were rare. Nocturnal desaturations were associated with a lower baseline FEV_1 and resting oxygenation as well as greater alveolar-arterial oxygen gradients. Based on these observations, current recommendations are to perform nocturnal polysomnography in all PAH patients suspected of having OSA. Given that nocturnal oxygen desaturations are so common and may just be a reflection of pulmonary hypertension, screening nocturnal oximetry can be done as an initial study, but the sensitivity of this study for sleep-disordered breathing has not been established and findings are likely to be nonspecific. A "sawtooth" pattern on nocturnal oximetry suggests intermittent apneas and would indicate that a formal sleep study be obtained. Polysomnography is necessary to diagnose, characterize, and grade the severity of sleep-disordered breathing in PAH patients. Recommendations for a sleep evaluation in patients with PAH are summarized in Table 3.

Continuous positive airway pressure (CPAP) to treat OSA in patients with pulmonary hypertension reduced mean PA pressure from 25.6 to 19.5 mm Hg after six months of therapy in one study *(29)*. Patients with cor pulmonale related to diurnal hypoventilation and alveolar hypoxemia may have dramatic responses to CPAP after resolution of their hypoventilation and adequate oxygenation for several months. In some cases, the signs and symptoms of cor pulmonale resolve completely. Hypoventilation observed in these patients, often related to obesity hypoventilation syndrome, may not resolve with CPAP alone, however. Bilevel, noninvasive, positive pressure ventilation with relatively high inspiratory pressures or even tracheostomy ventilation may be necessary. Although CPAP is clearly the initial therapy of choice for OSA in patients with pulmonary hypertension, the response to CPAP of patients with severe PAH who have only mild to moderate OSA has never been formally studied. Anecdotally, however, their pulmonary hypertension is usually minimally responsive to CPAP therapy, suggesting that the OSA is not a significant contributing factor.

2.7. Pulmonary Vasoconstriction

2.7.1. Vasodilator Therapy

During the 1950s, Dresdale et al. *(30)* reported acute vasodilatory responses to the alpha blocker tolazoline in patients with "primary" pulmonary hypertension and speculated that pulmonary

Table 3
Recommendations for Sleep Evaluation in Patients Presenting with Pulmonary Hypertension

---

Presence of Risk Factors for Nocturnal Oxygen Desaturation
 Daytime hypoxemia (resting or exercise-induced)
 Pulmonary dysfunction (moderate or severe obstruction or restriction)
 Nocturnal desaturations very common in PAH; reported in up to 77%
  of patients *(28)*

Indications for Nocturnal Oximetry*
 If daytime resting O_2 sat ≤ 89%, prescribe round-the-clock oxygen
  supplementation Oximetry during exercise and nocturnally useful in
  titrating O_2 rate**
 If exercise-induced desaturation only, nocturnal oximetry useful in
  determining
  O_2 needs at night
 If "sawtooth" pattern (repeated intermittent dips) or other risk
  factors for sleep apnea, do nocturnal polysomnogram

Presence of Risk Factors for Obstructive Sleep Apnea
 History of snoring
 Daytime hypersomnolence
 Witnessed apneas
 Systemic hypertension
 Obesity (BMI > 30)
 Older age

Indications for Full Polysomnogram
 Any risk factors for sleep apnea
 "Sawtooth" pattern on nocturnal oximetry

---

 *Sensitivity and specificity of nocturnal oximetry in pulmonary hypertension patients have not been established, and study may be difficult to arrange because of low reimbursement rates.

 **Oximetry during oxygen supplementation is most useful in prescribing O_2 supplementation rate.

vasoconstriction was an important contributor to the pathophysiology of pulmonary hypertension. However, advances in therapy awaited the development of more effective oral vasodilators. In 1980, Rubin and Peter *(31)* raised hopes for more effective therapy when they reported on four patients with IPAH who responded acutely to hydralazine and had sustained benefit for several months, taking the drug orally four times daily. Over the subsequent decade, more reports appeared of patients responding favorably to one vasodilator drug or another. The list of such drugs lengthened, including beta- and alpha-antagonists, nitrates, angiotensin-converting enzyme inhibitors, centrally acting systemic vasodilators, and calcium channel blockers. Virtually all the reports consisted of short-term, uncontrolled, anecdotal series, usually demonstrating favorable acute pulmonary hemodynamic responses. The agents lacked specificity for the pulmonary circulation, often resulting in systemic hypotension, and longer-term outcomes were usually disappointing.

2.7.2. CALCIUM CHANNEL BLOCKER THERAPY

Reports began appearing during the late 1980s suggesting that calcium channel blockers might offer unique benefit to some patients with IPAH. In 1992, a seminal article by Rich et al. *(18)* demonstrated that patients who responded acutely to calcium channel blockers had excellent long-term survivals. In their study of 64 IPAH patients, 17 (26%) responded acutely to calcium channel blockers with PA pressures and pulmonary vascular resistances that dropped at least 20% (average decreases 39% for mean PA pressure and 53% for pulmonary vascular resistance). Responders were continued on high-dose calcium channel blocker therapy (average dose: 172 mg/day of nifedipine and 720 mg/day of diltiazem). After five years, 94% of the responders were still alive, compared with only 55% of the nonresponders ($p = 0.003$) (Fig. 3). The survival among responders was also much better than among physiologically matched patients in the National Institutes of Health Registry *(32)*. These results offered new hope for patients with this heretofore virtually untreatable disease.

The findings also encouraged the performance of acute vasodilator trials during right heart catheterizations using calcium channel blockers to determine which patients should receive subsequent therapy with long-term high-dose calcium channel blocker therapy. Although this aggressive approach identified potential responders to long-term therapy, it was also potentially hazardous, because some patients experienced recalcitrant systemic hypotension and died, and some of those discharged on oral calcium channel blocker therapy had sudden deaths soon thereafter *(33)*.

Subsequently, the clinical availability of intravenous epoprostenol, intravenous adenosine, and inhaled nitric oxide (NO) during the late 1990s provided a quicker and safer means of testing acute pulmonary vasoreactivity than with the calcium channel blockers. Sitbon et al. *(34)* demonstrated that inhaled NO could be used as a screening agent to test for possible calcium channel blocker responsiveness. Among 33 patients undergoing right heart catheterizations, 10 had decreases of at least 20% in both mean PA pressure and pulmonary vascular

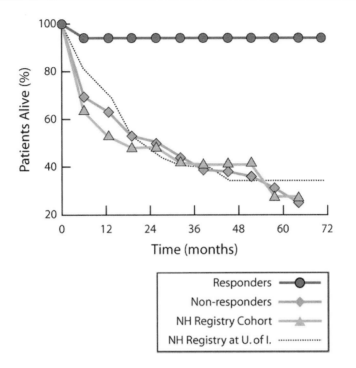

Fig. 3. Survival is shown among patients responding to calcium channel blocker therapy compared to those who failed to respond and the survival of the NIH Registry cohort and the NIH Registry cohort followed at the University of Illinois, where the study was performed. Patients who responded to calcium channel blockers had excellent survivals. [From reference *(18)*, with permission.]

resistance in response to inhaled NO. Of these, nine responded to calcium channel blockers acutely and six (19% of total) had favorable long-term responses. Of the remaining 23 patients, none responded to calcium channel blockers or NO. Also, 38% of patients had serious adverse events in response to the acute challenge with calcium channel blockers, whereas none had adverse events with inhaled NO. This important study demonstrated that short-acting vasodilator agents could effectively and safely screen for the responsiveness of calcium channel blockers.

More recently, Sitbon et al. *(35)* reported on the characteristics and prevalence of IPAH patients who manifest long-term responses to calcium channel blocker therapy, based on a population of 557 patients referred to a pulmonary vascular disease center in France. Of these, 70 (12.6%) had decreases in mean PA pressure and pulmonary vascular resistance of >20%. These responders were given long-term calcium channel blockers; after at least one year, only 38 (6.8%) had long-term improvement as evidenced by a functional capacity of class I or II on calcium channel blocker monotherapy. After an average of seven years of follow-up, only 1 of these 38 responders had died. Of note, the long-term responders had less severe pulmonary hypertension at baseline and, in response to acute vasoreactivity testing, had greater decreases in mean PA pressure than nonresponders (39% vs. 26%) to lower absolute mean values (33 vs. 46 mm Hg). These observations confirm that long-term responders to calcium channel blockers have excellent survivals but also that they are much less common (5–10% of IPAH cases) than originally thought. These findings also serve as the foundation for the current ACCP recommendation that a favorable response to an acute vasodilator challenge be defined as a fall in mean PA pressure of at least 10 mm Hg to an absolute pressure of ≤40 mm Hg *(6)*.

This additional evidence has dimmed the initial enthusiasm for calcium channel blockers as a potential therapy for IPAH. In patients with severe pulmonary hypertension, these drugs have potentially lethal side effects (systemic hypotension) and must be used with extreme caution. They should not be used for acute vasodilator testing, and the high, aggressive dosing regimen based on the Rich study *(18)* is no longer recommended. It is now clear that calcium channel blockers are beneficial for only a small minority of patients. These patients should still be sought using acute vasodilator trials because of the potential for such favorable responses, but calcium channel blocker therapy should be reserved only for those manifesting responses that meet the ACCP criteria, and even then, doses should be increased gradually and cautiously over weeks.

The role of calcium channel blocker therapy in forms of PAH besides idiopathic has never been adequately assessed. Interestingly, patients with connective tissue disease are often already taking calcium channel blockers for their Raynaud's phenomenon when they present with PAH. Obviously, the calcium channel blocker therapy in these patients failed to prevent the development of PAH, but whether it prevents PAH in some patients is unclear. Patients with connective tissue disease are thought to be less likely to have a "significant" acute vasodilator response during right heart catheterization than IPAH patients, and long-term favorable responses to calcium channel blockers are considered to be very unusual in connective tissue disease patients with PAH. For these reasons, enthusiasm is low for using calcium channel blockers to treat forms of pulmonary hypertension other than idiopathic. Also, as more effective alternative therapies have been introduced, the role for calcium channel blockers in the therapy of pulmonary hypertension has continued to diminish.

Currently, the best candidates for calcium channel blocker therapy are class II to III IPAH patients who manifest a significant response to acute vasodilator testing and are clinically stable with adequate systemic blood pressure (Table 4). Obviously, these criteria apply to those not already being treated with calcium channel blockers.

Table 4
Recommendations for Vasodilator Testing and Use of Calcium Channel Blockers in PAH

Vasoreactivity Testing
  Indication
    IPAH patients undergoing right heart catheterization who are
      candidates for calcium channel blocker therapy (see below)
  Not indicated
    Calcium channel blocker not being considered
    Systemic blood pressure too low (<90–100 systolic)
    Class IV or III progressing over prior few months
    Already receiving calcium channel blocker therapy for other process
  Recommended agents and doses for vasoreactivity testing
    Inhaled nitric oxide (10–20 parts per minute for 10 minutes)
    Intravenous epoprostenol, increasing from 2 to 6–10 ng/kg/min by
      increments of 2 ng/kg/min every 10 minutes as tolerated*
    Intravenous adenosine 20 μ g/min, increasing by increments of
      20 μ g/min every 2 minutes as tolerated* or to a maximum of
      200 μ g/min
    Significant response to vasodilators
    Drop in mean PA pressure by $\geq$ 10 mm Hg to $\leq$ 40 mm Hg
Calcium Channel Blocker Therapy
  Indication
    Significant vasodilator response during acute testing
    Adequate systemic blood pressure
    Class I, II, or III stable over previous few months
  Agents and daily doses (start at lower doses and gradually increase
    depending on symptomatic response and tolerance)
      Nifedipine 30–240 mg
      Diltiazem 120–360 mg
      Amlodipine 5–10 mg
      Verapamil—not recommended because of negative inotropic effect

* May develop flushing, nausea, headache, restlessness.
Source: Adapted from N. Hill, Pulmonary Hypertension Therapy, Summit Publishers, New York, 2006.

The agents used most commonly in clinical practice are diltiazem, nifedipine, and amlodipine, although no direct comparisons have been made between agents. Diltiazem is preferred for patients needing rate control (such as those with chronic atrial fibrillation), and verapamil is avoided in light of its greater negative inotropic effects. Patients started on calcium channel blockers should be given a trial over several months, with frequent monitoring of symptoms, functional capacity, echocardiograms, and, possibly, BNP levels. If no improvement is apparent, additional or alternative therapy should be contemplated. Regarding vasoreactivity testing, although the ACCP Guidelines Committee recommended testing of all PAH patients, our opinion is that there is no need for acute vasodilator testing in patients who are not being contemplated for new calcium channel blocker therapy (i.e., unstable class III and IV patients or those already receiving calcium channel blockers).

2.8. Pulmonary Vascular Remodeling

Remodeling—the vessel-wall thickening and other related structural changes observed in patients with longstanding pulmonary hypertension—is receiving increasing attention as a potential therapeutic target (36). The belief is that the key to controlling the disease long-term is to learn how to prevent and even reverse remodeling as this is much more important to disease pathology than vasoconstriction. Intensive research is now aimed at understanding the remodeling process and learning ways to manipulate intracellular pathways regulating proliferation and apoptosis. The newer agents recently introduced to treat PAH, as well as many others currently undergoing investigation, have the ability to inhibit the remodeling process. A thorough discussion of this topic is beyond the scope of this chapter and is examined in more detail in subsequent chapters.

2.9. Deconditioning

The exercise intolerance of patients with PAH is clearly related to the limited capacity to increase cardiac output due to pulmonary vascular disease, but other factors like deconditioning often contribute, as well. In a prospective, randomized trial, 30 patients with PAH or chronic thromboembolic pulmonary hypertension were randomized to undergo exercise training with standard medical therapy or standard medical therapy alone (controls) (37). After 15 weeks, the exercise training group increased the 6 minute walk distance by 111 m compared to controls, and experienced greater improvements in quality of life,

WHO functional class and peak oxygen uptake. There were no changes in the severity of PAH or in medical therapy. These data highlight the potential therapeutic value of pulmonary rehabilitation programs in rehabilitating patients with PAH.

3. SUMMARY

The availability of newer, effective agents to treat pulmonary hypertension should not cause physicians to lose sight of the fact that many traditional therapies can still be useful. As part of the diagnostic evaluation, reversible contributing factors to pulmonary hypertension should be identified and treated as ways of palliating symptoms or even, in some cases, effectively treating the disease. Fluid overload, polycythemia, and hypoxemia are all factors that can be ameliorated, sometimes with dramatic symptomatic benefit. Treatment of presumed *in situ* thrombosis may slow progression of the disease. Sleep apnea and vasoconstriction can respond to appropriate therapy, sometimes with a near-curative effect. These factors should be sought with appropriate testing (sleep studies and vasoreactivity testing, respectively), because therapy can often bring amelioration. Routinely seeking out and treating all potentially reversible factors should be considered one of the fundamental principles of managing pulmonary hypertensive diseases.

REFERENCES

1. Moro C, Berlan M. Cardiovascular and metabolic effects of natriuretic peptides. Fundam Clin Pharmacol 2006; 20:41–9.
2. Marcy TR, Ripley TL. Aldosterone antagonists in the treatment of heart failure. Am J Health Syst Pharm 2006; 63:49–58.
3. O'Dell KM, Kalus JS, Kucukarslan S, Czerska B. Nesiritide for secondary pulmonary hypertension in patients with end-stage heart failure. Am J Health Syst Pharm 2005; 62:606–9.
4. Mehta S, Hill NS. Noninvasive ventilation. Am J Respir Crit Care Med 2001; 163:540–77.
5. Hauge A. Hypoxia and pulmonary vascular resistance. The relative effects of pulmonary arterial and alveolar PO_2. Acta Physiol Scand 1969; 76: 121–30.
6. Badesch DB, Abman SH, Ahearn GS, Barst RJ, McCrory DC, Simonneau G, McLaughlin VV; American College of Chest Physicians. Medical therapy for pulmonary arterial hypertension: ACCP evidence-based clinical practice guidelines. Chest 2004; 126(1 Suppl):35S–62S.
7. Paciocco G, Martinez FJ, Bossone E, Pielsticker E, Gillespie B, Rubenfire M. Oxygen desaturation on the six-minute walk test and

mortality in untreated primary pulmonary hypertension. Eur Respir J 2001; 17:647–52.

8. Roberts DH, Lepore JJ, Maroo A, Semigran MJ, Ginns LC. Oxygen therapy improves cardiac index and pulmonary vascular resistance in patients with pulmonary hypertension. Chest 2001; 120:1547–55.

9. Roos A. Poiseuille's law and its limitations in vascular systems. Med Thorac 1962; 19:224–38.

10. Murray JF, Karp RB, Nadel JA. Viscosity effects on pressure-flow relations and vascular resistance in dogs' lungs. J Appl Physiol 1969; 27:336–41.

11. Petit RD, Warburton RR, Ou LC, Brinck-Johnson T, Hill NS. Exogenous erythropoietin fails to augment hypoxic pulmonary hypertension in rats. Respir Physiol 1993; 91:261–70.

12. Petit RD, Warburton RR, Ou LC, Hill NS. Pulmonary vascular adaptation to augmented polycythemia during chronic hypoxia. J Appl Physiol 1995; 79:229–35.

13. Klinger JR, Hill NS. Right ventricular dysfunction in chronic obstructive pulmonary disease: Evaluation and management. Chest 1991; 99:715–23.

14. Bornstein R, Menon D, York E, Sproule B, Zak C. Effects of venesection on cerebral function in chronic lung disease. Can J Neurol Sci 1980; 7:293–6.

15. DeFilippis AP, Law K, Curtin S, Eckman JR. Blood is thicker than water: The management of hyperviscosity in adults with cyanotic heart disease. Cardiol Rev 2007; 15:31–4.

16. Wagenvoort CA, Mulder PG. Thrombotic lesions in primary plexogenic arteriopathy. Similar pathogenesis or complication? Chest 1993; 103: 844–9.

17. Fuster V, Steele PM, Edwards WD, Gersh BJ, McGoon MD, Frye RL. Primary pulmonary hypertension: Natural history and the importance of thrombosis. Circulation 1984; 70:580–7.

18. Rich S, Kaufmann E, Levy PS. The effect of high doses of calcium-channel blockers on survival in primary pulmonary hypertension. N Engl J Med 1992; 327:76–81.

19. Ogata M, Ohe M, Shirato K, Takishima T. Effects of a combination therapy of anticoagulant and vasodilator on the long-term prognosis of primary pulmonary hypertension. Jap Circ J 1993; 57:63–9.

20. Rich S, Seidlitz M, Dodin E, Osimani D, Judd D, Genthner D, McLaughlin V, Francis G. The short-term effects of digoxin in patients with right ventricular dysfunction from pulmonary hypertension. Chest 1998; 114:787–92.

21. Heerdt PM, Caldwell RW. The cardiovascular response to digoxin in conscious dogs with left atrial obstruction. J Cardiothorac Anesth 1990; 4:687–94.

22. Young T, Palta M, Dempsey J, et al. The occurrence of sleep-disordered breathing among middle-aged adults. N Engl J Med 1993; 328:1230–5.

23. Collop NA. Obstructive sleep apnea syndromes. Sem Respir Crit Care Med 2005; 26:13–24.

24. Atwood CW, McCrory D, Garcia JCN, Abman SH, Ahearn GS. Pulmonary artery hypertension and sleep-disordered breathing: ACCP evidence-based practice guidelines. Chest 2004; 126:72S–77S.

25. Apprill M, Weitzenblum E, Krieger J, Oswald M, Kurtz D. Frequency and mechanism of daytime pulmonary hypertension in patients with obstructive sleep apnoea syndrome. Cor Vasa 1991; 33:42–9.

26. Fung JW, Li TS, Choy DK, et al. Severe obstructive sleep apnea is associated with left ventricular diastolic dysfunction. Chest 2002; 121:422–9.

27. Laks L, Lehrhaft B, Grunstein RR, Sullivan CE. Pulmonary hypertension in obstructive sleep apnoea. Eur Respir J 1995; 8:537–41.

28. Rofanan AL, Golish JA, Dinner DS, et al. Nocturnal hypoxemia is common in pulmonary hypertension. Chest 2001; 120:894–9.

29. Alchanatis M, Tourkohoriti G, Kakouris S, et al. Daytime pulmonary hypertension in patients with obstructive sleep apnea. Respiration 2001; 68:566–72.

30. Dresdale DT, Michtom RF, Schultz M. Recent studies in primary pulmonary hypertension including pharmacodynamic observations on pulmonary vascular resistance. Bull NY Acad Med 1954; 30:195–207.

31. Rubin LJ, Peter RH. Oral hydralazine therapy for primary pulmonary hypertension. N Engl J Med 1980 Jan 10; 302(2):69–73.

32. Rich S, Dantzker DR, Ayres SM, et al. Primary pulmonary hypertension. A national prospective study. Ann Intern Med 1987; 107:216–23.

33. Farber HW, Karlinsky JB, Faling LJ. Fatal outcome following nifedipine for pulmonary hypertension. Chest 1983; 83:708–9.

34. Sitbon O, Humbert M, Jogot TL, et al. Inhaled nitric oxide as a screening agent for safely identifying responders to oral calcium channel blockers in primary pulmonary hypertension. Eur Respir J 1998; 12:265–70.

35. Sitbon O, Humbert M, Jais X, et al. Long-term response to calcium channel blockers in idiopathic pulmonary arterial hypertension. Circulation 2005; 111:3105–11.

36. Ito T, Ozawa K, Shimada K. Current drug targets and future therapy of pulmonary arterial hypertension. Curr Med Chem 2007; 14:719–33.

37. Mereles D, Eheken N, Kreuscher S, et al. Exercise and respiratory training improve exercise capacity and quality of life in patients with severe chronic pulmonary hypertension. Circulation 2006; 114:1448–9.

12 Prostacyclin Therapy for Pulmonary Arterial Hypertension

Nicholas S. Hill, Todd F. Vardas, and Vallerie McLaughlin

CONTENTS

INTRODUCTION
PHARMACOLOGICAL ACTIONS OF
   PROSTACYCLIN
CLINICAL APPLICATIONS OF PROSTACYLINS
SUMMARY
REFERENCES

Abstract

The first class of agents approved specifically for the therapy of pulmonary hypertension in the United States, the prostacyclins have assumed a key treatment role, especially via the intravenous route for class IV patients. The best established agent for efficacy and the only one shown to significantly improve survival is epoprostenol via continuous intravenous infusion. Epoprostenol also improves symptoms, exercise capacity, and pulmonary hemodynamics in IPAH patients. While the literature is not as voluminous in patients with PAH associated with other disorders, epoprostenol therapy improves the symptoms of PAH in many of these patients. Enthusiasm for epoprostenol must be tempered by its cumbersome intravenous delivery system and inherent risks. Newer prostacyclins include treprostinil, available in subcutaneous and intravenous forms, and inhaled iloprost. Each has established efficacy in randomized trials. Subcutaneous treprostinil has been plagued by infusion site pain but is a good

From: *Contemporary Cardiology: Pulmonary Hypertension*
Edited by: N. S. Hill and H. W. Farber © Humana Press, Totowa, NJ

alternative for those who can tolerate it. Inhaled iloprost is being used increasingly because the inhaled route has fewer systemic side effects and improves oxygenation compared to the intravenous route, and an improved administration system makes it more tolerable for patients. Whichever of the prostacyclins is chosen, patients are monitored closely thereafter because of the many potential complications and since most forms require timely dose increases because of tolerance.

Key Words: prostacyclin; epoprostenol; intravenous therapy; treprostinil; iloprost; beraprost; inhaled therapy; subcutaneous therapy; pulmonary hypertension pharmacotherapy.

1. INTRODUCTION

In order to frame an approach to treating pulmonary arterial hypertension (PAH), it may be helpful to contemplate the ideal therapy. In addition to alleviating the symptoms of PAH, including dyspnea, edema, and fatigue, and restoring functional capacity, the therapy would reverse the underlying vascular remodeling, thrombosis, and vascular damage, prevent myocardial dysfunction, and allow for repair of the hypertrophied myocardium. Its effects would be limited to the pulmonary vasculature, and it would be simple to administer, inexpensive, and without significant side effects or drug-drug interactions. While this ideal therapy is not yet available, the past decade has brought us closer to its realization.

Based on the imbalance of the prostaglandin metabolites prostacyclin and thromboxane that favors vasoconstriction in patients with primary pulmonary hypertension (1), now referred to as idiopathic pulmonary arterial hypertension (IPAH), investigators hypothesized that providing exogenous prostacyclin (PGI_2) to IPAH patients would be beneficial. Epoprostenol, the first prostacyclin to be studied for the treatment of IPAH in randomized, controlled trials (2,3), received Food and Drug Administration (FDA) approval for the treatment of IPAH in 1995 and for the treatment of PAH related to the scleroderma spectrum of diseases (SSD) in 1999 (4). Epoprostenol has also been used to treat PAH associated with other disorders including congenital heart disease (CHD) (5), human immunodeficiency virus (HIV) (6), portal hypertension (7), and distal thromboembolic disease (8), although these latter diseases have not been as rigorously studied. To date, epoprostenol has the longest track record and is the most thoroughly studied of the medications approved for the treatment of PAH. Despite its inherent complications and side effects, epoprostenol ameliorates symptoms in most PAH patients and is the only therapy shown to significantly prolong survival (3).

Randomized, controlled trials and cohort studies have established epoprostenol as a safe and effective therapy for PAH, and they permit a rational approach to the selection of patients who will derive the greatest benefit. Less information is available for other prostacyclins, but randomized, controlled trials have been performed, leading to FDA approval of subcutaneous treprostinil to treat class II to IV PAH subcutaneously in 2001 and intravenously in late 2004, and of iloprost as an inhaled agent in 2005. Oral beraprost failed to gain approval by the FDA after a 12-month, randomized, controlled trial showed no sustained benefit *(9)*.

This chapter reviews the pharmacology of PGI_2 and the results of salient studies pertaining to epoprostenol, treprostinil, iloprost, and beraprost in the therapy of PAH. It also examines practical aspects of dosing, follow-up monitoring, and long-term treatment goals.

2. PHARMACOLOGICAL ACTIONS OF PROSTACYCLIN

Prostacyclin [prostaglandin I_2 (PGI_2)] was first described in 1976 *(10)* by the Nobel prize-winning group led by Sir John Vane as a vasodilator product of cyclo-oxygenase-1-mediated arachidonic metabolism. In the pulmonary circulation, prostacyclin functions as an endogenous autoregulator, helping to maintain the low resistance of pulmonary vessels *(11)*. Prostacyclin is rapidly metabolized in the systemic circulation, with a half-life of only minutes. The synthesis of prostacyclin decreases in proportion to the diameter of the pulmonary vessel *(12)* and is thought to be regulated neurohumorally via control of the cholinergic system. Prostacyclins are synthesized from arachidonic acid-derived linoleic/cell membrane precursors via the phospholipase A2, cyclooxygenase, and peroxidase pathways *(13)*. Prostacyclin binds to specific cell membrane receptors, stimulating adenylate cyclase to increase intracellular cAMP. By virtue of its vasodilator actions, prostacyclin has numerous extrapulmonary effects, including blunting of systemic vasoconstriction induced by sympathetic nerve stimulation and angiotensin II release in hemorrhagic shock models, and inhibition of gastric acid secretion from the gastric mucosa *(14)*.

Levels of prostacyclin, prostaglandin synthase, and thromboxane are abnormal in patients with pulmonary hypertension *(1)*. Urinary excretion of 11-dehydro-thromboxane A_2 and 2,3-dinor-6-keto-prostaglandin-1 α, the stable metabolites of the vasoconstrictor prostaglandin, thromboxane A_2, and prostacyclin, respectively, are significantly altered in PAH patients. Urinary thromboxane metabolite levels are higher (3,224–5,392 pg/mg Cr vs. 1,145 pg/mg Cr), whereas prostacyclin metabolites are decreased (304–369 pg/mg Cr vs. 644 pg/mg Cr) in patients with PAH compared to normal controls, and the ratio of vasoconstrictor to vasodilator metabolites is much higher in patients than in normal controls *(1)*. In addition, prostacyclin synthase, measured by western blot, was absent in four patients with PAH, CREST, or congenital heart disease as compared to two normal controls *(15)*. The percentage of arteries expressing prostacyclin synthase was also decreased throughout large, medium-sized, and small pulmonary arteries in patients with PAH as compared to controls *(15)*.

Platelet abnormalities and a prothrombotic state also contribute to the pathogenesis of PAH, with highly abnormal platelet function detectible in up to 87% of adults and 79% of children with PAH *(16)*. These abnormalities, which likely contribute to the arterial injury and pathogenesis of PAH, have been shown to correct after one year of prostacyclin therapy in 80% to 83% of patients *(16)*. After one week, prostacyclin also significantly lowers levels of thrombomodulin and p-selectin *(17)*, important mediators of thrombin and platelet activation. The ability of prostacyclin to reverse these abnormalities is likely to be at least partly responsible for its therapeutic efficacy in PAH.

3. CLINICAL APPLICATIONS OF PROSTACYLINS

3.1. Epoprostenol

3.1.1. EARLY CASE REPORT

Long-term continuous infusion of epoprostenol to treat IPAH was first reported in 1987 in a 27-year-old female *(18)*. She had experienced dyspnea on exertion for the previous 6.5 years but had acute worsening of her symptoms 11 weeks after parturition. She had no evidence of thromboembolic disease and had had a poor symptomatic response to treatment with hydralazine, coumadin, and nifedipine. Before treatment with epoprostenol, her systolic pulmonary arterial pressure (PAP) was 100 mm Hg and her pulmonary vascular resistance (PVR) was 27 Wood units. She was referred for heart-lung transplantation; epoprostenol was initiated on an experimental basis as a bridge to transplant. She responded well, with an improvement in her symptoms of dyspnea on exertion, angina, and syncope. Her exercise tolerance improved and her ability to live independently was restored.

3.1.2. RANDOMIZED, CONTROLLED TRIALS

Rubin et al. *(2)* reported substantial improvements in pulmonary hemodynamics, exercise tolerance, and symptoms in the first randomized, controlled trial of intravenous epoprostenol in IPAH patients in 1990. Among 18 patients from this cohort followed subsequently in an open-label and uncontrolled fashion, the six-minute walk distance improved significantly from a mean of 264 ± 160 m at baseline to 370 ± 119 m at 6 months and to 408 ± 138 m at 18 months *(19)*. Pulmonary hemodynamics also significantly improved, with decreases in mean PAP and PVR and an increase in cardiac index (CI). Kaplan–Meier estimates of one-, two-, and three-year survivals of these patients were 86.9%, 72.4%, and 63.3%, respectively, compared with 77.4%, 51.6%, and 40.6% for a historical control group *(20)*. Complications included seven episodes of nonfatal sepsis, two deaths that were attributed to the infusion system (thrombus and sepsis), and a rapid deterioration in one patient after delivery system malfunction. Five patients had temporary interruption of drug infusion leading to worsening of pulmonary hypertension symptoms. While demonstrating that intravenous epoprostenol is a cumbersome and challenging therapy, these results also encouraged its use as a "bridge" to lung transplantation and paved the way for the pivotal trial of epoprostenol as a definitive PAH therapy.

The pivotal prospective, controlled trial of epoprostenol in IPAH randomized 81 patients with functional class III or IV symptoms who had failed calcium channel blocker therapy, to receive intravenous epoprostenol plus conventional therapy or conventional therapy alone *(3)*. The mean epoprostenol dose at the end of the 12-week study was 9.2 ng/kg/min. The six-minute walk distance (6MWD), the main outcome variable, significantly improved in the 41 patients randomized to epoprostenol plus conventional therapy (median: 315 m at baseline vs. 362 m at 12 weeks), but worsened in the 40 patients randomized to conventional therapy alone (median: 270 m at baseline vs. 204 m at 12 weeks, $p < 0.002$). There were also significant improvements in pulmonary hemodynamics and quality of life in the epoprostenol group, but not in the conventional therapy group. Functional class improved in 40%, worsened in 5%, and showed no change in 48% of the patients treated with epoprostenol. Of those randomized to maximal conventional therapy, functional class improved in 3% of cases, worsened in 10%, and did not change in 87% of cases. Eight patients died during the 12-week study, all in the conventional therapy group, yielding a 20% mortality compared to none in the epoprostenol group ($p < 0.003$). To date, this is the only randomized, controlled trial to demonstrate a survival benefit for PAH. Serious complications in the treatment group included sepsis in four patients and nonfatal thromboembolism in one patient. This landmark study led to the FDA approval of intravenous epoprostenol for IPAH later in 1996.

Epoprostenol has also been studied systematically in patients with PAH associated with the scleroderma spectrum of diseases. Badesch et al. *(4)* reported the results of a randomized, controlled trial of epoprostenol plus conventional therapy, versus conventional therapy alone, in 111 functional class III or IV patients with PAH associated with the scleroderma spectrum of diseases but without significant interstitial lung disease. Fifty-five patients were randomized to receive conventional therapy and 56 to continuous infusion of epoprostenol. Dosing was titrated according to a symptom-based scheme, and the mean dose of epoprostenol at the end of the 12-week study was 11.2 ng/kg/min. Median 6MWD, again the major outcome variable, increased significantly more in the epoprostenol patients, from 270 m at baseline to 316 m at 12 weeks, as compared to a decline in the control group from 240 m at baseline to 192 m at 12 weeks ($p < 0.001$). Hemodyamic improvements were noted in mean PAP, PVR, and CI and were similar in magnitude to improvements noted in the IPAH study. Improvement in functional class was seen in 38% of patients randomized to epoprostenol, while none of the patients randomized to conventional treatment experienced an improvement in functional class ($p < 0.001$). Mortality occurred with equal frequency in both groups: four patients in the epoprostenol group and five in the control group. Additionally, a trend toward improvement in the Raynaud's symptom score was observed in those treated with epoprostenol. There were 36 new digital ulcers in the epoprostenol group, compared with 72 in the conventional group. This trial led the FDA to expand the indications for intravenous epoprostenol to include PAH related to the scleroderma spectrum of diseases.

3.1.3. LONG-TERM STUDIES

3.1.3.1. Functional and Hemodynamic Effects.   The randomized trials described above were relatively brief, but longer-term open-label and retrospective studies of intravenous epoprostenol in PAH patients have been reported. Shapiro et al. *(21)* observed a significant reduction in PAP in 69 patients with IPAH treated with epoprostenol, 18 of whom were treated for more than 330 days. McLaughlin et al. *(22)* used repeated right heart catheterizations to provide a more detailed analysis of pulmonary hemodynamic responses in patients treated long-term with epoprostenol. Twenty-seven PAH patients with functional class III or IV at baseline were treated with epoprostenol and underwent invasive hemodynamic analysis at baseline and after a mean of 16.7 ± 5.2 months of therapy. Dosing of epoprostenol started at 2 ng/kg/min and increased to the maximum symptom-limited dose during the index hospitalization. The dose was then increased during outpatient follow-up based on the symptoms of PAH and the side effects of the drug. The mean dose of epoprostenol at the end of follow-up was 40 ± 15 ng/kg/min. Treadmill exercise time, as measured by the Naughton–Balke protocol, improved from a mean of 261 seconds to 631 seconds. Symptoms improved in all of the patients. Hemodynamic improvements at the end of the follow-up period actually exceeded those noted acutely at the time of baseline vasoreactivity testing with adenosine, conducted before the initiation of chronic epoprostenol therapy. There were a 22% reduction in mean PAP (67 ± 10 mm Hg to 52 ± 12 mm Hg, $p < 0.001$) and a 67% increase in cardiac output (3.75 ± 1.19 L/min to 6.29 ± 1.97 L/min, $p < 0.001$). The PVR fell by 53%, from 16.7 ± 5.4 Wood units to 7.9 ± 3.8 Wood units ($p < 0.001$). Twenty-six of the 27 patients had a reduction in PVR of at least 20%. Pulmonary vascular resistance at baseline did not predict a clinical response to epoprostenol ($r = 0.56$), nor did the baseline vasodilator response. The authors speculated that because the hemodynamic improvements with chronic epoprostenol therapy exceeded those of acute vasodilator testing, the response to long-term therapy might reflect a reduction in chronic vascular remodeling with a regression of vessel wall thickening.

Favorable changes in peak work and maximal oxygen consumption as measured by cardiopulmonary exercise testing in 16 IPAH patients treated with intravenous epoprostenol have also been reported *(23)*. These improvements complement those observed in the 6MWD and treadmill tests as reported in other studies.

The above randomized, controlled, and long-term trials have focused on IPAH and PAH related to the scleroderma spectrum of diseases, but investigators have also reported the use of epoprostenol in small series of patients with PAH related to a variety of other disorders. One such case series included 33 patients with PAH of functional class III or IV (39% and 61%, respectively) with a number of associated conditions including congenital heart disease ($n = 7$), connective tissue disease ($n = 14$), sarcoidosis ($n = 2$), distal thromboembolic disease ($n = 3$), and portopulmonary hypertension ($n = 7$) *(7)*. After a mean obser-vation period of 12.7 months, there were significant improvements in exercise capacity, functional class, and hemodynamic parameters such as mean PAP, CO, and PVR. Rosenzweig et al. *(5)* described 20 patients with PAH associated with congenital heart disease who had a 21% reduction in mean PAP, a 62% increase in cardiac index, and a 52% decrease in PVR index after one year of epoprostenol therapy. Functional class also significantly improved and there was a trend toward improvement in the six-minute walk distance. Kuo et al. *(24)* observed similar responses in a group of four patients with portopulmonary hypertension, who had reductions in mean PA pressure (from 60 to 40 mm Hg) and PVR (from 8.9 to 5.1 Wood units) after six months of epoprostenol therapy. Aguilar and Farber *(6)* reported favorable responses to intravenous epoprostenol in a cohort of six HIV patients with PAH, with improvements in functional class in all and a drop in cardiac output of 55% on average after a year of therapy. These and other studies support the notion that epoprostenol is an important treatment option in patients with PAH related to a variety of disorders.

3.1.4. LONG-TERM SURVIVAL WITH EPOPROSTENOL

Three large series have confirmed the long-term survival benefit of epoprostenol therapy for IPAH patients. In a retrospective analysis of 162 IPAH patients followed at a single center in the United States for a mean of 36.3 months, McLaughlin et al. *(25)* observed improvements in functional class, hemodynamics, exercise tolerance, and survival. Functional class improved from a mean of 3.5 to 2.5 (p > 0.001), exercise time as measured by the Naughton–Balke treadmill test increased from 217 seconds to 432 seconds at 17 ± 15 months, and pulmonary hemodynamic improvements included decreases in mPAP (61 to 53 mm Hg), PVR (16.7 to 10.2 Wood units), and mean right atrial pressure (13 to 10 mm Hg) and increases in CO (3.4 to 5.5 L/min) and mixed venous oxygen saturation (54 to 62%) (all $p < 0.05$). These measures improved most during the first six months of therapy but then had a tendency to plateau (Fig. 1). Survival at one, two, and three years was 87.8%, 76.3%, and 62.8%, respectively, compared to the expected survival of 58.9%, 46.3%, and 35.4% based on the National Institutes of Health equation *(21)* (Fig. 2). Survival at four and five years was 56% and 47%, respectively. Baseline characteristics that predicted poor survival included functional class IV symptoms and elevated right atrial pressure. After approximately one year of therapy, factors that portended a worse prognosis included persistence of functional class III or IV symptoms, elevated right atrial pressure, and low cardiac index. Complications attributed to the delivery system observed during the study period included 119 infections localized to the catheter site (0.24 per person-year), 70 episodes of sepsis (0.14 per person-year), 72 catheter replacements (0.15 per person-year), 4 deaths related to sepsis, and 1 death related to infusion interruption. These

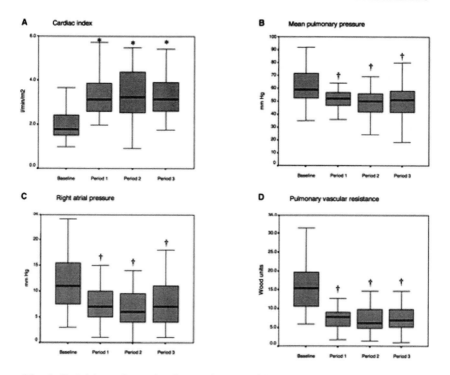

Fig. 1. Serial hemodynamics for a subgroup of 35 patients who underwent right heart catheterization at baseline and periods 1 (17 months), 2 (30 months), and 3 (43 months). *$P < 0.05$; ≢$P < 0.001$ compared to baseline.

complications underscore the need for vigilant monitoring of this effective but complicated therapy.

The long-term experience with intravenous epoprostenol in France is remarkably similar to that in the United States *(26)*. One hundred seventy-eight patients were observed for a mean of 26 ± 21 months and compared to 135 historical controls. Patients were reassessed after three months of therapy, at which time the 6MWD increased in 90% of patients from an average of 251 m at baseline to 376 m. Functional class improved in 75% of patients, was unchanged in 24% of patients, and had worsened in one patient. At three months, 55% of patients had improved to NYHA functional class I or II, while 45% remained in functional class III or IV. Survival at one, two, three, and five years was 85%, 70%, 63%, and 55%, respectively. Baseline factors associated with poor survival included RV failure, class IV symptoms, 6 MWD < 240 m, RAP > 12 mm Hg, and, interestingly, mean PA pressure < 65 mm Hg. At three months, NYHA class III or IV (odds ratio = 4.58 to 16.7), 6 MWD < 380 m, right atrial pressure > 10 mm Hg, mean PA

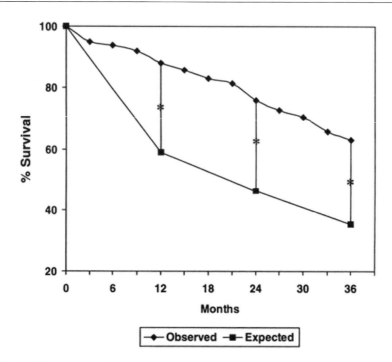

Fig. 2. Three-year survival observed with epoprostenol and predicted by the NIH equation using baseline hemodynamics. $P < 0.001$ at one, two, and three years. [From *(25)*, with permission.]

pressure < 59 mm Hg, mixed oxygen saturation at rest < 62%, and, compared to baseline, an increase in CI < 0.5 L/m/m^2 or a decrease in total pulmonary resistance < 30% were significantly associated with increased mortality.

Kuhn and colleagues described the long-term survival of a cohort of 91 patients treated with epoprostenol including both IPAH ($n = 49$) and PAH associated with other disorders including scleroderma ($n = 19$), SLE ($n = 5$), and congenital heart disease ($n = 11$) *(27)*. They noted improvements in functional class, exercise tolerance, and hemodynamics. Survival at one, two, and three years was 79%, 70%, and 59%, respectively. When stratified based on etiology, survival was greatest in those with PAH related to congenital heart disease and least in those with PAH related to systemic sclerosis. Consistent with the U.S. and French studies, functional class IV status at baseline predicted a worse prognosis, although in this study no hemodynamic variables were predictive of outcome.

All of these studies show comparable survival rates, in the range of 60% at three years. This is a substantial improvement over survival observed in the NIH Registry for pulmonary hypertension accumulated during the 1980s *(20)*. Although the relevance of this 20-year-old data set to studies conducted more than a decade later has been questioned, the more recent outcome studies strongly support the inference that epoprostenol infusion therapy prolongs long-term survival in PAH patients. These studies also underline the importance of functional status in predicting outcomes to therapy, not only at baseline but also after several months of therapy. Some investigators have even proposed using functional status after three months of therapy to decide whether or not to consider patients for lung transplantation; those with a persisting class III or IV status are evaluated for listing *(28)*. The finding from the French study that a lower mean PA pressure predicts mortality seems paradoxical but is probably related to the decline in the pressure-generating capacity of the failing right ventricle.

3.1.5. Practical Aspects of Epoprostenol Use

3.1.5.1. Patient Selection. Intravenous epoprostenol therapy is labor-intensive and complicated and, in the authors' opinion, is best managed by a pulmonary hypertension center with expertise in the management of PAH patients and parenteral therapies. Indicated for functional class III and IV patients, patient recipients should be selected carefully, based not only on the severity of the illness but also on patient willingness and ability to manage this invasive therapy. Patients who fail to keep appointments or to adhere to simpler regimens are poor candidates for epoprostenol therapy. With the recent availability of oral therapies for PAH, some centers initiate epoprostenol only after oral therapies have failed to improve clinical status significantly. While this is appropriate for many patients, patients in functional class IV or in functional class III with progressive symptoms, particularly those with short 6 MWD, high right atrial pressure, and/or low cardiac indexes, should be started promptly on intravenous epoprostenol as the initial therapy.

Epoprostenol is contraindicated in patients with left ventricular dysfunction and an ejection fraction < 30%. An earlier trial of epoprostenol to treat left-sided heart failure was terminated early because of excess mortality in the treatment group, thought possibly related to coronary steal *(29)*. Also, epoprostenol should be used with caution, if at all, in patients with active coronary artery disease.

3.1.5.2. Administration and Dosage. Epoprostenol therapy is delivered via a transcutaneous tunneled intravenous catheter, preferably with a single lumen to minimize the risk of line infection. With a half-life of approximately six minutes, epoprostenol is rapidly hydrolyzed to 2 active and 14 inactive metabolites that are subsequently cleared by the biliary and renal systems *(30)*. The patient (or surrogate) must reconstitute epoprostenol daily from a dry powder and diluent, injecting the mixture into a pump cassette. A portable, battery-operated infusion pump along with ice packs and carrying case are most often worn on a belt (or fanny pack), although some patients have become very creative in finding ways to hide the delivery system under their clothes. The pump is positive-pressure driven and has low-battery, end-of-infusion, and occlusion alarms. Intervals between pulses are not to exceed three minutes to deliver the medication at the prescribed rate and avoid excessive swings in drug concentration.

Therapy is usually initiated in the hospital, but insurance approval for initiation of the drug should be obtained prior to hospitalization, except in emergencies, and patients should bring the drug and equipment with them. Epoprostenol is distributed via specialty pharmacies that offer comprehensive services including home nurses for training. Whenever possible, our practice is to have the patient receive home teaching sessions from a skilled nurse with extensive training in the use of epoprostenol prior to hospitalization, to facilitate the patient's ability to mix the medication in a sterile fashion and operate the ambulatory infusion pump.

Many different epoprostenol dosing regimens have been described. Initially, clinicians thought that the epoprostenol dose had to be increased on a regular basis indefinitely, and a "more-is-better" attitude was pervasive. In 1999, Rich and McLaughlin reported on a series of 12 IPAH patients who experienced a high cardiac output syndrome related to excessive doses of epoprostenol *(31)*. As the dose of epoprostenol was lowered, cardiac output fell without deleterious effects on PA pressure or clinical status and, in some cases, with less intractable fluid retention. This report has led to the use of more "moderate" doses of epoprostenol. Currently, for elective initiation, we begin epoprostenol as an inpatient at 2 ng/kg/min and increase the dose by 2 ng/kg/day on a daily basis until the patient experiences adverse effects such as intolerable jaw pain, headache, or diarrhea (see Table 1). At the time of hospital discharge, most patients tolerate a dose between 4 and 8 ng/kg/min. The inpatient hospitalization is typically three to five days in duration, depending on the patient's ability to mix the medicine in a sterile fashion, operate the ambulatory infusion pump, care for the central venous catheter, and troubleshoot emergencies. We also

Table 1
Suggested Dosing Regimen for Epoprostenol Infusion

Starting dose	2 ng/kg/min*
Routine in hospital	Increase by 2 ng/kg/min daily
Emergent in hospital	Increase by 2 ng/kg/min multiple times daily
Hospital discharge	4–8 ng/kg/min
First three months	15–20 ng/kg/min
First year	25–35 ng/kg/min
Subsequent doses as dictated by symptoms, hemodynamic response**	

*Dosing is always "as tolerated," balancing symptoms of PAH (dyspnea, exertional chest pain or dizziness, fatigue) against symptoms of prostacyclin excess (Table 2).

**Some centers perform right heart catheterization after the first year and adjust dosing according to changes in cardiac index (see text for details).

require that a "mixing partner," generally a family member or close friend, learn the same mixing techniques as a backup for the patient. After discharge, a nurse clinician contacts the patient on a weekly basis for the first month or two, and then twice monthly thereafter. The dose of epoprostenol is increased to control symptoms of PAH and without causing excessive adverse side effects of the drug. Based on our experience, our target dose for most patients at one year is between 25 and 35 ng/kg/min.

3.1.5.3. Monitoring. Patients are monitored in the outpatient clinic every three months, at which time a six-minute walk test is performed to objectively assess the response to therapy (Table 2). Our standard practice also includes a repeat right heart catheterization after one year of therapy. As discussed above, one of the expected hemodynamic changes with epoprostenol therapy is an improvement in cardiac index. The repeat measurement of cardiac index assists us in deciding on further epoprostenol dose adjustments. If the cardiac index remains less than 2.5 L/min/m^2, we continue to increase the dose of epoprostenol. If the cardiac index is in the normal range of 2.5–4.5 L/min/m^2, we no longer increase the dose of epoprostenol on a regular basis. Rather, dose increases are as dictated by the patient's symptoms. With our more moderate dosing regimens, cardiac indexes over 4.5 L/min/m^2 are rare, but we adjust the dose downward if we encounter them. For those patients who are critically ill, in whom we start epoprostenol "emergently," the dose is initiated at 2 ng/kg/min but may be uptitrated several times per day based on clinical status. While these dosing strategies have served our patients well, they have

Table 2
Suggested Outpatient Monitoring for Epoprostenol Infusion

Initiation

Frequent visits from specialty pharmacy nurse until patient and "mixing
partner" demonstrate competency in mixing medication and managing
pump
Frequent phone contact with specialized pulmonary hypertension staff

Maintenance
Visits every 2 to 3 months
Assess:
    PAH symptoms: exertional dyspnea, chest pain, dizziness, etc.
    Symptoms of prostacyclin excess: intolerable jaw ache, headache,
      nausea, diarrhea, leg pain
    Problems with administration of system: pain, leaking, redness at
      catheter insertion site, dislodgement or movement of catheter,
      pump malfunction, fevers, chill, sweats, changes in mental status*
Examine vital signs:
    Cardiac findings: intensity of pulmonic component of second heart
      sound (P2), right ventricular lift or heave, tricuspid murmur, neck
      vein distension
    Leg edema
Examine functional capacity: six-minute walk or similar test; New York
  Heart Association class
Labs:
    CBC with platelet count
    Cardiac echo
    BNP or troponin 1*
Hemodynamics:
    Cardiac echo
    Right heart catheterization to assess pressures and cardiac index**

* Optional tests, whose value in long-term management has not been established.
** May be useful in assessing responses to therapy or altering management.

not been subjected to validation in controlled prospective trials, and
each experienced PAH center has individualized approaches to dosing.

3.1.5.4. Side Effects and Complications. Side effects and
complications of epoprostenol infusion are shown in Table 3. Jaw
pain, typically described as affecting the first bite or two during
eating, is commonly the first side effect. Nearly universal, some use
it as an indicator that at least some epoprostenol effect is being
achieved. Additional chronic side effects include thrombocytopenia,

Table 3
Side Effects and Complications of Epoprostenol Infusion

Prostacyclin Excess:	*Prostacyclin Deficiency:*
Flushing	Dyspnea
Restlessness	Chest pain
Jaw ache	Fatigue
Headache	Malaise
Nausea, vomiting	
Diarrhea	
Leg pain	

Complications:
Line infection
Line sepsis
Accidental discontinuation
    Occlusion, breakage, or removal of line
    Pump malfunction
    Syncope or sudden death
Hemorrhage from insertion site
Paradoxical embolism
Thrombocytopenia (particularly in SLE)

rash, sometimes with intense erythema that may be intermittent, weight loss, ascites, and leg and foot pain. Other adverse events related to the delivery system include catheter infection, thrombosis, and rebound symptoms due to abrupt discontinuation. Despite extensive teaching of catheter care, local central line infections are common, occurring at a rate of 0.22 to 0.68 infections per patient-year *(25)*. Most centers have an "infection protocol," which should be instituted at the first sign of a local infection. The incidence of sepsis, or positive blood cultures as a result of the delivery system, is approximately 0.39 infections per patient-year, with occasionally fatalities *(25)*. Because of prostacyclin's short half-life, patients may experience rebound pulmonary hypertension when the infusion is abruptly discontinued, such as by catheter dislodgement or pump malfunction. Patients should be instructed to keep a backup pump with them at all times. In the event of catheter dislodgement, patients should seek immediate medical attention. In such an emergency, peripheral access should be established and epoprostenol delivered via a peripheral line until more stable access can be established.

3.2. Treprostinil

3.2.1. SUBCUTANEOUS ADMINISTRATION

The shortcomings of intravenous epoprostenol have stimulated the search for alternative therapies. One is treprostinil, a prostacyclin analogue with a half-life of several hours that requires no cold packs and can be administered subcutaneously using a continuous infusion pump that approximates the size of a pager. In addition, the obviation of continuous intravenous therapy eliminates the risks of line infection/sepsis and paradoxical embolism. These differences from epoprostenol bestow important convenience and safety advantages on subcutaneous treprostinil.

3.2.1.1. Randomized, Controlled Trials. An early study demonstrated that intravenous epoprostenol and treprostinil have similar beneficial acute effects on pulmonary hemodynamics *(32)*. A pilot phase II arm of the study randomized 25 PAH patients in a two-to-one distribution to eight weeks of subcutaneously infused treprostinil versus placebo *(32)*. Treprostinil increased 6MWD by 37 ± 17 m compared to a drop of 6 ± 28 m in controls. Pulmonary vascular resistance dropped 20% in the treprostinil group, although this was not significantly different from controls. Patients treated with treprostinil frequently had site pain and erythema that were intolerable in some patients.

Two subsequent international pivotal randomized trials that were combined *(33)* used lower initial doses than in the pilot study, with the hope that infusion site reactions would be less problematic. Four hundred seventy patients with functional class II to IV IPAH or PAH related to connective tissue disease or congenital pulmonary to systemic shunts were randomized to receive subcutaneous treprostinil or placebo. At the end of the 12-week trial, the median difference in the 6MWD between the two groups was only 16 m, raising questions about the drug's efficacy. However, the main outcome variable, the 6MWD, revealed a clear dose-response relationship, with patients who received more than 13.8 ng/kg/min increasing their walk distance by 36 m and patients given less than 10 ng/kg/min manifesting virtually no increase (Fig. 3). Thus, the relatively meager average increase in six-minute walk distance in this study appears to have been related to underdosing in many of the enrolled patients because of concerns about site pain. Follow-up studies have shown that with dose escalation, improvements in the 6MWD in patients treated with treprostinil approach 50 m, the same range as with epoprostenol.

Other statistically significant improvements observed with treprostinil included a reduction in dyspnea, a slight drop in mean PA pressure

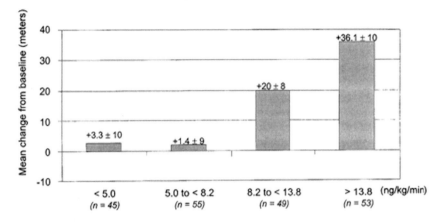

Fig. 3. Mean change in the six-minute walk distance from baseline to week 12 versus week 12 trepostinil dose quartile. [From *(33)*, with permission.]

(−2.3 vs. +0.7 mm Hg in controls), and a slight increase in cardiac output (−0.12 vs. −0.06 L/min in controls) *(33)*. Quality of life tended to improve but did not reach statistical significance, perhaps related to diminished mobility related to site pain. A follow-up study showed that the subgroup of 90 patients with connective tissue disease from the original randomized trials manifested similar benefits in response to subcutaneous treprostinil, with the same dose-response issues *(34)*. Based on these findings, in 2002 the FDA approved subcutaneous treprostinil for use in class II to IV patients with IPAH or PAH associated with connective tissue disease or congenital heart disease. Because of its subcutaneous route of administration, no need for mixing, and the highly portable pump system, subcutaneous treprostinil has substantial safety and convenience advantages over intravenous epoprostenol. Unfortunately, many patients encounter pain at the infusion site, and a significant minority of patients finds the drug intolerable. Various topical formulations and narcotics bring some alleviation, but this pain has limited the appeal of the therapy.

3.2.2. Practical Aspects of Treprostinil Use

3.2.2.1. Patient Selection. Indications for subcutaneous treprostinil are similar to those of epoprostenol, but unlike epoprostenol, the FDA also approved the use of treprostinil in class II patients. The substantial safety and convenience advantages over the intravenous route make it desirable for patients who value those advantages. For example, some patients with scleroderma may find it difficult to mix

epoprostenol daily but may be able to use subcutaneous treprostinil successfully. Unfortunately, because of its tendency to cause infusion site pain, it is generally not used as a first-line therapy. Rather, it is most often offered to patients thought to be too ill or poor candidates for an oral therapy and who have a high pain threshold. A patient with portopulmonary hypertension and class III PAH, deemed to be a poor candidate for an endothelin-receptor antagonist because of potential liver toxicity, might do well with subcutaneous treprostinil. Another common indication is as a substitute for intravenous prostacyclin when patients have had complications of intravenous therapy such as repeated bouts of line sepsis.

3.2.2.2. Administration and Dosage. Treprostinil dosing is similar to epoprostenol dosing, but infusion rates are often higher. The initial infusion rate is 1.25 ng/kg/min, or 0.625 ng/kg/min in patents with severe liver disease, and gradually increases at twice-weekly intervals, perhaps 1.25 ng/kg/min each time, as tolerated. Increases might be more or less rapid, depending on the clinical response. Typical doses after the first year of therapy range from 30–80 ng/kg/min. Unlike epoprostenol, subcutaneous treprostinil can be started at home because of its greater safety. The drug is supplied by specialty pharmacies, and the insurance approval process and costs are similar to those of epoprostenol. Patients (and surrogates) are taught to self-administer the drug in their homes by infusion therapy nurses. Delivery is via a system first developed to infuse insulin consisting of a pager-sized pump (Minimed) and a 27 gauge subcutaneous cannula. The drug is aspirated into a syringe from premixed vials and loaded into the pump. The infusion site is usually changed every three to four days, although some patients use the same site for up to a few weeks if it is a "good" one. The abdomen is the most commonly used site for infusion, although some patients prefer the thighs, flanks, or medial or lateral aspects of the upper arms.

3.2.2.3. Side Effects and Complications. In the pivotal trial, jaw ache and diarrhea were encountered in 13% and 25% of patients, respectively—significantly more often than in controls *(33)*. These rates are lower than those associated with epoprostenol use, perhaps because many patients were underdosed in the pivotal treprostinil trial. Infusion site pain occurred in 85% of patients, however, leading to withdrawal from the trial in 8% of patients. Infusion site pain has been the major drawback of subcutaneous treprostinil therapy, causing some specialized centers to avoid using it.

Numerous strategies have been tried to minimize site pain, including topical lidocaine, capsaicin and corticosteroids, oral nonsteroidal or steroidal anti-inflammatory drugs, and narcotics. Plogel, a topical compound that enhances penetration into the skin, has met with some success when combined with lidocaine, ketamine, ibuprofen, and corticosteroids and infiltrated under artificial skin placed over the infusion site. However, plogel has been more successful at shortening the duration of pain at postinfusion sites rather than treating active sites. Oral ibuprofen, gabapentin or even corticosteroids for brief periods of time may be helpful. Unfortunately, no approach has met with consistent success in controlling infusion site pain. Some patients cannot tolerate the drug and stop, while others can be maintained on therapy only if they use oral narcotics concomitantly, sometimes at high doses.

3.2.2.4. Intravenous Administration. The FDA approved treprostinil for intravenous administration in late 2004. Although this therapy shares with epoprostenol the risks of line infection/sepsis and paradoxical embolism, it offers a safety advantage over epoprostenol in that its longer half-life [approximately 4.5 hours *(35)*] allows more time to seek medical attention in the event of sudden discontinuation. In addition, intravenous treprostinil is more convenient because it requires no mixing and the pump cassette is changed every other day rather than daily. Limited data on pulmonary hemodynamics and functional status after transitions from epoprostenol and *de novo* starts suggest that both intravenous forms of therapy have similar efficacy *(32,36)*.

A recent Centers for Disease Control (CDC) investigation into bloodstream infections associated with IV treprostinil found that although infections were infrequent for both agents, they occurred 2.4 times as often with IV treprostinil compared to IV epoprostenol *(37)*. The infections associated with IV treprostinil were largely Gram-negative bacteria (pseudomonas and enterobacter) in contrast to the predominance of Gram-positives with IV epoprostenol infections. The differences in bloodstream infections are considered hypothetical, because the CDC investigation was preliminary and not designed to be conclusive. The drug itself was thought not to be the source of the infections, but handling of the drug and some effect of the drug on the immune system were proposed as possible explanations. Clinicians are encouraged to cover for the possibility of Gram-negative infections when selecting antibiotics for presumed bloodstream infections in patients receiving IV treprostinil.

The dosing of intravenous treprostinil has been controversial. In a recent study of 27 patients with PAH transitioned from epoprostenol, the treprostinil dose immediately following the transition was roughly the same as the initial epoprostenol dose of 40 ng/kg/min. Twelve weeks later, average dose of treprostinil was 83 ng/kg/min after adjustments had been made for symptoms *(36)*. This suggests that an appropriate comparable dose of treprostinil is at least twice that of epoprostenol.

3.2.2.5. Inhaled and Oral Administration. Inhaled and oral forms of treprostinil are currently under investigation. In a sheep model, inhaled treprostinil had greater beneficial pulmonary hemodynamic effects than equivalent intravenous doses *(38)*. A preliminary report on acute inhalation in humans suggests that a few inhalations of treprostinil improve pulmonary hemodynamics for at least several hours, longer than with inhaled iloprost, raising the possibility of four-time daily administration *(39)*. A phase III trial of inhaled treprostinil has recently reported a preliminary finding of a 20 m median improvement in 6 minute walk distance compared to placebo, and a phase III trial of oral treprostinil is underway.

3.3. Iloprost

Iloprost, another prostacyclin analogue with a half-life intermediate between those of epoprostenol and treprostinil [approximately 20–25 minutes *(40)*], has been available in some European countries and New Zealand in inhaled and intravenous forms for several years. The FDA approved iloprost by inhalation during late 2004. The inhalational route is attractive because it delivers medication to gas-exchanging areas of the lungs, potentially dilating blood vessels in ventilated areas and thereby improving ventilation–perfusion matching and enhancing oxygenation, all with minimal systemic side effects.

3.3.1. CLINICAL STUDIES

Early trials demonstrated that inhaled iloprost acutely dilates pulmonary vessels, increases cardiac output, and improves oxygenation and that these effects are sustained for three months *(41)*. Duration of the hemodynamic effect is approximately 90 minutes. A randomized, controlled European trial of inhaled iloprost enrolled 203 patients with class III and IV IPAH, PAH associated with connective tissue disease, appetite-suppressant use, or chronic thromboembolic disease *(42)* (AIR trial). More patients on iloprost treatment reached the study goal that combined improvements in functional class and 6MWD (of at least 10%) with the lack of deterioration or death (16.8% vs. 4.9% in controls). The iloprost-treated patients walked 36.4 m farther than controls ($p < 0.01$) (Fig. 4) and a higher percentage improved by one NYHA class (23.8% vs. 12.7% in controls, $P = 0.03$). Other iloprost

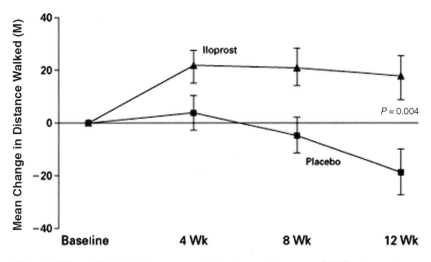

Fig. 4. Effect of inhaled iloprost and placebo on the mean (±SE) change from baseline in the distance walked in six minutes, according to an intention-to-treat analysis. [From *(42)*, with permission.]

benefits included better dyspnea and quality of life scores and greater improvement in pulmonary hemodynamics, at least after iloprost inhalation. Survival did not differ significantly between the groups. Although iloprost was well tolerated (cough, headache, flushing, and jaw pain occurring more frequently in the iloprost group), there was a trend toward more syncope in patients receiving iloprost, perhaps because of excessive exercise after too long a period between treatments. The mean frequency of inhalations was 7.5 per day.

Iloprost appears to have long-term sustained beneficial effects on exercise capacity and pulmonary hemodynamics. In 24 patients treated with aerosolized iloprost for at least one year, the six-minute walk distance remained increased (363 vs. 278 m at baseline, $p < 0.001$) and mean PA pressure was lower, even before iloprost inhalation (52 vs. 59 mm Hg at baseline, $p < 0.006$) *(43)*. However, other studies suggest that iloprost has limitations. One using an implantable continuous hemodynamic monitor noted that iloprost had beneficial effects on resting pulmonary hemodynamics but not at maximal workload *(44)*. In a five-year follow-up study using death, transplantation, or addition of or switching to another therapy as endpoints, only 29% of patients had not reached an endpoint at three years and only 13% at five years *(45)*. Furthermore, there are some reports of patients with severe pulmonary hypertension deteriorating when switched from intravenous epoprostenol to inhaled iloprost, presumably because the hemodynamic benefits of iloprost were abbreviated in them (20-minute duration) *(46)*. These patients restabilized when returned to intravenous epoprostenol or iloprost.

Another application for inhaled iloprost has been in patients with pulmonary hypertension associated with idiopathic pulmonary fibrosis. In eight patients with idiopathic fibrosis and pulmonary hypertension, inhaled iloprost and epoprostenol brought about pulmonary selective vasodilation and improved oxygenation, whereas intravenous epoprostenol and oral calcium channel blockers were not pulmonary-selective, and intravenous prostacyclin substantially increased shunting *(47)*. Long-term therapy with inhaled iloprost in one patient with right heart failure brought about a sustained improvement in functional status.

Recently, results of the phase II STEP (iloprost inhalation solution Safety and pilot efficacy Trial in combination with bosentan for Evaluation in Pulmonary arterial hypertension) trial were reported *(48)*. Sixty-five patients were enrolled into this double-blind, multicenter trial that added inhaled iloprost versus inhaled placebo to oral bosentan. After 12 weeks of combination therapy, the 6MWD increased by 26 m versus placebo, New York Heart Association functional class and pulmonary hemodynamics improved, and time to clinical worsening was prolonged. Based on these findings, the FDA has expanded labeling of iloprost to include its addition to oral bosentan.

3.3.2. Practical Application of Inhaled Iloprost

3.3.2.1. Patient Selection. Inhaled iloprost is indicated for *de novo* patients or those on oral bosentan with PAH (WHO group 1) and a functional class III or IV. Contraindications other than hypersensitivity to prostacyclins are not known.

3.3.2.2. Administration and Dosing. After initial release, the drug was administered using an aerosolization device that weighed 3 kg, had no battery backup, and took up to 15 minutes for each dose. Presently, a much more portable, pocket-sized, battery-operated inhalation device that weighs less than a pound permits dosing in roughly 10 minutes. Dosing with inhaled iloprost starts with a 2.5-µg dose and, if tolerated, advances to a 5-µg dose administered every 3 hours during the daytime, for a total of at least six nebulizer treatments per 24 hours. Overdosing has not been reported, but the usual symptoms of prostacyclin excess including headache, flushing, hypotension, nausea, vomiting, and diarrhea can develop, necessitating a reduction in dose. Although the inhaled route has obvious safety advantages over the intravenous route and avoids the pain of subcutaneous administration, many patients find the frequency of treatments cumbersome, and cough is an additional potential side effect.

3.4. Beraprost

Beraprost, another stable prostacyclin analogue with a longer half-life than epoprostenol, is suitable for oral administration. Uncontrolled trials in Japan, where the drug is currently available, have suggested beneficial actions in patients with pulmonary hypertension related to congenital heart disease as well as in chronic thromboembolic pulmonary hypertension (49). One nonrandomized Japanese trial of IPAH patients found a survival of 76% at 3 years in 24 patients treated with beraprost, and only 44% in patients treated conventionally (50). A three-month, randomized, controlled trial in Europe on class II and III PAH patients showed significant improvements in the 6MWD (25.1 m), functional class, and dyspnea, although pulmonary hemodynamics did not improve (51). A subsequent 12-month, randomized, controlled trial on 116 patients with IPAH or PAH related to connective tissue disease or congenital systemic to pulmonary shunts in the United States failed to show sustained benefit, even though there was significant improvement in the six-minute walk distance at three and six months (9) (Fig. 5). For this reason, an application for beraprost to the

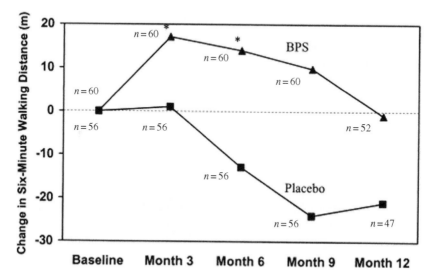

Fig. 5. Median change in six-minute walking distance from baseline to months 3, 6, 9, and 12 in the placebo and beraprost sodium (BPS) groups; $P = 0.010$ at 3 months, 0.016 at 6 months, 0.098 at 9 months, and 0.180 at 12 months (adjusted for center, etiology, and baseline peak oxygen consumption, six-minute walk, Borg dyspnea score, and vasodilator use). [From (9), with permission.]

FDA was not filed. Further work will be needed to determine whether the lack of the sustained effects of oral prostacyclins might be related to insufficient dose escalation or another remediable problem.

4. SUMMARY

The efficacy of continuous infusion epoprostenol treatment in patients with IPAH functional class III or IV is better established than with other agents. Epoprostenol improves symptoms, exercise capacity, hemodynamics, and survival in IPAH patients. While the literature is not as voluminous in patients with PAH associated with other disorders, epoprostenol therapy improves the symptoms of PAH in many of these patients. Enthusiasm for epoprostenol must be tempered by its cumbersome delivery system and inherent risks. Newer prostacyclins include treprostinil, available in subcutaneous and intravenous forms, and inhaled iloprost. Each has established efficacy in randomized trials. Subcutaneous treprostinil has been plagued by infusion site pain but is a good alternative for those who can tolerate it. Inhaled iloprost is being used increasingly because the inhaled route has fewer systemic side effects and improves oxygenation compared to the intravenous route. Whichever agent is chosen, patients are monitored closely thereafter regarding timely adjustment in doses and potential complications.

REFERENCES

1. Christman BW, McPherson CD, Newman JH, et al. An imbalance between the excretion of thromboxane and prostacyclin metabolites in pulmonary hypertension. N Engl J Med 1992; 327:70–7.
2. Rubin LJ, Mendoza J, Hood M, et al. Treatment of primary pulmonary hypertension with continuous intravenous prostacyclin (epoprostenol). Results of a randomized trial. Ann Intern Med 1990; 112(7):485–91.
3. Barst RJ, Rubin LJ, Long WA, et al. A comparison of continuous intravenous epoprostenol (prostacyclin) with conventional therapy for primary pulmonary hypertension. N Engl J Med 1996; 334:296–301.
4. Badesch DB, Tapson VF, McGoon MD, et al. Continuous intravenous epoprostenol for pulmonary hypertension due to the scleroderma spectrum of disease: A randomized, controlled trial. Ann Intern Med 2000; 132:425–34.
5. Rosenzweig EB, Kerstein D, Barst RJ. Long-term prostacyclin for pulmonary hypertension with associated congenital heart defects. Circulation 1999; 99:1858–65.

6. Aguilar RV, Farber HW. Epoprostenol (prostacyclin) therapy in HIV-associated pulmonary hypertension. Am J Respir Crit Care Med 2000; 162(5):1846–50.

7. McLaughlin VV, Genthner DE, Panella MM, Hess DM, Rich S. Compassionate use of continuous prostacyclin in the management of secondary pulmonary hypertension: A case series. Ann Intern Med 1999; 130:740–3.

8. Bresser P, Fedullo PF, Auger WR, et al. Continuous intravenous epoprostenol for chronic thromboembolic pulmonary hypertension. Eur Respir J 2004 Apr; 23(4):595–600.

9. Barst RJ, McGoon M, McLaughlin V, et al. Beraprost therapy for pulmonary arterial hypertension. J Am Coll Cardiol 2003; 41:2119–25.

10. Moncada S, Gryglewski R, Bunting S, Vane JR. An enzyme isolated from arteries transforms prostaglandin endoperoxides to an unstable substance that inhibits platelet aggregation. Nature 1976; 263:663–5.

11. Moncada S. Prostacyclin, EDRF and atherosclerosis. Adv Exp Med Biol 1988; 243:1–11.

12. Dinh-Xuan AT. Endothelial modulation of pulmonary vascular tone. Eur Respir J 1992 Jun; 5(6):757–62.

13. Chen YF, Oparil S. Endothelial dysfunction in the pulmonary vascular bed. Am J Med Sci 2000; 320:223–32.

14. Skoglund ML, Nies AS, Gerber JG. Inhibition of acid secretion in isolated canine parietal cells by prostaglandins. J Pharmacol Exp Ther 1982; 220:371–4.

15. Tuder RM, Cool CD, Geraci MW, et al. Prostacyclin synthase expression is decreased in lungs from patients with severe pulmonary hypertension. Am J Respir Crit Care Med 1999; 159:1925–32.

16. Friedman R, Mears G, Barst RJ. Continuous infusion of prostacyclin normalizes plasma markers of endothelial cell injury and platelet aggregation in primary pulmonary hypertension. Circulation 1997; 96:2782–4.

17. Sakamaki F, Kyotani S, Nagaya N, et al. Increased plasma P-selectin and decreased thrombomodulin in pulmonary arterial hypertension were improved by continuous prostacyclin therapy. Circulation 2000; 102:2720–5.

18. Jones DK, Higenbottam TW, Wallwork J. Treatment of primary pulmonary hypertension intravenous epoprostenol (prostacyclin). Br Heart J 1987; 57:270–8.

19. Barst RJ, Rubin LJ, McGoon MD, Caldwell EJ, Long WA, Levy PS. Survival in primary pulmonary hypertension with long-term continuous intravenous prostacyclin. Ann Intern Med 1994; 121:409–15.

20. Rich S, Dantzker DR, Ayres SM, et al. Primary pulmonary hypertension: A national prospective study. Ann Intern Med 1987; 107:216–23.

21. Shapiro SM, Oudiz RJ, Cao T, et al. Primary pulmonary hypertension: Improved long-term effects and survival with continuous intravenous epoprostenol infusion. J Am Coll Cardiol 1997; 30:343–9.

22. McLaughlin VV, Genthner DE, Panella MM, Rich S. Reduction in pulmonary vascular resistance with long-term epoprostenol (prostacyclin)

therapy in primary pulmonary hypertension. N Engl J Med 1998; 338: 273–7.

23. Wax D, Garofano R, Barst RJ. Effects of long-term infusion of prostacyclin on exercise performance in patients with primary pulmonary hypertension. Chest 1999; 116:914–20.

24. Kuo PC, Johnson LB, Plotkin JS, Howell CD, Bartlett ST, Rubin LJ. Continuous intravenous infusion of epoprostenol for the treatment of portopulmonary hypertension. Transplantation 1997 Feb 27; 63(4):604–6.

25. McLaughlin V, Shillington A, Rich S. Survival in primary pulmonary hypertension: The impact of epoprostenol therapy. Circulation 2002; 106:1477–82.

26. Sitbon O, Humbert M, Nunes H, et al. Long-term intravenous epoprostenol infusion in primary pulmonary hypertension: Prognostic factors and survival. J Am Coll Cardiol 2002; 40(4):780–8.

27. Kuhn KP, Byrne DW, Arbogast PG, Doyle TP, Loyd JE, Robbins IM. Outcome in 91 consecutive patients with pulmonary arterial hypertension receiving epoprostenol. Am J Respir Crit Care Med 2003; 167: 580–6.

28. Conte JV, Gaine SP, Orens JB, Harris T, Rubin LJ. The influence of continuous intravenous prostacyclin therapy for primary pulmonary hypertension on the timing and outcome of transplantation. J Heart Lung Transplant 1998; 17(7):679–85.

29. Sueta CA, Gheorghiade M, Adams KF Jr., et al. Safety and efficacy of epoprostenol in patients with severe congestive heart failure. Epoprostenol Multicenter Research Group. Am J Cardiol 1995 Jan 19; 75(3):34A–43A.

30. Oates, JA, Fitzgerald GA, Branch RA, Jackson EK, Knapp HR, Roberts LJ. Clinical implications of prostaglandin and thromboxane A2 formation. N Engl J Med 1998; 319: 761–7.

31. Rich S, McLaughlin VV. The effects of chronic prostacyclin therapy on cardiac output and symptoms in primary pulmonary hypertension. J Am Coll Cardiol 1999; 34:1184–7.

32. McLaughlin VV, Gaine SP, Barst RJ, et al. Efficacy and safety of treprostinil: An epoprostenol analog for primary pulmonary hypertension. J Cardiovasc Pharmacol 2003; 41:293–9.

33. Simonneau G, Barst RJ, Galie N, et al. Continuous subcutaneous infusion of treprostinil, a prostacyclin analogue, in patients with pulmonary arterial hypertension: A double-blind, randomized, placebo-controlled trial. Am J Respir Crit Care Med 2002; 165:800–4.

34. Oudiz RJ, Schilz RJ, Barst RJ, et al. Treprostinil, a prostacyclin analogue, in pulmonary arterial hypertension associated with connective tissue disease. Chest 2004; 126:420–7.

35. Laliberte K, Arneson C, Jeffs R, et al. Pharmacokinetics and steady state bioequivalence of treprostinil sodium (Remodulin) administered by the intravenous and subcutaneous routes to normal volunteers. J Cardiovasc Pharmacol 2004; 44:209–14.

36. Gomberg-Maitland M, Tapson VF, Benza RL, et al. Transition from intravenous epoprostenol to intravenous treprostinil in pulmonary hypertension. Am J Respir Crit Care Med 2005; 172:1586–9.

37. Bloodstream infections among patients treated with intravenous epoprostenol or intravenous treprostinil for pulmonary arterial hypertension —Seven sites 2003–2006. Morb Mort Wkly Rep 2007; 56:170–2.
38. Sandifer BL, Brigham KL, Lawrence EC, Mottola D, Cuppels C, Parker RE. Potent effects of aerosol compared to intravenous treprostinil on the pulmonary circulation. J Appl Physiol 2005; 99:2363–8.
39. Voswinckel R, Enke B, Reichenberger F, et al. Favorable effects of inhaled treprostinil in severe pulmonary hypertension: Results from randomized controlled pilot studies. J Am Coll Cardiol 2006 Oct 17; 48(8):1672–81.
40. Krause W, Krais T. Pharmacokinetics and pharmacodynamics of the prostacyclin analogue iloprost in man. Eur J Clin Pharmacol 1986; 30: 61–8.
41. Olschewski H, Walmrath D, Schermuly R, Ghofrani A, Grimminger F, Seeger W. Aerosolized prostacyclin and iloprost in severe pulmonary hypertension. Ann Intern Med 1996; 124:820–4.
42. Olschewski H, Simonneau G, Galie N, et al. Inhaled iloprost for severe pulmonary hypertension. N Engl J Med 2002; 347:322–9.
43. Hoeper MM, Schwarze M, Ehlerding S, et al.. Long-term treatment of primary pulmonary hypertension with aerosolized iloprost, a prostacyclin analogue. N Engl J Med 2000 Jun 22; 342(25):1866–70.
44. Wonisch M, Fruhwald FM, Maier R, et al. Continuous haemodynamic monitoring during exercise in patients with pulmonary hypertension. Int J Cardiol 2005; 101:415–20.
45. Opitz CF, Wensel R, Winkler J, et al. Clinical efficacy and survival with first-line inhaled iloprost therapy in patients with idiopathic pulmonary arterial hypertension. Eur Heart J 2005; 26:1895–902.
46. Schenk P, Petkov V, Madl C, et al. Aerosolized iloprost therapy could not replace long-term IV epoprostenol (prostacyclin) administration in severe pulmonary hypertension. Chest 2001; 119:296–300.
47. Olschewski H, Ghofrani HA, Walmrath D, et al. Inhaled prostacyclin and iloprost in severe pulmonary hypertension secondary to lung fibrosis. Am J Respir Crit Care Med 1999; 160:600–7.
48. McLaughlin VV, Oudiz RJ, Frost A, et al. Randomized study of adding inhaled iloprost to existing bosentan in pulmonary arterial hypertension. Am J Respir Crit Care Med 2006; 174:1257–63.
49. Suzuki H, Sato S, Tanabe S, Hayasaka K. Beraprost sodium for pulmonary hypertension with congenital heart disease. Pediatr Int 2002; 44:528–9.
50. Nagaya N, Uematsu M, Okano Y, et al. Effect of orally active prostacyclin analogue on survival of outpatients with primary pulmonary hypertension. J Am Coll Cardiol 1999; 34:1188–92.
51. Galie N, Humbert M, Vachiery JL, et al. Effects of beraprost sodium, an oral prostacyclin analogue, in patients with pulmonary arterial hypertension: A randomized, double-blind, placebo-controlled trial. J Am Coll Cardiol 2002; 39:1496–502.

13 Endothelin and Its Blockade in Pulmonary Arterial Hypertension

David Langleben

CONTENTS

INTRODUCTION
PULMONARY VASCULAR ENDOTHELIN
   RECEPTORS IN HEALTH AND DISEASE
CLINICAL STUDIES OF ENDOTHELIN-RECEPTOR
   ANTAGONISTS IN PAH
SELECTION OF AN ENDOTHELIN-RECEPTOR
   ANTAGONIST
CONCLUSION AND FUTURE DIRECTIONS
REFERENCES

Abstract

Endothelin-1, a potent vasoconstrictor and mitogenic peptide manufactured by endothelial cells, has been identified as an important mediator in human pulmonary arterial hypertension. Endothelin-1 binds to two different receptors, termed ET_A and ET_B. While it is generally agreed that the ET_A receptor is the predominant receptor responsible for constriction and proliferation, it is unclear whether the net effect of ET_B-receptor activation is beneficial or detrimental. In the past decade, the development of both nonspecific and specific ET_A endothelin-receptor antagonists has offered hope of benefit for patients with PAH. These agents have the advantage of permitting oral administration with once- or twice-daily dosing. They improve functional status and capacity as well as pulmonary hemodynamics and slow the time to clinical worsening. Elevation of liver enzymes appears to be a class effect, although some agents may be less liver-toxic than others. However, many questions remain to be answered about the role of endothelin and its receptors in the pathogenesis and therapy of PAH.

From: *Contemporary Cardiology: Pulmonary Hypertension*
Edited by: N. S. Hill and H. W. Farber © Humana Press, Totowa, NJ

Key Words: pulmonary arterial hypertension; endothelin receptors; bosentan; sitaxsentan; ambrisentan; BREATHE trials.

1. INTRODUCTION

Endothelin-1 (ET-1) is a 21 amino acid peptide related to the sarafotoxin family of peptides found in the venom of a variety of predatory animals. These peptides act to immobilize prey by inducing rapid and severe cardiovascular collapse. Endothelial cells are the main source of ET-1, although other cells can express it in disease states *(1)*. ET-1 is an extremely potent vasoconstrictor and also acts as a mitogen for a variety of cells, mainly of mesenchymal origin. At the time of its discovery in 1988, ET-1 was identified as a likely mediator of vascular diseases including pulmonary hypertension *(1)*. A subsequent study in patients found increased plasma ET-1 levels in types of pulmonary hypertension that are now included in the category of PAH *(2)*. Shortly thereafter, using immunohistochemical techniques and *in situ* hybridization, Giaid et al. found increased ET-1 expression and synthesis in lung tissue from patients with PAH, with the levels being greatest at the postulated primary site of the disorder, i.e., in the precapillary microvasculature and plexiform lesions *(3)*. This evidence, as well as other evidence for ET-1 as a mediator of pulmonary hypertension in a variety of animal models, provides a strong impetus for the development of endothelin-receptor antagonists for therapeutic applications.

2. PULMONARY VASCULAR ENDOTHELIN RECEPTORS IN HEALTH AND DISEASE

The actions of ET-1 in humans are transduced via two classic G protein-coupled receptors, termed A- and B-type endothelin receptors (ET_A and ET_B) *(4,5)*. Second messenger systems related to ET-receptor activation include suppression of voltage-gated K channels, activation of calcium channels, alteration of intracellular calcium, phospholipase A_2 and arachidonic acid, phospholipase C, and the phosphoinositol system *(6–9)*. A tyrosine kinase-independent pathway resulting in myofilament calcium sensitization may also be present, mediated via the ET_A receptor *(10)*. In vitro activation of the ET_A receptor on smooth muscle cells, pericytes, and fibroblasts results in vasoconstriction and proliferation. There are conflicting reports as to whether activation of the ET_B receptor on these cells of mesenchymal origin also induces vasoconstriction and proliferation, depending on the cell type and the experimental model as well as the chosen agonist and its concentration *(11,12)*. In isolated perfused lungs, stimulation of the pulmonary ET_B receptor with a selective agonist results in vasoconstriction only if the counterbalancing nitric oxide mechanism is inhibited *(13)*. However, the biologically relevant molecule for disease states is ET-1, not a receptor-specific agonist. When the effects of selective receptor antagonists on vasoconstriction were studied in an animal model of PAH in the presence of endogenous levels of ET-1, ET_A-receptor blockade decreased pulmonary vascular resistance by 25%, but ET_B-receptor blockade did not decrease pulmonary vascular resistance *(14)*. Although there have been no corresponding studies in human PAH, the experimental data support a predominant role for the ET_A receptor over the ET_B receptor in constrictive and proliferative responses to biologically relevant concentrations of endogenous ET-1.

Although the predominant effects of ET-1 are to cause vasoconstriction and cellular proliferation, the vascular actions of ET-1 are not all deleterious. ET_B receptors are found in abundance on endothelial cells, particularly in the distal lung microvasculature *(11)*. Their actions may moderate some of the detrimental effects of ET-1 on smooth muscle and other mesenchymal cells. Activation of endothelial ET_B receptors leads to the release of nitric oxide and prostacyclin, both potent vasodilators and inhibitors of smooth muscle proliferation *(15)*. Moreover, the endothelial ET_B receptor is responsible for clearance of ET-1 from the circulation, thereby lowering ET-1 levels *(15–18)*. By virtue of its large surface area and abundant ET_B receptors, the lung circulation normally clears 47 ± 7% of circulating ET-1 on a first-pass basis. Furthermore, in many patients with PAH, this endothelial ET_B-mediated clearance is intact, despite a reduced microvascular surface area from vascular remodeling *(19)*. Thus, when treating PAH with endothelin-receptor antagonists, the preservation of endothelial ET_B receptor's vasodilatory and clearance activity by the use of selective ET_A-receptor antagonists may be beneficial, but this hypothesis requires confirmation in clinical studies.

The expression of ET_B receptors can be induced in vitro and in disease states *(20)*. Numerous studies of ET receptors have been performed in animal models of disease, but their relevance to human PAH is unclear since their pathogenesis and histopathology are different from PAH, and significant interspecies variation exists in patterns of response of the pulmonary vasculature to injury. Several studies have described the upregulation of ET_B receptors in pulmonary hypertension, but the clinical significance of these findings is unclear.

Although an animal model of high pulmonary blood flow in lambs showed an increase in smooth muscle cell ET_B-receptor expression and ET_B-mediated vasoconstriction with time, the investigators employed receptor-specific agonists rather than ET-1 itself *(14)*. However, when the animals were studied in their baseline state, the vasoconstriction seen was almost entirely mediated by ET_A receptors, and not by the upregulated ET_B receptors *(14)*. In an animal model of hypoxic pulmonary hypertension, ET_B receptors were upregulated, but mainly on endothelial cells, not smooth muscle cells *(21)*. ET_B receptors are upregulated in patients with scleroderma-induced lung fibrosis, but without pulmonary hypertension, and the clinical relevance of this finding is unclear *(22)*. Indeed, much of the increased ET_B-receptor expression was in the interstitium and microvessels, but not in the smooth muscle cells *(22)*. Furthermore, a study of the effects of ET-1 on in vitro contraction of cultured lung fibroblasts from patients with scleroderma revealed that all the contraction was mediated through the ET_A receptor and not through the ET_B receptor, suggesting that even if fibroblast ET_B receptors are upregulated in scleroderma, this has little functional significance.

In patients with chronic thromboembolic pulmonary hypertension (CTEPH), which does not fall under the broad category of PAH, increased gene and protein expression of the ET_B receptor was found in the media of pulmonary arteries *(23)*. However, these were large preacinar arteries rather than arteries of the more distal precapillary microvasculature that may be more clinically relevant. Also, although the level of ET_B-receptor expression was increased in patients with CTEPH, those levels were still much lower than ET_A-receptor levels. In another study, an elegant autoradiographic technique showed an increase in both ET_A- and ET_B-receptor binding in the media of pulmonary arteries with diameters of approximately 100 μm from patients with idiopathic PAH and PAH related to congenital heart disease *(11)*. However, the technique lacked the resolution needed to assess levels of the endothelial ET_B receptor separately.

The increased autocrine ET-1 production in pulmonary hypertensive states could also downregulate endothelial ET receptors *(24)*, and this could render moot the argument that preservation of endothelial ET_B function by selective ET_A-receptor blockade is advantageous in PAH. However, first-pass clearance studies of trace doses of radiolabeled ET-1 injected into the pulmonary circulation show preservation of ET_B receptor-mediated ET-1 clearance in most patients with idiopathic PAH and patients with PAH related to connective tissue disease *(19)*.

Preservation of these receptors during endothelin-receptor antagonist therapy may be worthwhile because of their ability to clear ET-1. On the other hand, these studies examined only the clearance function of the ET_B receptors, and it remains unknown whether these receptors in patients with PAH retain any vasodilator activity and whether preservation of ET_B function using specific ET_A-receptor blockade is clinically advantageous over nonspecific inhibition.

3. CLINICAL STUDIES OF ENDOTHELIN-RECEPTOR ANTAGONISTS IN PAH

Endothelin-receptor antagonists are divided broadly into two groups: ETA receptor-selective and dual ET_A- and ET_B-receptor antagonists. The agents that are clinically approved, or that are currently in phase III trials, include bosentan (Tracleer®), which is nonselective (ET_A:ET_B 20:1); sitaxsentan (Thelin®), which is highly ETA-selective (ET_A:ET_B 6500:1); and ambrisentan, which is more ET_A-selective than bosentan (ET_A:ET_B 77:1) but which falls under the nonselective category when compared to one of the molecules traditionally used for the selectivity threshold, BQ-123 (ET_A:ET_B 2465:1). All are oral agents that are potentially hepatotoxic to varying degrees, but the hepatotoxicity is usually reversible upon discontinuation of therapy. The mechanisms of this toxicity are unknown, but the various agents interact more or less with the hepatic cytochrome P450 enzyme systems. Bosentan-induced hepatotoxicity may partly be due to inhibition of the canalicular bile salt export pump *(25)*.

3.1. Trials with Bosentan

In the initial clinical study of ET-receptor blockade, pulmonary vascular resistance fell by 25% when bosentan was infused intravenously into seven patients with PAH *(26)*. Plasma ET-1 levels rose consistent with blockade of the ET_B receptor. Unfortunately, two of the seven patients died within 36 hours of entering the second phase of the study, and several others had clinical deteriorations. Both patients who died were in advanced WHO functional class IV at the time of entry into the study, and their deaths were not unexpected. Despite this setback, the belief and determination of pioneering clinicians led to the continued evaluation and eventual approval of clinically effective endothelin-receptor antagonists for PAH.

The first randomized, double-blind, placebo-controlled trial of an endothelin-receptor antagonist (study 351) showed that over a 12-week period, oral bosentan (62.5 mg bid for 4 weeks, then 125 mg bid) provided significant benefit to patients with idiopathic PAH or PAH related to scleroderma *(27)*. All patients were in WHO functional class III at baseline. The six-minute walk distance improved by a mean of 70 m compared to baseline, and there were concordant improvements in pulmonary vascular resistance and WHO functional class and a significant delay in the time to clinical worsening. However, pulmonary arterial pressure did not change, and there was a 10% incidence of hepatotoxicity in bosentan-treated patients, which resolved upon discontinuation of the drug.

3.1.1. BREATHE-1

The success of this initial trial stimulated a large double-blind, placebo-controlled study, the Bosentan Randomized trial of Endothelin receptor Antagonist THERapy of pulmonary hypertension (BREATHE-1) *(28)*, which randomized 213 patients to placebo or bosentan for 16 weeks. In the bosentan group, after 4 weeks of 62.5 mg bid, patients were randomized to 125 mg bid or 250 mg bid. Over 90% of the patients were in WHO functional class III at baseline, and the remainder was in functional class 4. Once again, patients treated with bosentan (both doses combined) had improved six-minute walk distance (mean 36 m over baseline) (Fig. 1) and WHO functional class and had a delayed time to clinical worsening. Despite the significant improvements, the majority of patients were still in functional class III

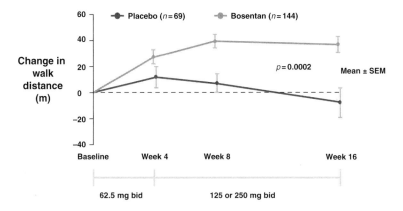

Fig. 1. Increase in six-minute walk distance (m) in BREATHE-1, the major outcome variable in the pivotal trial testing the clinical efficacy of bosentan in PAH. The two doses of bosentan (125 and 250 mg bid) were combined in this analysis. The difference compared to placebo was statistically significant at the weeks 12 and 16 time points. (From [28], with permission.) (To view this figure in color, see insert.)

or IV at the end of the study, and the combined bosentan group had a 9% incidence of abnormal hepatic function. Although there was no significant dose-response relationship for efficacy, there was a trend toward greater treatment effect as compared to placebo in the 250-mg bid group. However, the incidence of hepatotoxicity was found to be dose-dependent, with an incidence of abnormal hepatic function in 14% and severe hepatic aminotransferase elevations (>8 times the limit for upper normal) in 7% of patients treated with 250 mg bid. Therefore, the recommended maintenance dose was set at 125 mg bid. Compared to baseline, bosentan therapy increased the six-minute walk distance (6MWD) by 46 m in patients with idiopathic PAH, but only by 3 m in those with scleroderma. On the other hand, bosentan prevented a deterioration in walk distance in patients with scleroderma, whereas the distance declined in the placebo control group. In addition, an echocardiographic substudy showed that bosentan improved right ventricular size and systolic function as well as left ventricular filling *(29)*. BREATHE-1 was a landmark study and led to the U.S. Food and Drug Administration approval of bosentan and to its clinical availability in 2002.

The durability of bosentan was evaluated in a one-year follow-up study of patients receiving open-label bosentan. The six-minute walk distance, pulmonary hemodynamics, and functional class all improved compared to baseline *(30)*. At initiation, 97% of patients were in functional class III. By 12 months, only 55% were in class III, whereas 38% were in class II. Liver function abnormalities developed in 9% of patients but did not necessitate discontinuation. One patient deteriorated and was switched to epoprostenol therapy. In a survival analysis on a different cohort of 169 bosentan-treated patients with idiopathic PAH, two-year survival was approximately 92% *(31)*. While these data are very encouraging, the figure of 92% must be interpreted with caution, since 9% of the patients were in functional class II at baseline and would have an expected high survival and another 10% of the patients failed bosentan therapy alone. They required concurrent epoprostenol therapy and should not be considered "survival successes" for bosentan. Thus, the actual failure-free survival for functional class III patients is probably closer to 80%. These results are still impressive for an oral agent. By comparison, the survival for a similar group with functional class III idiopathic PAH treated with continuous intravenous epoprostenol was 88% *(32)*.

The relative ease and safety of an oral endothelin antagonist as compared to intravenous epoprostenol have led to attempts to wean patients off epoprostenol and onto bosentan. In a small study, four patients were successfully transitioned from epoprostenol to bosentan *(33)*. All had achieved normal pulmonary artery pressures on epoprostenol and then had clinical stability when on bosentan. In a series of three children who also had normal pulmonary artery pressures while on epoprostenol, it was successfully changed to bosentan, with clinical stability for up to one year *(34)*. In a larger series of carefully selected, stable adults with PAH, only 65% could be successfully transitioned from epoprostenol or treprostinil to bosentan over a 12-week period; due to hepatotoxicity, other side effects, or failure of bosentan therapy, only 39% of the cohort remained on bosentan 3 to 16 months after stopping the prostaglandins *(35)*. Unlike the patients in the two previous studies, the pulmonary arterial pressure (as assessed by Doppler echocardiography) was moderately to severely elevated while on the prostaglandin therapy. Patients who failed transition tended to have higher pulmonary arterial pressures. On the basis of these data, it has been suggested that transition from prostaglandins to bosentan not be attempted unless the pulmonary arterial pressure has reached normal levels while on prostaglandin therapy.

3.1.2. BREATHE-2

The use of bosentan in combination with prostanoids as therapy for PAH has been explored *(36,37)*. In an open-label study, the use of bosentan as an add-on therapy was studied in patients already receiving either inhaled iloprost or oral beraprost *(36)*. After three months of combination therapy, the mean 6MWD increased by 58 m. In a subsequent study (BREATHE-2), 33 patients with PAH received epoprostenol, and also bosentan or placebo, in a double-blind fashion for 16 weeks *(37)*. There was a nonsignificant trend to greater hemodynamic improvement with combined therapy than with epoprostenol alone, but this did not translate into improved exercise tolerance or functional class. Two of the patients on combination therapy died, and another had worsening PAH; the possibility of a negative interaction of combination therapy could not be excluded. It was appropriately suggested that larger trials of combination therapy are needed to properly address the question.

3.1.3. BREATHE-3

The BREATHE-3 trial *(38)* was an open-label, 12-week trial that tested dosing and pulmonary hemodynamic effects of bosentan in a pediatric population, approximately half of whom had idiopathic and the remainder congenital heart disease-related PAH. Nineteen patients were enrolled, half of whom were receiving concomitant intravenous epoprostenol. A weight-adjusted dosing regimen resulted in bosentan levels in the desired range, and pulmonary hemodynamics significantly improved, with drops in mean PA pressure of 8.0 mm Hg and in pulmonary vascular resistance index of 300 dyne/sec/cm^{-5}/m^{-2} compared to baseline.

3.1.4. BREATHE-4

BREATHE-4 was an open-label, 16-week trial of the efficacy and safety of bosentan in a group of 16 patients with HIV-related PAH *(39)*. The six-minute walk distance increased from 333 m at baseline to 424 m at 16 weeks, NYHA class improved in 14 of the patients, quality of life improved, and the drug was well-tolerated. The expected frequency of liver toxicity was encountered (9%), and there were no adverse interactions with concomitant antiretroviral therapy.

3.1.5. BREATHE-5

BREATHE-5 was a randomized, placebo-controlled trial of PAH therapy for patients with Eisenmenger's syndrome *(40)*. Fifty-four patients were randomized to bosentan or placebo for 16 weeks. Bosentan-treated patients had no significant change in oxygen saturation (+1.0%), the major outcome variable. Pulmonary hemodynamics improved significantly, in that pulmonary vascular resistance index decreased by 472 dyne/s/cm^{-5}/m^{-2} and the 6MWD increased by 34 m compared to baseline ($p < 0.01$). The side effect profile was comparable to prior studies of bosentan.

3.2. Trials with Sitaxsentan

Clinical studies with the highly selective ET$_A$-receptor antagonist sitaxsentan have also provided extremely encouraging results. In a 12-week, open-label pilot study *(41)*, at doses of 100 to 500 mg bid, the mean 6MWD increased by 50 m in patients with functional class II, III, and IV PAH, with concomitant improvements in hemodynamics. There were two cases of acute hepatitis during the study extension phase, one of which was fatal, and which, in retrospect, may have been related to the dose and nonlinear pharmacokinetics of sitaxsentan at high doses.

3.2.1. STRIDE-1

A subsequent large, placebo-controlled, double-blind trial of sitaxsentan at lower doses (100 mg and 300 mg daily) showed significant efficacy with low toxicity *(42)*. That study, STRIDE-1, had inclusion criteria that were different from those of earlier trials of endothelin-receptor antagonist therapy in PAH, which have traditionally included patients with functional class III and IV PAH, idiopathic or related to connective disease only, and with a baseline six-minute walk distance between 150 and 450 m *(28)*. STRIDE-1 also included patients with functional class II PAH and with PAH related to congenital heart disease, and it had no minimum or maximum 6MWD. Instead, it utilized the peak V_{O2} on cardiopulmonary exercise testing as an inclusion criterion and an endpoint. In retrospect, this technique of assessing functional capacity carried too much interhospital variability to be able to detect meaningful differences, a problem that had also been seen in a study of beraprost for PAH *(43)*. Nonetheless, STRIDE-1 showed that sitaxsentan significantly improved the six-minute walk distance (treatment effects of 22 m for 100 mg daily and 20 m for 300 mg daily), functional class, and pulmonary hemodynamics *(42)*. The U.S. FDA has recognized the difficulties with cardiopulmonary exercise testing as a primary endpoint and has accepted STRIDE-1 as a pivotal trial toward approval. The incidence of elevated hepatic aminotransferase levels at more than three times the upper limit of normal was 0% for 100 mg daily and 10% for 300 mg daily. Pharmacokinetic studies demonstrated a 1.3-fold increase in the area under the curve at week 12 versus baseline for 100 mg daily, and a 3.1-fold increase for 300 mg daily, confirming the nonlinearity of sitaxsentan elimination when given at a dose of 300 mg daily. In the study extension trial, the incidence of liver enzyme abnormalities was 5% for 100 mg daily and 21% for 300 mg daily, with a median exposure of 26 weeks up to a maximum of 58 weeks. With these data, 100 mg was chosen as the preferred maximum dose for further evaluation. Sitaxsentan inhibits the CYP2C9 cytochrome P450 enzyme, which is involved in the metabolism of warfarin. This drug interaction was easily managed by reducing the warfarin dose and following the INR levels.

A small, single-center, open-label study has demonstrated a durable effect for sitaxsentan over a one-year period *(43)*. Out of 11 patients with PAH, one worsened at seven months of therapy and failed a transition to epoprostenol. The other patients all improved and stabilized at functional class II. The six-minute walk distance improved by 50 m, and there were significant improvements in pulmonary vascular resistance and cardiac output. There were no serious adverse events over the year, nor instances of hepatotoxicity or complications related to the sitaxsentan–warfarin interaction.

3.2.2. STRIDE-2 AND -2X

A second pivotal study of sitaxsentan in PAH, STRIDE-2, was performed *(44)*. An 18-week multicenter trial randomized 245 patients to four groups: placebo, sitaxsentan 50 or 100 mg daily, or bosentan 62.5 mg twice daily for a month and then 125 mg twice daily as long as liver function test results were acceptable. As per the FDA-mandated design, bosentan was included as a "standard therapy" arm and was "open-label." Both the 100-mg sitaxsentan and bosentan arms showed statistically significant increases in the 6MWD (the major outcome variable) of 25 and 23 m, respectively, but the increase in the 6MWD for the 50-mg sitaxsentan group did not reach statistical significance (Fig. 2). There were also significant improvements in functional class for the 100-mg sitaxsentan and bosentan groups. The incidence of hepatic transaminase levels above three times the upper limit of normal was 3% in the 100-mg sitaxsentan group versus 5% in placebo versus 11% in the bosentan group.

STRIDE-2X *(45)*, the open-label extension trial for STRIDE-2, investigated sitaxsentan 100 mg once daily (145 pts) and bosentan 125 mg twice daily (84 pts). The two arms consisted of patients continued on sitaxsentan 100 mg daily or bosentan, and placebo patients, who were randomized to receive one or the other. Patients begun on the 50-mg-daily sitaxsentan dose in STRIDE-2 were increased to

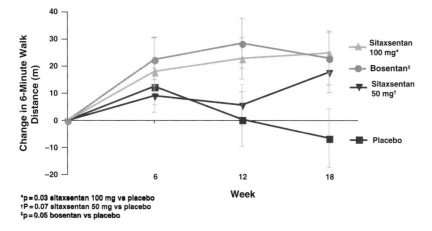

*p = 0.03 sitaxsentan 100 mg vs placebo
†P = 0.07 sitaxsentan 50 mg vs placebo
‡p = 0.05 bosentan vs placebo

Fig. 2. Increase in six-minute walk distance, the major outcome variable in the STRIDE-2 study. Both sitaxsentan (100 mg) and bosentan (125 mg bid) showed significant improvements over placebo at 12 and 18 weeks, although they were not different from each other. (To view this figure in color, see insert.)

100 mg sitaxsentan for STRIDE-2X. Because of potential method-
ological pitfalls related to the failure to randomize patients receiving
the 50-mg sitaxsentan dose to the 100-mg dose or bosentan, a conservative analysis of the data has been performed that excludes this patient
group and also considers only "hard" deterioration endpoints such as
death, hospitalization, transplantation, change in functional class and
exercise duration, and need for epoprostenol rescue therapy. Interim
results for patients with up to a year of follow-up revealed a significant therapeutic benefit in the time to clinical worsening and survival
in the sitaxsentan compared to the bosentan group (Fig. 3). Most of
this difference was attributable to the connective tissue disease group.
Only 1% of patients receiving sitaxsentan discontinued because of
liver toxicity, whereas 9% of patients receiving bosentan did so ($p <$
0.01). Also, 79% of the sitaxsentan group continued on monotherapy,
compared to 63% in the bosentan group ($p < 0.01$). These results

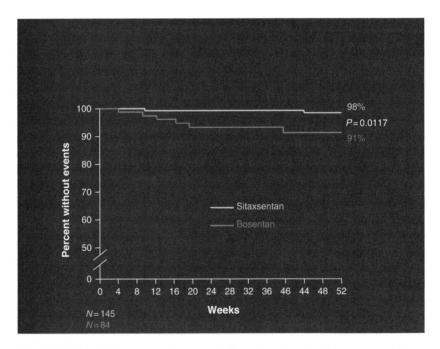

Fig. 3. Kaplan–Meier curves for rate of discontinuation for liver enzyme elevations (larger than fivefold elevation over normal) in the STRIDE-2X study. At
the end of 52 weeks of follow-up, the sitaxsentan group had significantly fewer
discontinuations than the bosentan group. (From Barst et al., presented at Annual
Meeting of the American Thoracic Society, San Diego, CA, 2005.) (To view this
figure in color, see insert.)

have not yet been subjected to peer review and must be considered preliminary.

3.2.3. STRIDE-3

STRIDE-3 is an ongoing trial that consists of patients completing STRIDE-2X and others entered *de novo* in this long-term safety trial. Over 800 patients are now being monitored, but as of yet no results have been reported.

3.2.4. STRIDE-4

Conducted in Latin America, Poland, and Spain, STRIDE-4 was an additional dose-ranging trial that compared 50- and 100-mg daily doses of sitaxsentan *(46)*. Among 98 patients randomized 1:1:1 to the two doses and a placebo arm, the 6MWD, the primary endpoint, improved 58 m for the 100-mg dose versus 22 m for the 50-mg dose ($p = 0.014$) and 34 m with placebo ($p = 0.2$). The unusual increase in the 6MWD in the placebo group was ascribed to improved medical care after enrollment among South American patients. Other variables that suggested improvement at the 100-mg dose versus placebo included WHO functional class ($p = 0.038$), time to clinical worsening ($p = 0.09$), and Borg dyspnea scale ($p = 0.016$). As with STRIDE-2, the 50-mg dose showed no significant efficacy. The drug was well tolerated, with only one patient in each group (3%) experiencing liver enzyme increases exceeding three times the upper limit of normal.

3.2.5. STRIDE-6

STRIDE-6 tested the efficacy and toxicity of sitaxsentan in patients discontinued from bosentan because of liver enzyme elevation (13 patients) or lack of efficacy (35 patients) *(47)*. After 12 weeks, only one of the 13 patients experiencing liver function abnormalities on bosentan developed transaminase elevations on sitaxsentan. Of 15 patients discontinued because of lack of efficacy and placed on the 100-mg dose, 33% increased the 6MWD by more than 15%, compared to 10% for 20 patients receiving the 50-mg dose. These findings demonstrate that during the initial 12 weeks, sitaxsentan is unlikely to cause liver toxicity in patients with previous bosentan-induced liver enzyme elevation and may still bring about clinical improvement in some patients in whom bosentan lacked efficacy.

3.3. Trials with Ambrisentan

A phase II clinical study in PAH has been reported with the slightly ET_A-selective antagonist ambrisentan (48). In a 12-week blinded study that was not placebo-controlled, ambrisentan at 1, 2.5, 5, or 10 mg daily increased the mean six-minute walk distance by 33.9–38.1 m as compared to baseline. There was a dose relationship for the subgroup with idiopathic PAH, where the mean 6MWD increased by 54 m at the 10-mg dose. Significant improvements were also seen in WHO class, Borg dyspnea score, and pulmonary hemodynamics, with the mean PA pressure dropping by 5.2 mm Hg and the cardiac index increasing by 0.33 L/min. This study was followed by a 12-week, open-label uptitration phase, after which 48% of patients were receiving 10 mg per day by week 24. Elevated liver enzymes (more than three times the normal level) occurred in 3.1% of patients, and the medication was stopped in only one patient.

3.3.1. ARIES-1 AND ARIES-2

Two large placebo-controlled phase III trials of ambrisentan—ARIES-1 and ARIES-2—have been completed (49,50). In ARIES-1, 202 patients, mainly from North America, were randomized to receive placebo or 5 or 10 mg of ambrisentan daily for 12 weeks. The major outcome variable, the 6MWD, showed a 44-m improvement for the 10-mg dose and a 23-m improvement for the 5-mg dose, both statistically significant. There were also improvements in WHO functional class, the Borg dyspnea score, and the SF-36 quality-of-life scale. ARIES-2 randomized 192 patients, mainly from Europe, to placebo, 2.5 mg, and 5 mg, respectively. The mean 6MWD improved by 49 m and 22 m in the 5- and 2.5-mg daily dosage groups, respectively. Improvements in time to clinical worsening compared to placebo were observed for both the 5-mg and 2.5-mg dosage groups.

Ambrisentan was generally well tolerated in both trials. In ARIES-2, the most frequent adverse event was headache in 12.7% of patients in the 5-mg dose group and 7.8% in the 2.5-mg dose group, compared to 6.2% in the placebo group. No patients treated with ambrisentan developed serum aminotransferase concentrations greater than three times the upper limit of the normal range, compared to one patient in the placebo group. Ambrisentan had no apparent interaction with warfarin.

4. SELECTION OF AN ENDOTHELIN-RECEPTOR ANTAGONIST

With the approval of ambrisentan by the FDA in June 2007, clinicians now have the welcome predicament there are now 2 endothelin-receptor antagonists available in the US. Sitaxsentan received an "approveable" rating from the FDA, but has not yet been formally approved (see Table 1). Although approved in Europe, Australia, New Zealand and Canada, sitaxsentan has not yet been approved by the FDA for marketing in the US. In 12- to 18-week trials, all three agents—bosentan, sitaxsentan, and ambrisentan—appear to have similar efficacy (see Table 1). A post hoc comparison between the STRIDE-1 and BREATHE-1 studies analyzing only the subset of PAH patients that met inclusion criteria of both endothelin antagonist trials, i.e., PAH that was idiopathic or related to connective tissue disease, functional classes III and IV, and baseline 6MWD < 450 m, suggested a greater effect with sitaxsentan *(51)*. The placebo-subtracted treatment effect was 65 m, exceeding that in the BREATHE-1 trial of bosentan, despite the fact that the treatment duration in BREATHE-1 was four weeks longer *(28)*. There were also highly significant improvements in hemodynamics and functional class in this STRIDE-1 cohort. In BREATHE-1, the benefit of bosentan in connective tissue disease patients was to prevent the deterioration seen in the placebo group; the mean six-minute walk distance in the bosentan-treated patients improved by only 3 m as compared to their baseline distance. In STRIDE-1, the 6MWD in the placebo group with connective tissue disease declined to almost an identical degree to that of the placebo group with connective tissue disease in BREATHE-1; sitaxsentan not only prevented the decline, but it actually resulted in a mean 20-m improvement in 6MWD as compared to baseline *(42)*.

Other potential advantages of sitaxsentan and ambrisentan are that they are dosed once daily as compared to twice daily for bosentan and they appear to have less liver toxicity. On the other hand, monthly liver enzyme monitoring will probably be required for all three drugs, and the liver toxicity of bosentan is reversible as long as the drug is stopped promptly in the face of more than a fivefold elevation. Sitaxsentan has a greater interaction with warfarin than the others, but this can be easily managed with a downward adjustment of the warfarin dose and appropriate monitoring of the INR until stabilized. Bosentan has a greater interaction with sildenafil, but the clinical significance of this effect is unclear.

Table 1
Comparison of Endothelin-Receptor Antagonists

	Bosentan (Tracleer)	Sitaxsentan (Thelin)	Approved 2007
FDA approval status	Approved 2001	"Approveable"	Approved 2007
Selectivity (ET_A:ET_B)	20:1	6500:1	77:1
Dosing	bid	Once daily	Once daily
Clinical efficacy: Six-minute walk distance (change from baseline in placebo-controlled trials)	↑ 29–70 m	↑ 20–39 m	↑ 23–49 m
Improved WHO class[1]	Yes	Yes	Yes
Delay of worsening[2]	Yes	Maybe[3]	Yes
Liver toxicity[4]	7–10%	3–5%	3–5%
Drug interactions: Warfarin	↑ metabolism	↓ metabolism	None
Sildenafil	↑ metabolism	None	None

[1] World Health Organization/New York Heart Association functional class.
[2] Delay in clinical worsening.
[3] Delay of clinical worsening compared to bosentan in preliminary study.
[4] At least a threefold elevation in aminotransferases.

Long-term follow-up data are available for bosentan, showing excellent survival rates, although some patients require additional therapies over time. In addition, approximately 60% of bosentan-treated patients remain in functional class III or IV after one year of therapy, indicating the need for more effective oral therapy. As discussed above, a preliminary analysis of STRIDE-2X data suggests that after one year of follow-up, the sitaxsentan-treated PAH group had more benefit than a matched bosentan-treated PAH group *(45)*. Thus, all three drugs have relative advantages and disadvantages, and clinicians will have to decide among them based on a careful assessment of the evidence. Current evidence raises the possibility that there may be merit to the hypothesis of clinical superiority of selective ET_A-receptor antagonism versus nonselective antagonism, particularly for the connective tissue disease subgroup, but the hypothesis remains to be confirmed in properly designed comparison trials.

5. CONCLUSION AND FUTURE DIRECTIONS

In the 18 years since its discovery *(1)*, and in the 15 years since increased levels were identified in PAH *(2)*, the recognition that ET-1 is a mediator of PAH has provided an invaluable opportunity to modify the disease through endothelin-receptor blockade. Pathophysiological studies to date have demonstrated that the ET_A receptor contributes to pulmonary hypertension, but the clinical significance of increased smooth muscle and fibroblast ET_B-receptor expression in disease states is unclear. Functional studies published thus far using selective ET_B-receptor blockers suggest that the excess ET_B receptors do not contribute to vasoconstriction or proliferation. However, many unanswered questions remain to be resolved: Will selective ET_A-receptor blockade be superior to nonselective ET_A- and ET_B-receptor blockade? How important is the degree of selectivity? Will ET-1-receptor antagonists have the long-term effectiveness of prostaglandins? Which medication combinations will be the most effective? Can we identify, using pharmacogenomic analyses, subsets of patients who will benefit the most from ET-1-receptor blockade, and can we prospectively identify nonresponders? Will we be able to identify PAH etiologies that respond better to selective ET_A-receptor blockade, and others that respond better to nonselective blockade? Careful study of well-characterized patient populations should provide us with answers, and we hope to be able to offer increasingly effective therapy for this infrequent but devastating group of diseases.

REFERENCES

1. Yanagisawa M, Kurihara H, Kimura S, Tomobe Y, Kobayashi M, Mitsui Y, et al. A novel potent vasoconstrictor peptide produced by vascular endothelial cells. Nature 1988; 332:411–5.
2. Stewart DJ, Levy RD, Cernacek P, Langleben D. Increased plasma endothelin-1 in pulmonary hypertension: Marker or mediator of disease? Ann Intern Med 1991; 114:464–9.
3. Giaid A, Yanagisawa M, Langleben D, Michel RP, Levy RD, Shennib H, et al. Expression of endothelin-1 in the lungs of patients with pulmonary hypertension. N Engl J Med 1993; 328:1732–9.

4. Arai H, Hori S, Aramori I, Ohkubo H, Nakanishi S. Cloning and expression of a cDNA encoding an endothelin receptor. Nature 1990; 348:730–2.

5. Sakurai T, Yanagisawa M, Takuwa Y, Miyazaki H, Kimura S, Goto K, et al. Cloning of a cDNA encoding a non-isopeptide-selective subtype of the endothelin receptor. Nature 1990; 348:732–4.

6. Sham JK, Crenshaw BR, Deng LH, Shimoda LA, Sylvester JT. Effects of hypoxia in porcine pulmonary arterial myocytes: Role of Kv channel and endothelin-1. Am J Physiol (Lung Cell Mol Physiol) 2000; 279: L262–L272.

7. Kawanabe Y, Okamoto Y, Nozaki K, Hashimoto N, Miwa S, Masaki T. Molecular mechanisms for endothelin-1-induced stress fiber formation: Analysis of G proteins using a mutant endothelin (A) receptor. Mol Pharmacol 2002; 61:277–84.

8. Kedzierski RM, Yanagisawa M. Endothelin system: The double-edged sword in health and disease. Ann Rev Pharmacol Toxicol 2001; 41:851–76.

9. Iwamuro Y, Miwa S, Zhang XF, Minowa T, Enoki T, Okamoto Y, et al. Activation of three types of voltage-independent Ca^{2+} channel in A7r5 cells by endothelin-1 as revealed by a novel Ca^{2+} channel blocker LOE 908. Br J Pharmacol 1999; 126:1107–14.

10. Evans AM, Cobban HJ, Nixon GF. ET_A receptors are the primary mediators of myofilament calcium sensitization induced by ET-1 in rat pulmonary artery smooth muscle: A tyrosine kinase independent pathway. Br J Pharmacol 1999; 127:153–60.

11. Davie N, Haleen SJ, Upton PD, Polak JM, Yacoub MH, Morrell NW. ET_A and ET_B receptors modulate the proliferation of human pulmonary artery smooth muscle cells. Am J Respir Crit Care Med 2002; 165:398–405.

12. Shi-Wen X, Chen Y, Denton CP, Eastwood M, Renzoni EA, Bou-Gharios G, et al. Endothelin-1 promotes myofibroblast induction through the ETA receptor via a rac/phosphoinositide 3-kinase/Akt-dependent pathway and is essential for the enhanced contractile phenotype of fibrotic fibroblasts. Mol Biol Cell 2004; 15:2707–19.

13. Muramatsu M, Rodman DM, Oka M, McMurtry IF. Endothelin-1 mediates nitro-L-arginine vasoconstriction of hypertensive rat lungs. Am J Physiol (Lung Cell Mol Physiol) 1997; 272:L807–L812.

14. Black SM, Mata-Greenwood E, Dettman RW, Ovadia B, Fitzgerald RK, Reinhartz O, et al. Emergence of smooth muscle cell endothelin B-mediated vasoconstriction in lambs with experimental congenital heart disease and increased pulmonary blood flow. Circulation 2003; 108: 1646–54.

15. De Nucci G, Thomas R, D'Orleans-Juste P, Antunes E, Walder C, Warner TD, et al. Pressor effects of circulating endothelin are limited by its removal in the pulmonary circulation and by the release of prostacyclin and endothelium-derived relaxing factor. Proc Natl Acad Sci USA 1988; 85:9797–800.

16. Dupuis J, Stewart DJ, Cernacek P, Gosselin G. Human pulmonary circulation is an important site for both clearance and production of endothelin-1. Circulation 1996; 94:1578–84.

17. Dupuis J, Goresky CA, Fournier A. Pulmonary clearance of circulating endothelin-1 in dogs *in vivo*: Exclusive role of ETB receptors. J Appl Physiol 1996; 81:1510–5.

18. Dupuis J, Goresky CA, Stewart DJ. Pulmonary removal and production of endothelin in the anesthetized dog. J Appl Physiol 1994; 76:694–700.

19. Langleben D, Dupuis J, Langleben I, Hirsch AM, Baron M, Senecal JL, et al. Etiology-specific endothelin-1 clearance in human precapillary pulmonary hypertension. Chest 2006; 129:689–95.

20. Adner M, Geary GG, Edvinsson L. Appearance of contractile endothelin-B receptors in rat mesenteric arterial segments following organ culture. Acta Physiol Scand 1998; 163:121–9.

21. Muramatsu M, Oka M, Morio Y, Soma S, Takahashi H, Fukuchi Y. Chronic hypoxia augments endothelin-B receptor-mediated vasodilation in isolated perfused rat lungs. Am J Physiol (Lung Cell Mol Physiol) 1999; 276:L358–L364.

22. Abraham DJ, Vancheeswaran R, Dashwood MR, Rajkumar VS, Pantelides P, Shi-Wen X, et al. Increased levels of endothelin-1 and differential endothelin type A and B receptor expression in scleroderma-associated fibrotic lung disease. Am J Pathol 1997; 151:831–41.

23. Bauer M, Wilkens H, Langer F, Schneider SO, Lausberg H, Schafers HJ. Selective upregulation of endothelin B receptor gene expression in severe pulmonary hypertension. Circulation 2002; 105:1034–6.

24. Clozel M, Loffler BM, Breu V, Hilfiger L, Maire JP, Butscha B. Downregulation of endothelin receptors by autocrine production of endothelin-1. Am J Physiol (Cell Physiol) 1993; 265:C188–C192.

25. Fattinger K, Funk C, Pantze M, Weber C, Reichen J, Stieger B, et al. The endothelin antagonist bosentan inhibits the canalicular bile salt export pump: A potential mechanism for hepatic adverse reactions. Clin Pharmacol Ther 2001; 69:223–31.

26. Williamson DJ, Wallman LL, Jones R, Keogh AM, Scroope F, Penny R, et al. Hemodynamic effects of bosentan, an endothelin receptor antagonist, in patients with pulmonary hypertension. Circulation 2000; 102:411–8.

27. Channick RN, Simonneau G, Sitbon O, Robbins IM, Frost A, Tapson VF, et al. Effects of the dual endothelin-receptor antagonist bosentan in patients with pulmonary hypertension: A randomised placebo-controlled study. Lancet 2001; 358:1119–23.

28. Rubin LJ, Badesch DB, Barst RJ, Galie N, Black CM, Keogh A, et al. Bosentan therapy for pulmonary arterial hypertension. N Engl J Med 2002; 346:896–903.

29. Galie N, Hinderliter AL, Torbicki A, Fourme T, Simonneau G, Pulido T, et al. Effects of the oral endothelin-receptor antagonist bosentan on echocardiographic and Doppler measures in patients with pulmonary arterial hypertension. J Am Coll Cardiol 2003; 41:1380–6.

30. Sitbon O, Badesch DB, Channick RN, Frost A, Robbins IM, Simonneau G, et al. Effects of the dual endothelin receptor antagonist bosentan in patients with pulmonary arterial hypertension. Chest 2003; 124:247–54.
31. McLaughlin V, Sitbon O, Rubin LJ, Levy P, Barst R, Badesch D, et al. The effect of first-line bosentan on survival of patients with primary pulmonary hypertension. Am J Resp Crit Care Med 2003; 167:A442.
32. McLaughlin VV, Shillington A, Rich S. Survival in primary pulmonary hypertension: The impact of epoprostenol therapy. Circulation 2002; 106:1477–82.
33. Kim NH, Channick RN, Rubin LJ. Successful withdrawal of long-term epoprostenol therapy for pulmonary arterial hypertension. Chest 2003; 124:1612–5.
34. Ivy DD, Doran A, Claussen L, Bingaman D, Yetman A. Weaning and discontinuation of epoprostenol in children with idiopathic pulmonary arterial hypertension receiving concomitant bosentan. Am J Cardiol 2004; 93:943–6.
35. Suleman N, Frost AE. Transition from epoprostenol and treprostinil to the oral endothelin receptor antagonist bosentan in patients with pulmonary hypertension. Chest 2004; 126:808–15.
36. Hoeper MM, Taha N, Bekjarova A, Gatzke R, Spiekerkoetter E. Bosentan treatment in patients with primary pulmonary hypertension receiving nonparenteral prostanoids. Eur Respir J 2003; 22:330–4.
37. Humbert M, Barst RJ, Robbins IM, Channick RN, Galie N, Boonstra A, et al. Combination of bosentan with epoprostenol in pulmonary arterial hypertension: BREATHE-2. Eur Respir J 2004; 24:353–9.
38. Barst RJ, Dunbar I, et al. Pharmacokinetics, safety, and efficacy of bosentan in pediatric patients with pulmonary arterial hypertension. Clin Pharmacol Ther 2003; 73:372–82.
39. Sitbon O, Gressin V, Speich R, et al. Bosentan for the treatment of human immunodeficiency virus-associated pulmonary arterial hypertension. Am J Respir Crit Care Med 2004; 170:1212–7.
40. Galie N, Beghetti M, Gatzoulis MA, Granton J, Berger RMF, Lauer A, et al. Bosentan therapy in patients with Eisenmenger syndrome: A multi-center, double-blind, randomized, placebo-controlled study. Circulation 2006; 114:48–54.
41. Barst RJ, Rich S, Widlitz A, Horn EM, McLaughlin V, McFarlin J. Clinical efficacy of sitaxsentan, an endothelin-A receptor antagonist, in patients with pulmonary arterial hypertension: Open-label pilot study. Chest 2002 Jun; 121(6):1860–8.
42. Barst RJ, Langleben D, Frost A, Horn EM, Oudiz RJ, Shapiro SM, et al. Sitaxsentan therapy for pulmonary arterial hypertension. Am J Respir Crit Care Med 2004; 169:441–7.
43. Langleben D, Hirsch AM, Shalit E, Lesenko L, Barst RJ. Sustained symptomatic, functional, and hemodynamic benefit with the selective endothelin-A receptor antagonist, sitaxsentan, in patients with pulmonary arterial hypertension. Chest 2004; 126:1377–81.

44. Barst RJ, Langleben D, Badesch D, Frost A, Lawrence EC, Shapiro S, et al. Treatment of pulmonary arterial hypertension with the selective endothelin-A receptor antagonist sitaxsentan. J Am Coll Cardiol 2006; 47:2049–56.

45. Benza R, Frost A, Girgis R, Langleben D, Lawrence EC, Naeije R. Chronic treatment of pulmonary arterial hypertension with sitaxsentan and bosentan. Proc Am Thorac Soc 2006; 3:A729.

46. Pulido T, Kurzyna M, Souza R, Ramirez A, Sandoval J. Sitaxsentan 100 mg proves more effective than sitaxsentan 50 mg in patients with pulmonary arterial hypertension. Proc Am Thorac Soc 2006; 3:A417.

47. Benza R, Mehta S, Keogh A, Lawrence EC, Oudiz R, Barst RJ. Sitaxsentan treatment for patients with pulmonary arterial hypertension failing bosentan treatment. Proc Am Thorac Soc 2005; 2:A201.

48. Galie N, Badesch D, Oudiz R, Simonneau G, McGoon MD, Keogh AM, Frost AE, Zwicke D, Naeije R, Shapiro S, Olschewski H, Rubin LJ. Ambrisentan therapy for pulmonary arterial hypertension. J Am Coll Cardiol 2005 Aug 2; 46(3):529–35.

49. ARIES-1 News Release, April 10, 2006.

50. Olschewski H, Galie N, Ghofrani HA, Kramer MR, Rubin LJ. Ambrisentan improves exercise capacity and time to clinical worsening in patients with pulmonary arterial hypertension: Results of the ARIES-2 study. Proc Am Thorac Soc 2006; 3:A728.

51. Langleben D, Brock T, Dixon R, Barst R. STRIDE-1: Effects of the selective ET-A receptor antagonist, sitaxsentan sodium, in a patient population with pulmonary arterial hypertension that meets traditional inclusion criteria of previous pulmonary arterial hypertension trials. J Cardiovasc Pharmacol 2004; 44:S80–S84.

14 PDE5 Inhibitors and the cGMP Pathway in Pulmonary Arterial Hypertension

Ioana R. Preston

CONTENTS

INTRODUCTION
MODULATION OF CGMP IN THE PULMONARY
    VASCULATURE
PDE5 INHIBITION IN OTHER WHO PH
    SUBGROUPS
COMBINATION THERAPY
COMPARING PAH THERAPIES
CONCLUSIONS
REFERENCES

Abstract

Agents that raise the intracellular cGMP are effective pulmonary vasodilators and smooth muscle antimitogens. Compelling evidence supports the acute and long-term efficacy of PDE5 inhibition in different forms of PAH, both experimental and clinical. In these studies, sildenafil at doses ranging from 20 mg to 100 mg tid or the equivalent consistently improved pulmonary hemodynamics, reduced evidence of remodeling (in experimental models), and, in clinical studies, enhanced functional capacity. Preliminary reports also suggest that the combination of PDE5 inhibitors with other therapies that either enhance cGMP elevation (NO, natriuretic peptides) or increase cAMP (prostacyclins), or even act on a different pathway altogether (endothelin-receptor blockers), may be beneficial in the treatment of this complex disease. However, much additional

From: *Contemporary Cardiology: Pulmonary Hypertension*
Edited by: N. S. Hill and H. W. Farber © Humana Press, Totowa, NJ

work is needed to better establish the mechanisms of efficacy, demonstrate the durability of beneficial effects, and establish that combination therapy will live up to its promise.

Key Words: phosphodiesterase inhibitors; nitric oxide; natriuretic peptides; pulmonary hypertension; pulmonary hemodynamics; cyclic guanine monophosphate; sildenafil; tadalafil; vardenafil.

1. INTRODUCTION

Cyclic guanosine monophosphate (cGMP) is an intracellular second messenger that relaxes smooth muscle and inhibits smooth muscle cell proliferation. Accordingly, one approach to the therapy of pulmonary hypertension is to manipulate the cGMP pathway to augment intracellular levels and exploit these beneficial effects. Nitric oxide and natriuretic peptides stimulate the production of cGMP, but long-term clinical use of these agents is impractical. The only practical, currently available long-term therapy for pulmonary hypertension that acts via increasing cGMP levels is sildenafil, the oral phosphodiesterase-5 (PDE5) inhibitor that slows cGMP metabolism. Thus, this chapter focuses on the pharmacology, clinical efficacy, and use of PDE5 inhibitors, mainly sildenafil, while briefly examining other possible approaches to raising cGMP levels.

2. MODULATION OF CGMP IN THE PULMONARY VASCULATURE

Intracellular cGMP mediates pulmonary vascular relaxation and inhibits proliferation by activating cGMP-related protein kinases and K-channels *(1,2)*. cGMP is produced through the action of either nitric oxide (NO), which stimulates soluble guanylyl cyclase, or natriuretic peptides (atrial and brain natriuretic peptides, ANP and BNP), which stimulate particulate guanylyl cyclase via either the natriuretic A or B receptors (Fig. 1). NO is a continuously released vasodilator in many vascular beds via the cleavage of L-arginine by endothelial cell nitric oxide synthase (eNOS). A reduction in the expression of eNOS and a presumed decrease in the synthesis of NO have been implicated in the pathogenesis of PAH *(3,4)*. The natriuretic peptides also play a physiological role in modulating pulmonary vascular and right ventricular hypertrophic responses during both the acute and chronic experimental forms of pulmonary hypertension *(5,6)* but have not yet been implicated as contributors to PAH.

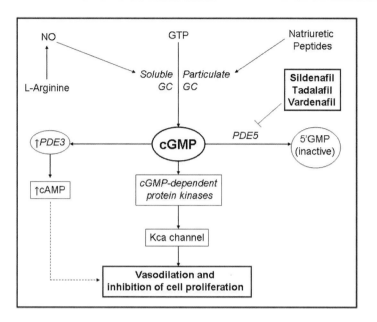

Fig. 1. Schema depicting components of the cGMP pathway. Nitric oxide and natriuretic peptides act on guanylate cyclase to stimulate the production of cGMP, which acts through calcium-dependent potassium channels to vasodilate. cGMP is metabolized by PDE5. The resulting increase in cGMP enhances vasodilator actions and feeds back on PDE3, slowing the metabolism of cAMP and intensifying the vasodilator effect. Sildenafil, tadalafil, and tardenafil block the action of PDE5 and increase cGMP levels. GC = guanylyl cyclase; NO = nitric oxide; cAMP = cyclic adenosine monophosphate; cGMP = cyclic guanosine monophosphate; PDE = phosphodiesterase.

PDEs comprise a superfamily of enzymes that inactivate cyclic adenosine monophosphate (cAMP) and cGMP *(7)*. Most families contain several distinct genes that are expressed in different tissues as functionally unique alternative splice variants. Among the 11 families of PDEs thus far described, PDE5 is the isoenzyme that selectively degrades cGMP into the inactive form. Pulmonary arteries have a large amount of PDE5 activity *(8)* that further increases in experimental forms of pulmonary hypertension *(9,10)* as well as in patients with PAH *(11)*. In addition to vasodilation, PDE5 inhibition also reduces DNA synthesis and cell proliferation in human pulmonary artery smooth muscle cells *(12)* and stimulates apoptosis *(11)*, suggesting that PDE5 inhibition also has antiremodeling effects on the pulmonary vasculature. In addition to PDE5, lungs have abundant PDE3 activity, which specifically inactivates cAMP. In a phenomenon referred to as "cross-talk" *(13)*, cGMP negatively feeds back on PDE3 and slows the inactivation of cAMP. Like cGMP, cAMP also has vasodilatory and antiproliferative pulmonary vascular actions. Thus, the pulmonary vasodilatory effects of cGMP are achieved not only via cGMP-related protein kinases but also via increasing cAMP, and it is unclear whether either messenger or the combination is most important.

The increased expression of PDE5 in pulmonary hypertensive states suggests that increased cGMP degradation contributes to the pathogenesis of pulmonary hypertension. Therefore, the salutary effects of cGMP on pulmonary vasculature might be restored in disease states by *(1)* increasing cGMP production via the nitric oxide or natriuretic peptides and/or *(2)* blocking PDE5 activity to slow cGMP degradation. Nitric oxide and natriuretic peptides ameliorate pulmonary hypertension in experimental models of pulmonary hypertension, but they require continuous delivery by the inhaled or intravenous routes, respectively, rendering them technically challenging and very expensive for clinical purposes. On the other hand, three oral PDE5 inhibitors to slow cGMP metabolism in patients with erectile dysfunction have been approved by the FDA. These include sildenafil (Viagra™), which has been available for nearly a decade, tadalafil (Cialis™), and vardenafil (Levitra™). The following examines studies on the effects of PDE5 inhibition, mainly sildenafil, which has been the most studied, in experimental and clinical forms of pulmonary hypertension.

2.1. PDE5 Inhibition Reduces Experimental PAH

Several experimental models of pulmonary hypertension have been developed to evaluate mechanisms of disease and responses to potential therapies. These include acute and chronic hypoxia, injection with oleic acid, which produces acute lung injury complicated by pulmonary hypertension, injection of the plant-derived alkaloid monocrotaline pyrrole, and acute infusion of the pulmonary vasoconstrictor thromboxane mimetic U46619.

2.1.1. Acute Pulmonary Hypertension

Several dozen experimental studies have shown that PDE5 inhibitors, alone or in combination with PDE3 inhibitors, effectively dilate pulmonary arteries *(14–17)*, regardless of the species or whether the route of administration is intravenous, oral, or inhaled. Furthermore, augmentation of cGMP by a combination of inhaled NO and inhaled sildenafil *(18)*, or intravenous atrial natriuretic peptide and oral sildenafil *(14)*, produces more pulmonary vasodilation than sildenafil alone.

2.1.2. Chronic Pulmonary Hypertension

PDE5 inhibition also attenuates pulmonary hypertension and reduces the proportion of distal pulmonary arteries that are muscularized in chronically hypoxic rats *(10,19)*. When administered for six weeks in the drinking water of rats with monocrotaline (MCT)-induced pulmonary hypertension, sildenafil increased cGMP and reduced pulmonary hypertension, muscularization of the peripheral pulmonary arteries, and right ventricular hypertrophy. It also improved survival but had no effect on gas exchange or systemic arterial pressure *(20)*. These findings indicate that PDE5 inhibitors have both acute vasodilator and chronic antiproliferative actions on the pulmonary circulation of animals with experimental pulmonary hypertension.

The vasodilator and antiremodeling effects of PDE5 inhibition also depend on the preservation of the NO/natriuretic peptide-cGMP pathways. Compared to wild-type controls, sildenafil achieved less reduction in the mean pulmonary artery (PA) pressure in chronically hypoxic mice with targeted disruption of the gene encoding endothelial NO synthase (eNOS) *(21)* and failed to reduce RV hypertrophy or pulmonary vascular muscularization. Similarly, chronically hypoxic mice with gene-targeted disruption of the guanylyl cyclase-linked natriuretic peptide A receptor (NPR-A) manifested less blunting of the rise in mean PA pressure, RV hypertrophy, and pulmonary vascular remodeling than wild-type controls *(22)*. These findings indicate that endogenous natriuretic peptides and NO synthesis are involved in the pulmonary vascular effects of sildenafil.

2.2. Effects of PDE5 Inhibition on Clinical PAH

2.2.1. Acute Effects of PDE5 Inhibition on Pulmonary Hypertension

Several studies have shown that sildenafil is a potent and rapidly acting pulmonary vasodilator in PAH patients. One compared acute responses to oral sildenafil (total dose: 100 mg), iNO (40 ppm), and aerosolized iloprost (15 to 20 µg) in 10 consecutive patients with idiopathic PAH *(23)*. All three significantly lowered the mean PA pressure and pulmonary vascular resistance (PVR), but iloprost reduced PVR > 20% in 7 of the 10 patients compared to 4 of 10 for each of the other agents and was the only one to significantly improve oxygenation. In 13 PAH patients, all but one with NYHA class III or IV, sildenafil (75 mg) and iNO (80 ppm) reduced the PVR similarly (-27% and -19% for sildenafil and iNO, respectively) *(24)*, but the response to sildenafil was considered more favorable because, in contrast to iNO, it increased the cardiac index without raising the wedge pressure. When combined, the two agents reduced the PVR and increased the cardiac index more than either agent alone and sildenafil prolonged the effect of inhaled NO *(24)*. In other PAH cohorts of 20 patients and 5 patients, respectively, sildenafil proved to be a potent acute pulmonary vasodilator, an effect that was potentiated by combination with inhaled NO *(25)* or iloprost *(26)*. These findings confirm the acute efficacy of sildenafil and suggest that certain drug combinations that elevate both cAMP as well as cGMP may be particularly attractive.

Although little is known about the acute pulmonary hemodynamic effects of the other commercially available PDE5 inhibitors, one clinical study compared the acute effects of sildenafil, tadalafil, and vardenafil in 60 consecutive PAH patients. The three differed markedly in their kinetics for pulmonary vasorelaxation (vardenafil had the most rapid effect), their selectivity for the pulmonary circulation (sildenafil and tadalafil were pulmonary-selective; vardenafil was not), and their impact on arterial oxygenation (sildenafil was the only one to improve it) *(27)*. These differences raise the possibility that long-term effects of the drugs in patients with PAH could differ, but this possibility has yet to be tested.

2.2.2. Chronic PDE5 Inhibition in Patients with Pulmonary Hypertension

Several uncontrolled studies have suggested that PDE5 inhibition has salutary effects on the pulmonary circulation of PAH patients. A single-center study of five PAH patients treated with sildenafil for three months (50 mg orally three times daily) *(8)* found that functional class improved by at least one class in all patients, the six-minute walk distance increased from 376 ± 30 to 504 ± 27 m ($p < 0.0001$), the mean PA pressure fell from 70 ± 3 to 52 ± 3 mm Hg ($p < 0.007$), the PVR index dropped from 1702 ± 151 to 996 ± 92 dyne $\cdot$ s $\cdot$ cm$^{-5} \cdot$ m^{-2} ($p < 0.006$), and the right ventricular mass as measured by MRI decreased. The drug was well tolerated, systemic arterial pressure was unchanged, and no adverse effects occurred. A subsequent prospective study of 10 patients placed on long-term sildenafil found symptomatic improvement in 9, and the drug was well tolerated *(25)*.

Subsequently, two placebo-controlled crossover trials have shown functional benefit. One found that two weeks of therapy (25 mg three times daily) *(28)* improved six-minute walk distance (267 vs. 170 m), Borg dyspnea score during exercise (3.56 vs. 5.11), and PA systolic pressure estimated by echocardiogram (55 vs. 75 mm Hg), all $p < 0.05$, compared to placebo. These findings suggest that favorable responses to sildenafil can occur quite rapidly, within two weeks. The second trial used six-week crossover periods *(29)* in 22 PAH patients treated with sildenafil (25–100 mg three times daily) or placebo. Compared to placebo, sildenafil significantly improved the treadmill exercise time (686 vs. 475 s), cardiac index (3.45 vs. 2.80 L/m^2), and dyspnea and fatigue components of the QOL questionnaire. Pulmonary artery systolic pressure decreased insignificantly, from 105.23 to 98.50 mm Hg. The effect on treadmill walking time was dramatic and showed the expected decline during the placebo period when it followed the active treatment phase (Fig. 2). Because of their controlled design, these studies strongly support the idea that sildenafil is effective at improving functional capacity and symptoms in PAH patients, at least temporarily.

The pivotal trial of sildenafil (SUPER-1) randomized 278 patients to receive 20, 40, or 80 mg of sildenafil three times daily or placebo for 12 weeks *(30)*. Patients with idiopathic, connective tissue-, and congenital heart-related forms of PAH were eligible if they were in functional class II–IV and their six-minute walk distances (6MWD) were between 100 and 450 m. Sildenafil increased the 6MWD (the main outcome variable) significantly more than placebo (45, 46, and 50 m for the three doses, respectively), but there were no significant dose-related effects (Fig. 3). Pulmonary hemodynamics also improved significantly, although once again, there were no statistically significant differences between doses. Mean PA pressure changes were +0.6, -2.1, -2.6, and -4.7 mm Hg, and mean PVR changes were +49, -122, -143, and -261 dyne $\cdot$ s $\cdot$ cm^{-5} for placebo and the three different doses, respectively. Time to clinical worsening was not significantly delayed compared to placebo, although there was a trend toward more hospitalizations in the placebo group *(30)*. Among the 222 patients completing the one-year extension trial of sildenafil (most of whom had the 80-mg dose), the improvement from baseline in 6MWD was 54 m *(31)*, essentially unchanged from the 12-week distance.

The combined results of the above studies, especially the pivotal trial, provide convincing evidence that sildenafil improves symptoms, functional capacity, and pulmonary hemodynamics in PAH patients. These benefits are comparable to those reported for prostacyclins and endothelin-receptor antagonists, except that, compared to bosentan, no significant effect on the time to clinical worsening was apparent. The latter may be explained by the relatively short duration of the trial (12 weeks) and the low occurrence of clinical worsening events in the placebo group (10%). On the basis of the above studies, the FDA approved sildenafil for the therapy of PAH in June 2005, but only at the

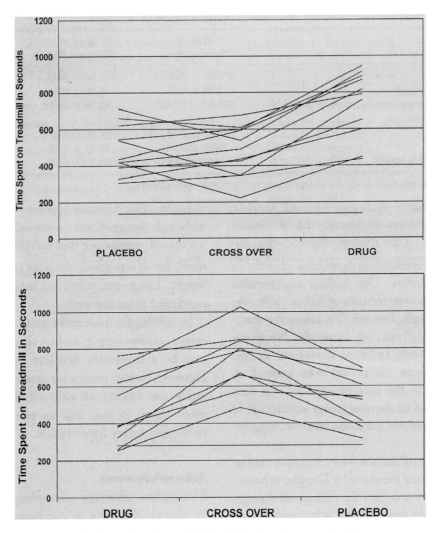

Fig. 2. Treadmill walking times (s) in individual patients enrolled in a six-week crossover trial who began on placebo (top panel) and sildenafil (bottom panel). [From *(29)*, with permission.]

dose of 20 mg three times daily, with higher doses "not recommended." A recent letter to the editor of the New England Journal of Medicine *(32)* pointed out that the FDA recommendation failed to consider that the trial was only 12 weeks in length and that higher doses may be more efficacious later on, that there may be a subgroup of patients who respond to higher doses, and that there was a strong trend toward better hemodynamic responses to the higher 80-mg tid dose in the pivotal

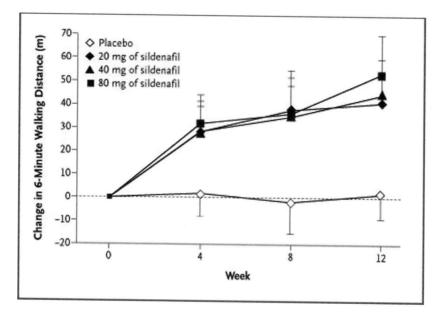

Fig. 3. Mean changes from baseline, with 95% confidence intervals, in the six-minute walking distance at week 12 in the placebo and sildenafil groups. [From *(30)*, with permission.]

trial. The unfortunate consequence of this ruling is that coverage for the cost of dosage escalation in patients not responding well to the 20-mg tid dose or losing efficacy after an initial favorable response may be denied by insurance companies.

The newer and longer-acting PDE5 inhibitors tadalafil and vardenafil are also promising and, by virtue of their longer half-lives, offer the possibility of once-daily or even less frequent administration. However, no long-term controlled trials of tadalafil or vardenafil to treat PAH have yet been reported, although a pivotal randomized, controlled trial is currently underway for tadalafil. A case report *(33)* has described a dramatic symptomatic response to tadalafil (20 mg qod) in an elderly woman who had become hypotensive on intravenous epoprostenol. With tadalafil, she improved from functional class IV to class II to III over a six-month period.

2.3. Side Effects and Tolerance

Sildenafil has been well tolerated in clinical trials. In the pivotal trial *(30)*, only headache and epistaxis occurred significantly more often than in controls (Table 1). Several other side effects occurred more often than in controls and might have been statistically significantly in

Table 1
Side Effects of Sildenafil Versus Placebo in the SUPER-1 Pivotal Trial*

Sildenafil Dose	Placebo	20 mg	40 mg	80 mg
Number	70	69	67	71
Headache	27(39)	32(46)	28(42)	35(49)
Back pain	8(11)	9(13)	9(13)	6(8)
Flushing	3(4)	7(11)	6(9)	11(15)
Dyspepsia	5(7)	9(13)	6(9)	9(13)
Diarrhea	4(6)	6(9)	8(12)	7(10)
Myalgia	3(4)	5(7)	4(6)	10(14)
Epistaxis	1(1)[†]	6(9)	5(7)	3(4)
Visual disturbances	0	0	3(4)	5(7)
Insomnia	1(1)	5(7)	4(6)	3(4)

* Number in parentheses is percentage of patients.
[†] $P < 0.05$ compared to pooled treatment groups. Mainly in CTD or patients on warfarin.
Source: Adapted from *(30)*.

a larger study. These include flushing, dyspepsia, diarrhea, myalgia, and visual disturbances (Table 1). Concerns have been raised about the visual side effects, in particular, nonischemic arteritic optic neuropathy (NIAON). This has been encountered with sildenafil use in patients with risk factors like diabetes, hypertension, or peripheral vascular disease but has not been reported in patients being treated for pulmonary hypertension. Pulmonary hypertension patients do occasionally notice a bluish haze in the periphery (11% of patients), but this does not affect visual acuity.

2.4. Drug Interactions

Caution should be exercised when combining PDE5 inhibitors with agents that stimulate production of cGMP, because this may intensify systemic side effects, especially systemic hypotension. For this reason, nitrates are considered contraindicated in patients taking sildenafil. Of course, one of the aims of combination therapy is to take advantage of synergies like this, and studies have shown that inhaled NO *(25)* and natriuretic peptides *(34)* have additive effects on pulmonary hemodynamics. It is conceivable that when applied cautiously, PDE5 inhibitors and nitrates could manifest similar additive beneficial effects on pulmonary hemodynamics, but this has not been tested.

Another interaction of potential importance is that between silde-nafil and bosentan. Bosentan speeds the metabolism of sildenafil and lowers circulating sildenafil levels by some 50%. Conversely, sildenafil slows the metabolism of bosentan by approximately 50% and doubles circulating bosentan levels *(35)*. Although concerns have been raised that the liver toxicity of bosentan might thereby be exacerbated, this has not been substantiated and at the present time, no dosage adjustment is recommended when the two drugs are combined.

3. PDE5 INHIBITION IN OTHER WHO PH SUBGROUPS

PDE5 inhibitors, specifically sildenafil, have been tested in other WHO PH subgroups. For example, treatment with sildenafil improves pulmonary hemodynamics and exercise capacity in healthy subjects with both acute hypoxic PH at rest *(36)* or with exercise *(37)*, as well as during exposure to chronic high altitude *(38)*. In a group of 11 patients with PH secondary to left ventricular systolic dysfunction due to coronary artery disease or idiopathic dilated cardiomyopathy, PDE5 inhibition with sildenafil lowered the mean PA pressure by 12%, increased the cardiac index by 14%, and decreased the pulmonary artery wedge pressure by 12% *(39)*. In combination with iNO, it increased the cardiac index more than with either agent alone (30%), lowered the PVR by 50%, and prolonged the hemodynamic effects of inhaled NO *(39)*.

Sildenafil *(40)* has also been tested as a therapy for chronic thromboembolic pulmonary hypertension in patients who are not candidates for thromboendarterectomy. Administered at a dose of 50 mg three times daily over approximately six months, sildenafil reduced the mean PA pressure and PVR by 15% and 30%, respectively, raised the cardiac index by 17%, and increased the 6MWD by 54 m. The pulmonary hemodynamic improvement seen in this study as well as in several prior studies using inhaled NO and iloprost *(41,42)* supports the notion that CTEPH responds favorably to vasodilator/antiremodeling therapy. Sildenafil also caused acute pulmonary vasodilation in 16 patients with severe lung fibrosis and secondary pulmonary hypertension *(43)*. Notable in this study was the favorable effect sildenafil had on oxygenation, which can deteriorate significantly with other vasodilators. This makes sildenafil a potentially attractive agent to try in patients with interstitial lung disease and pulmonary hypertension. Overall, the consistently favorable pulmonary hemodynamic effects of sildenafil, not only in idiopathic but also in other forms of pulmonary hypertension, suggest that repression of the cGMP pathway by increased PDE5 activity is a common contributing mechanism.

4. COMBINATION THERAPY

Experimental data indicate that treatment of PAH by manipulating multiple pathways concurrently may produce additive benefits. The current monotherapy for PAH is not curative, nor does it normalize pulmonary hemodynamics or functional capacity in the vast majority of cases. Thus, investigators are interested in the possibility that combinations of a PDE5 inhibitor with agents that act on either the endothelin pathway (bosentan) or the cAMP-prostacyclin pathway (epoprostenol, iloprost, beraprost) might offer more therapeutic efficacy. As discussed in detail in Chapter 16, preliminary studies suggest that combinations of sildenafil with prostacyclins, iNO, natriuretic peptides, and bosentan improve pulmonary hemodynamics more than monotherapy, although definitive randomized prospective trials have not yet been completed.

5. COMPARING PAH THERAPIES

Only one randomized, controlled trial thus far has attempted to directly compare the efficacy of a PDE5 inhibitor (sildenafil) and an endothelin-receptor antagonist (bosentan) (SERAPH study). In this double-blind study, 26 WHO/NYHA functional class III PAH patients were randomized to receive sildenafil (50 mg twice daily for four weeks, then 50 mg three times daily) or bosentan (62.5 mg twice daily for four weeks, then 125 mg twice daily) *(44)*. After 16 weeks, both groups manifested similar improvements in the cardiac index and exercise capacity. Compared to baseline, sildenafil significantly increased quality-of-life scores and decreased plasma brain natriuretic peptide levels, RV mass (by MRI), and systolic left ventricular eccentricity index, suggesting an improvement in cardiac function. Bosentan achieved favorable trends in these variables, but there were no statistically significant differences. In addition, sildenafil increased the 6MWD by 114 m compared to 59 m for bosentan, but the difference was not statistically significant. Despite the favorable trends, the study was inadequately powered and the authors rightly concluded that their data showed no clear superiority of one treatment over the other.

6. CONCLUSIONS

Agents that raise the intracellular cGMP are effective pulmonary vasodilators and smooth muscle antimitogens, Compelling evidence supports the acute and long-term efficacy of PDE5 inhibition in different forms of PAH, both experimental and clinical. In these studies, sildenafil at doses ranging from 20 mg to 100 mg tid or the equivalent consistently improved pulmonary hemodynamics, reduced evidence of remodeling (in experimental models), and, in clinical studies, enhanced functional capacity. Preliminary reports also suggest that the combination of PDE5 inhibitors with other therapies that either enhance cGMP elevation (NO, natriuretic peptides) or increase cAMP (prostacyclins), or even act on a different pathway altogether (endothelin-receptor blockers), may be beneficial in the treatment of this complex disease. However, much additional work is needed to better establish the mechanisms of efficacy, demonstrate the durability of beneficial effects, and establish that combination therapy will live up to its promise.

REFERENCES

1. Archer SL, et al. Nitric oxide and cGMP cause vasorelaxation by activation of a charybdotoxin-sensitive K channel by cGMP-dependent protein kinase. Proc Natl Acad Sci USA 1994; 91(16):7583–7.
2. Dhanakoti SN, et al. Involvement of cGMP-dependent protein kinase in the relaxation of ovine pulmonary arteries to cGMP and cAMP. J Appl Physiol 2000; 88(5):1637–42.
3. Adnot S, et al. Loss of endothelium-dependent relaxant activity in the pulmonary circulation of rats exposed to chronic hypoxia. J Clin Invest 1991; 87(1):155–62.
4. Dinh-Xuan AT, et al, Impairment of pulmonary-artery endothelium-dependent relaxation in chronic obstructive lung disease is not due to dysfunction of endothelial cell membrane receptors nor to L-arginine deficiency. Br J Pharmacol 1993; 109(2):587–91.
5. Klinger JR, et al. Cardiopulmonary responses to chronic hypoxia in transgenic mice that overexpress ANP. J Appl Physiol 1993; 75(1):198–205.
6. Abman SH, Accurso FJ. Sustained fetal pulmonary vasodilation with prolonged atrial natriuretic factor and GMP infusions. Am J Physiol 1991; 260(1 Pt 2):H183–92.
7. Soderling SH, Bayuga SJ, Beavo JA. Identification and characterization of a novel family of cyclic nucleotide phosphodiesterases. J Biol Chem 1998; 273(25):15553–8.
8. Michelakis ED, et al. Long-term treatment with oral sildenafil is safe and improves functional capacity and hemodynamics in patients with pulmonary arterial hypertension. Circulation 2003; 108(17):2066–9.
9. MacLean MR, et al. Phosphodiesterase isoforms in the pulmonary arterial circulation of the rat: Changes in pulmonary hypertension. J Pharmacol Exp Ther 1997; 283(2):619–24.
10. Sebkhi A, et al. Phosphodiesterase type 5 as a target for the treatment of hypoxia-induced pulmonary hypertension. Circulation 2003; 107(25):3230–5.

11. Wharton J, et al. Antiproliferative effects of phosphodiesterase type 5 inhibition in human pulmonary artery cells. Am J Respir Crit Care Med 2005; 172(1):105–13.

12. Tantini B, et al. Antiproliferative effect of sildenafil on human pulmonary artery smooth muscle cells. Basic Res Cardiol 2005; 100(2):131–8.

13. Degerman E, Belfrage P, Manganiello VC. cGMP-inhibited phosphodiesterases (PDE3 gene family). Biochem Soc Trans 1996; 24(4):1010–4.

14. Preston IR, et al. Synergistic effects of ANP and sildenafil on cGMP levels and amelioration of acute hypoxic pulmonary hypertension. Exp Biol Med 2004; 229:920–5.

15. Schermuly RT, et al. Coaerosolization of phosphodiesterase inhibitors markedly enhances the pulmonary vasodilatory response to inhaled iloprost in experimental pulmonary hypertension. Maintenance of lung selectivity. Am J Respir Crit Care Med 2001; 164(9):1694–700.

16. Schermuly RT, et al. Combination of nonspecific PDE inhibitors with inhaled prostacyclin in experimental pulmonary hypertension. Am J Physiol Lung Cell Mol Physiol 2001; 281(6):L1361–8.

17. Weimann J, et al. Sildenafil is a pulmonary vasodilator in awake lambs with acute pulmonary hypertension. Anesthesiology 2000; 92(6):1702–12.

18. Ichinose F, et al. Nebulized sildenafil is a selective pulmonary vasodilator in lambs with acute pulmonary hypertension [see comment]. Crit Care Med 2001; 29(5):1000–5.

19. Hanasato N, et al. E-4010, a selective phosphodiesterase 5 inhibitor, attenuates hypoxic pulmonary hypertension in rats. Am J Physiol 1999; 277(2 Pt 1):L225–32.

20. Schermuly R, et al. Chronic sildenafil treatment inhibits monocrotaline-induced pulmonary hypertension in rats [see comment]. Am J Respir Crit Care Med 2004; 169(1):39–45.

21. Zhao L, et al. Sildenafil inhibits hypoxia-induced pulmonary hypertension. Circulation 2001; 104(4):424–8.

22. Zhao L, et al. Beneficial effects of phosphodiesterase 5 inhibition in pulmonary hypertension are influenced by natriuretic peptide activity. Circulation 2003; 107(2):234–7.

23. Michelakis E, et al. Oral sildenafil is an effective and specific pulmonary vasodilator in patients with pulmonary arterial hypertension: Comparison with inhaled nitric oxide. Circulation 2002; 105(20):2398–403.

24. Leuchte HH, et al. Hemodynamic response to sildenafil, nitric oxide, and iloprost in primary pulmonary hypertension. Chest 2004; 125(2):580–6.

25. Preston IR, et al. Acute and chronic effects of sildenafil in patients with pulmonary arterial hypertension. Respir Med 2005; 99(12):1501–10.

26. Wilkens H, et al. Effect of inhaled iloprost plus oral sildenafil in patients with primary pulmonary hypertension. Circulation 2001; 104(11):1218–22.

27. Ghofrani HA, et al. Differences in hemodynamic and oxygenation responses to three different phosphodiesterase-5 inhibitors in patients with

pulmonary arterial hypertension: A randomized prospective study. J Am Coll Cardiol 2004; 44(7):1488–96.

28. Bharani A, Mathew V, Sahu A, Lunia B. The efficacy and tolerability of sildenafil in patients with moderate-to-severe pulmonary hypertension [see comment]. Ind Heart J 2003; 55(1):55–9.
29. Sastry BKS, et al. Clinical efficacy of sildenafil in primary pulmonary hypertension: A randomized, placebo-controlled, double-blind, crossover study. J Am Coll Cardiol 2004; 43(7):1149–53.
30. Galie N, et al. Sildenafil citrate therapy for pulmonary arterial hypertension. N Engl J Med 2005; 353(20):2148–57.
31. Rubin L, Burgen G, Parpia T, Simomeau G, the SUPER-1 team. Effects of Sildenafil on 6-Minute Walk Distance and WHO Functional class after 1 year of Treatment. Proceedings of the ATS 2005; A299.
32. Hoepper MM, Welte T. Sildenafil citrate for pulmonary arterial hypertension. N Engl J Med 2006; 354:1091.
33. Palmieri EA, Affuso F, Fazio S. Lembo D. Tadalafil for primary pulmonary arterial hypertension (letter). Ann Intern Med 2004; 141:743.
34. Klinger JR, Thaker S, Houtchens J, Preston IR, Hill NS, Farber HW. Pulmonary hemodynamic responses to brain natriuretic peptide and sildenafil in patients with pulmonary arterial hypertension. Chest 2006 Feb; 129(2):417–25.
35. Paul GA, Gibbs JS, Boobis AR, Abbas A, Wilkins MR. Bosentan decreases the plasma concentration of sildenafil when coprescribed in pulmonary hypertension. Br J Clin Pharmacol 2005; 60:107–12.
36. Richalet JP, et al. Sildenafil inhibits altitude-induced hypoxemia and pulmonary hypertension. Am J Respir Crit Care Med 2005; 171(3):275–81.
37. Ricart A, et al. Effects of sildenafil on the human response to acute hypoxia and exercise. High Alt Med Biol 2005; 6(1):43–9.
38. Aldashev AA, et al. Phosphodiesterase type 5 and high altitude pulmonary hypertension. Thorax 2005; 60(8):683–7.
39. Lepore JJ, et al. Hemodynamic effects of sildenafil in patients with congestive heart failure and pulmonary hypertension: Combined administration with inhaled nitric oxide. Chest 2005; 127(5):1647–53.
40. Ghofrani H, et al. Sildenafil for long-term treatment of nonoperable chronic thromboembolic pulmonary hypertension. Am J Respir Crit Care Med 2003; 167(8):1139–41.
41. Ghofrani H, et al. Combination therapy with oral sildenafil and inhaled iloprost for severe pulmonary hypertension. Ann Intern Med 2002; 136(7):515–22.
42. Olschewski H, et al. Inhaled iloprost for severe pulmonary hypertension. N Engl J Med 2002; 347(5):322–9.
43. Ghofrani HA, et al. Sildenafil for treatment of lung fibrosis and pulmonary hypertension: A randomised controlled trial. Lancet 2002; 360(9337): 895–900.
44. Wilkins MR, et al. Sildenafil versus Endothelin Receptor Antagonist for Pulmonary Hypertension (SERAPH) study. Am J Respir Crit Care Med 2005; 171(11):1292–7.

15 Statins for Treatment of Pulmonary Hypertension

John L. Faul, Peter N. Kao, Toshihiko Nishimura, Arthur Sung, Hong Hu, and Ronald G. Pearl

CONTENTS

INTRODUCTION
RATIONALE FOR THE BENEFIT OF STATINS
   IN PULMONARY HYPERTENSION
EXPERIMENTAL EVIDENCE SUPPORTING
   THE HYPOTHESIS THAT STATINS
     AMELIORATE PULMONARY HYPERTENSION
CLINICAL APPLICATIONS OF STATINS
   TO TREAT PULMONARY HYPERTENSION
CONCLUSIONS
REFERENCES

Abstract

By virtue of their multiple actions, including anti-inflammatory, antiproliferative, and pro-apoptotic traits and the ability to restore endothelial vasoactive mediator production, statins have been proposed as potential therapies for pulmonary hypertension. In experimental studies in rats with pulmonary hypertension induced either by either monocrotaline or hypoxia, statins have blunted the severity of pulmonary hypertension, right ventricular hypertrophy, and pulmonary vascular remodeling, sometimes in association with the restoration of the endothelial cell production of nitric oxide. Pending

From: *Contemporary Cardiology: Pulmonary Hypertension*
Edited by: N. S. Hill and H. W. Farber © Humana Press, Totowa, NJ

trials that demonstrate the efficacy of statins in pulmonary arterial hypertension in humans, however, the clinical use of statins should be considered investigational.

Key Words: statins; pulmonary hypertension therapy; monocrotaline; chronic hypoxia; experimental pulmonary hypertension; simvastatin.

1. INTRODUCTION

Statins, inhibitors of HMG-CoA reductase, confer cardiovascular benefits that far exceed their capacity to lower serum cholesterol *(1)*. Some of the mechanisms through which statins confer benefit in vascular disease provide a rationale for their use in pulmonary arterial hypertension *(2,3)*. These effects include increases in circulating endothelial progenitor cells *(4–6)*, increased expression of endothelial antithrombotic modulators *(7–10)*, increases in endothelial nitric oxide production *(11,12)*, and suppression of vascular inflammation and vascular smooth muscle cell proliferation *(13–15)*. This brief review examines the potential role of statins in ameliorating pulmonary hypertension, focusing on our experimental work in pulmonary hypertension models and briefly discussing the currently available clinical data.

2. RATIONALE FOR THE BENEFIT OF STATINS IN PULMONARY HYPERTENSION

2.1. Possible Synergism with Bone Morphogenetic Protein Receptor 2

Pulmonary arterial hypertension is characterized by inappropriate proliferation of vascular endothelial and smooth muscle cells within the lumen of small pulmonary arterioles *(16–18)*. This neointimal formation leads to progressive increases in pulmonary vascular resistance, increased afterload for the right ventricle, congestive heart failure, and death. The identification of mutations in bone morphogenetic protein receptor type II (*BMPR2*) as the genetic basis for 50% to 70% of familial pulmonary hypertension *(19–22)*, in addition to the apparent loss of BMPR2 protein in the vessels of patients with PAH *(23,24)*, suggests a key role for the BMPR2 signaling pathway in maintaining homeostasis of the pulmonary vascular bed. Endothelial cells represent the principal site of expression of BMPR2 in the adult lung *(23,24)*, and signaling through BMPR2 is associated with the intracellular phosphorylation of SMAD coactivators and activation of gene expression, including Id1 *(25,26)*. The gene expression pattern triggered by BMPR2 signaling represents the activation of differentiated endothelial cell genes. A similar activation of Id1 and endothelial differentiation can be induced in vitro by treatment with fluvastatin *(27)*. Thus, statins might synergize with BMPR2 signaling to promote differentiated endothelial function.

2.2. Enhancement of Endothelial Cell Function

Endothelial dysfunction in PAH is believed to be caused by a combination of microthrombosis and an imbalance between vasodilating and vasoconstricting substances, with an impairment of vasodilators such as nitric oxide (NO) and prostacyclin (PGI$_2$) and a dominance of vasoconstrictors, such as endothelin-1 *(28)*. Statins are well placed as potential therapeutic candidates to redress the vascular imbalances that occur in pulmonary arterial hypertension. Simvastatin treatment of human subjects with stable coronary artery disease causes a significant decrease in platelet thrombus formation after only eight weeks *(29)*. Simvastatin also reduces platelet aggregation and thromboxane production after 4 to 24 weeks of therapy *(30,31)*. Statin-induced improvements in endothelial function might be achieved by both the enhancement of vasodilator activities and the attenuation of vasoconstrictor activities in the vascular wall.

2.3. Opposition to Endothelin-1 Actions

The dramatic clinical benefits of statins in patients with coronary artery disease may result, in part, from their effects on ET-1. Endothelin-1 is thought to have an even more important role in pulmonary vascular disease. Simvastatin inhibits resting and stimulated prepro-endothelin-1 (ET-1) gene transcription in endothelial cells *(32,33)*. Simvastatin, but not pravastatin, induces a concentration-dependent and endothelium-independent relaxation of tonic contraction mediated by ET-1 *(32)*. Simvastatin also prevents Rho activation caused by ET-1 in aortic homogenates, as assessed by a Rho pulldown assay *(33)*. In unstimulated vascular smooth muscle cells, simvastatin inhibits ET-1-induced DNA synthesis and Rho translocation *(33)*. These results show that statins potently inhibit ET-1-mediated contraction and DNA synthesis via multiple mechanisms *(32)*.

2.4. Effects of Statins on Nitric Oxide and Cytokine Pathways

Patients with PAH have reduced expression of eNOS in the lungs. Simvastatin activates the serine/threonine protein kinase Akt in endothelial cells, which in turn leads to phosphorylation of eNOS, resulting in an increase in its activity and enhanced NO production *(34)*. PAH is also associated with increases in circulating interleukin-1beta (IL-1beta) and IL-6 levels. In a recent study, simvastatin, but not pravastatin, reduced the production of (IL-6) and IL-1beta in human umbilical vein endothelial cells *(35)*.

2.5. Hypothesis

Statins are pluripotent agents that act at multiple levels to interfere with cellular pathways contributing to the pathogenesis of pulmonary hypertension or abet others that might have protective effects. Thus, the hypothesis would be that statin therapy should ameliorate PAH in humans by preventing or even reversing the vascular remodeling process that contributes to the disease, either as monotherapy or in combination with other agents.

3. EXPERIMENTAL EVIDENCE SUPPORTING THE HYPOTHESIS THAT STATINS AMELIORATE PULMONARY HYPERTENSION

3.1. Statins Potently Attenuate Proliferative Pulmonary Vascular Changes

The pathology of PAH is characterized by remodeling the accumulation of cells in the walls of small pulmonary arteries, which is related to increased proliferation, reduced apoptosis, or both. We recently evaluated a panel of antiproliferative, nonvasodilator agents (triptolide, a potent immunosuppressive and antiproliferative diterpenoid triepoxide, cyclosporine A, FK506, SDZ-RAD, a derivative of the macrolide rapamycin, and simvastatin) for their effects on an experimental pulmonary hypertension *(36–38)*. We used the rat monocrotaline/pneumonectomy model developed by Botney and colleagues *(39)*. In this model, pneumonectomy (day 0) precedes the administration of monocrotaline (day 7). The monocrotaline undergoes hepatic metabolism to monocrotaline pyrrole, which then causes first-pass endothelial injury in the pulmonary circulation. This endothelial injury leads to a neointimal proliferative response, marked by extensive vascular occlusion of small pulmonary arteries, and muscular hypertrophy of medium-sized and larger pulmonary arteries. Vessels are prominently lined by pathological, proliferating vascular smooth muscle cells that express alpha smooth muscle actin. Endothelial cells (marked by CD31 immunostaining) are present in a single layer lining the vascular lumen, and plexiform lesions are not seen. Physiological measurements at day 35 (28 days after monocrotaline injection) compared to controls reveal that mean pulmonary artery pressure rises from 17 ± 1 mm Hg to 53 ± 2 mm Hg, and the ratio of RV/LV+S rises from 0.25 ± 0.03 to 0.78 ± 0.09, indicative of right ventricular hypertrophy. Triptolide, FK506, cyclosporine, and RAD partially attenuated the disease, but low-dose simvastatin (2 mg/kg/d) potently inhibited the development of PAH and RVH (Table 1). Furthermore, we performed quantitative histology to characterize the neointimal formation in the form of a vascular occlusion score (VOS) that ranged between 0 (fully patent) and 2.0 (100% of vessels were more than 50% occluded). Normal vessels have a VOS of 0, and monocrotaline/pneumonectomy rats given placebo have scores that approach 2. As shown in Table 1, simvastatin therapy markedly reduced the VOS score, much more effectively than the other agents, consistent with a potent antiremodeling effect.

3.2. Statins as "Rescue" Therapy

In a later "rescue" study of the use of simvastatin in rats that had already developed PAH, rats underwent pneumonectomy on day 0 and then a single subcutaneous injection of monocrotaline on day 28 *(40)*.

Table 1
Effects of Different Immunomodulatory Compounds in the Monocrotaline/Pneumonectomy Model of Pulmonary Hypertension in Rats

	mPAP	*RV/LV+S*	*VOS*
Normal	17	0.25	0
M/P control	45–52	0.66–79	1.98
M/P + cyclosporineA	42	0.63	1.44
M/P + FK 506	34	0.41	1.27
M/P + rapamycin	25	0.42	1.57
M/P + triptolide	21	0.39	1.27
M/P + simvastatin	26	0.34	0.59

M/P = monocrotaline/pneumonectomy; mPAP = mean pulmonary arterial pressure; RV/LV+S = the ratio of right ventricular to left ventricular plus weight as an index of right ventricular hypertrophy; VOS = vascular occlusion score.

At 11 weeks, all rats underwent hemodynamic monitoring, which documented severe pulmonary hypertension: mPAP = 42 ± 2 mm Hg. Half the pulmonary hypertensive rats received placebo and the other half received treatment with simvastatin (2 mg/kg/d by oral gavage). By 13 weeks, all rats that received placebo showed progression of pulmonary hypertension: mPAP = 53 ± 2 mm Hg, whereas every rat treated with simvastatin showed reversal of pulmonary hypertension: mPAP = 36 ± 2 mm Hg. Rats that received placebo showed 0% survival beyond 15 weeks, while rats treated with simvastatin showed 100% survival until the time of scheduled physiological measurements. The reversal of pulmonary hypertension by simvastatin was complete by 6 weeks, when mPAP was 24 ± 2 mm Hg, and was maintained at 13 weeks, when mPAP was 22 ± 2 mm Hg. RV/LV+S, which was 0.71 ± 0.1 at the time of randomization, increased to 0.92 ± 0.1 in placebo-treated rats and regressed to 0.69 ± 0.05 at 2 weeks, 0.38 ± 0.05 at 6 weeks, and returned to normal (0.28 ± 0.03) by 13 weeks in simvastatin-treated rats. The quantitative histopathology analysis showed similar changes. The VOS was 1.85 at the time of randomization, increased to 1.95 in rats that received placebo for 2 weeks and regressed to 1.34 at 2 weeks, 0.83 at 6 weeks, and 0.65 at 13 weeks of simvastatin treatment, respectively *(40)* (Fig. 1).

Immunohistochemistry on the diseased lungs to investigate the mechanisms through which simvastatin conferred its profound benefit showed a reduction in the number of proliferating cells by PCNA (proliferating cell nuclear antigen) staining and an increased number of apoptotic cells in the neointima by TUNEL (terminal deoxynucleotidyl transferase-mediated dUTP-biotin nick end-labeling) staining 40. Transcriptional profiling in lung tissue revealed that simvastatin decreased the in vivo expression of inflammatory transcription factors c-fos and jun, as well as that of cyclin E, erb B3, acetylcholine receptor alpha 5 subunit, and nerve growth factor *(40,41)*. Furthermore, simvastatin-treated rats had increased expression of eNOS, the cell cycle inhibitor p27Kip1, and BMPR1a.

Another group of investigators has examined the effect of once-daily simvastatin (20 mg/kg ip) on pulmonary vascular responses to 14 days of hypoxia (10% FIO_2) in rats *(42)*. As anticipated, simvastatin blunted the rise in the mean PA pressure, the severity of right ventricular hypertrophy, and the degree of alveolar arterial muscularization. Simvastatin also blunted the severity of hypoxia-induced polycythemia. In this model of pulmonary hypertension, these multiple actions were

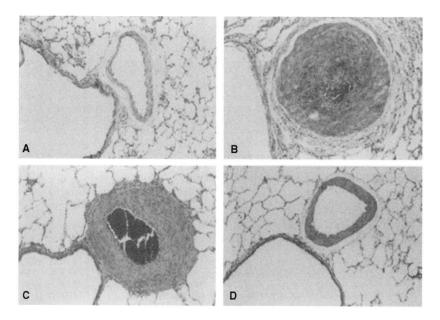

Fig. 1. Simvastatin reverses pulmonary artery medial hypertrophy in muscular pulmonary arteries. (a) Normal peribronchial muscular pulmonary artery in a normal rat. (b) Prominent thickened medial layer and neointimal lesion in control rats that received vehicle for two weeks (group PMV_{2w}). (c) Less thickened medial layer and neointimal lesion in rats rescued by simvastatin treatment for two weeks (group PMS_{2w}). (d) Regression of thickened medial wall in rats rescued by simvastatin treatment for six weeks (group PMS_{6w}). Hematoxylin and eosin staining; magnification ×400. (Courtesy of Circulation from Reference *(40)*)

not associated with a detectible increase in lung endothelial nitric oxide synthase expression. A gene array analysis of lung tissue from the hypoxic rats showed decreased expression of genes involved in mediation of inflammatory responses as well as cellular proliferation *(43)*.

Taken together, these results confirm the results of other in vitro and in vivo studies that demonstrate the anti-inflammatory, antiproliferative, and pro-apoptotic effects of statins, as well as their ability (at least in the monocrotaline model) to induce endothelial cell nitric oxide synthase gene expression and nitric oxide production. They are also strongly supportive of the hypothesis that statins are beneficial for clinical pulmonary hypertension, but with the caveat that the rat model of pulmonary hypertension used for these experiments may not reflect responses in humans with the disease.

4. CLINICAL APPLICATIONS OF STATINS TO TREAT PULMONARY HYPERTENSION

4.1. Favorable Toxicity Profile

One of the principal attractive features of statins as potential treatments for pulmonary hypertension is their widespread use and generally excellent toxicity profile. Simvastatin is well tolerated at the FDA-approved maximum dose of 80 mg/d for treatment of elevated cholesterol (44–46). A much higher maximum tolerable dose of 25–35 mg/kg/day of lovastatin was defined in phase I and II studies for cancer (47,48). Anorexia without evidence of liver inflammation was the main adverse effect of lovastatin; in one study, 2 of 14 patients developed muscle inflammation, while in another study no patients developed myalgias (49).

4.2. Open-Label Clinical Trial

We conducted an open-label observational trial of simvastatin for the treatment of pulmonary hypertension at Stanford University Medical Center. Sixteen patients with primary or secondary pulmonary hypertension completed the open-label follow-up period. Each patient served as his or her own control, and baseline and serial measurements of the six-minute walk exercise performance, echo Doppler estimates of right ventricular systolic pressure, hemodynamics, and laboratories were collected (50).

In this open-label trial of simvastatin, there was no detectable evidence of toxicity. Six of seven patients who died during the time of observation (up to 41 months) were WHO class IV when they entered the trial, and their deaths were due to the progression of pulmonary hypertension (Table 2). No patient treated with simvastatin in this study demonstrated liver function abnormalities or muscle inflammation.

Simvastatin treatment appeared to confer clinical benefits. Individual patients reported subjective and objective improvements in exercise capacity. Serial measurements of the six-minute walk distance (6MWD) showed that most patients experienced increases. Six patients had improvements of around 70 m, with one patient improving by 114 m after four to five months of treatment (Table 2). Most of the improvements in the 6MWD were *not* accompanied by significant decreases in right ventricular systolic pressure as assessed by echocardiogram. When invasive hemodynamic measurements were obtained, simvastatin treatment was associated with an improvement in cardiac index and corresponding decreases in pulmonary vascular resistance (50). Of course, the lack of controls and the observational nature of

Table 2
Individual Characteristics and Outcome of Patients in Open-Label Trial of Simvastatin for Pulmonary Arterial Hypertension (from Reference 50)

Pt/Age/Sex/WHO Classification	PAH Subtype	Epo (ng/kg/m)	mPAP (mm Hg)	C.I.	PVRI (WoodUnits)	RVSP (mm Hg)	Δ6MWm (Mo)	Outcome (Mo)
1/54/F/II Baseline	IPAH		48	1.9	18	84		
Treatment			51	2.7	15	100	76 (9)	Alive (41)
2/46/F/I Baseline	IPAH		40	1.8	17	57		
Treatment			28	2.1	11	44	0 (34)	Alive (37)
3/50/F/II Baseline	IPAH/cirrhosis					130		
Treatment						124	114 (4)	Alive (34)
4/21/M/I Baseline	CHD/ASD VSD closed		53	1.6	24	57		
Treatment			38	3.0	8.7	37	23 (11)	Alive (13)
5/72/F/IV Baseline	CTE/thromboendarter.					89		
Treatment						61	−61 (4)	Dead (19)
6/59/F/IV Baseline	IPAH/PVOD/CREST		50	1.4	30	118		
Treatment						80	NT	Dead (6)
7/70/F/III Baseline	IPAH/cirrhosis	26				162		
Treatment		12	45	2.6	8.8	109	69 (5)	Dead (31)

Table 2
Continued

Pt/Age/Sex/WHO Classification	PAH Subtype	Epo (ng/kg/m)	mPAP (mm Hg)	C.I.	PVRI (WoodUnits)	RVSP (mm Hg)	Δ6MWm (Mo)	Outcome (Mo)
8/46/F/IV Baseline	IPAH	10	85			71		
Treatment		10				71	76 (4)	Alive (35)
9/61/F/IV Baseline	IPAH/ scleroderma	12	47			77		
Treatment		12				75	37 (7)	Alive (38)
10/26/F/II Baseline	IPAH/ Graves	32	48			82		
Treatment		30				87	78 (5)	Alive (33)
11/41/F/III Baseline	IPAH/Graves cirrhosis	22		52				
Treatment		20				49	69 (5)	Alive (35)
12/58/M/IV Baseline	CHD/VSD R-to-L shunt	10	53	2.6	38	134		
Treatment		10	90			118	70 (3)	Dead (26)
13/49/F/III Baseline	IPAH/ FenPhen	38	65			42		
Treatment		38	60			110	46 (4)	Dead (17)
14/47/F/IV Baseline	IPAH	40				115		
Treatment		40				67	NT	Dead (4)

	Diagnosis	Treatment						Status
15/46/F/IV Baseline	IPAH		53	1.3	38/–	86		
Treatment		Tre 9				73	33 (13)	Alive (15)
16/54/M/II Baseline	CTE/	Epo14	37	3.5	6.0/+	67		
Treatment	cirrhosis	23	29			49	0 (3)	Dead (21)

IPAH = idiopathic pulmonary arterial hypertension; PVOD = pulmonary veno-occlusive disease; CTE = chronic thromboembolism; VSD = ventricular septal defect; ASD = atrial septal defect; Epo = epoprostenol dose; tre = treprostinil; mPAP = mean pulmonary arterial pressure; CI = cardiac index; PVRI = pulmonary vascular resistance index; RVSP = right ventricular systolic pressure by echocardiogram; Δ6MW = change in six-minute walk distance in meters.

the trial preclude any conclusions about the efficacy of simvastatin in this trial. The drug was well tolerated, and it is conceivable that the therapy benefited some patients.

4.3. Potential Adverse Side Effects of Statin Therapy

Potential adverse effects of long-term statin therapy include an increased occurrence of cancer, because angiogenesis and neovascularization might promote the development of malignant tumors. Indeed, an increased incidence of breast cancer was observed among women in the CARE trial. However, a meta-analysis of five large statin trials failed to detect an increased risk of fatal or nonfatal cancers associated with statin therapy *(51,52)*. Several recent reports also suggest that statins may eventually play a role in cancer prevention or even treatment. In particular, simvastatin has been shown to block leukemic cell growth *(53,54)*. The most serious side effect of statin therapy, which recently led to the removal of cerivastatin from the market, is rhabdomyolysis *(55–58)*. The cause of this is obscure, but the incidence might be increased in patients with deficiencies of co-enzyme Q10 or hypothyroidism. Considering that PAH has been associated with autoimmune thyroid disease and thyroid dysregulation, this is a potential concern *(59)*. These observations argue for caution and appropriate monitoring during statin therapy in patients with PAH.

5. CONCLUSIONS

By virtue of their multiple actions, including anti-inflammatory, antiproliferative, and pro-apoptotic qualities and the ability to restore endothelial vasoactive mediator production, statins have been proposed as potential therapies for pulmonary hypertension. In experimental studies in rats with pulmonary hypertension induced either by either monocrotaline or hypoxia, statins have blunted the severity of pulmonary hypertension, right ventricular hypertrophy, and pulmonary vascular remodeling, sometimes in association with the restoration of endothelial cell production of nitric oxide. Pending trials that demonstrate the efficacy of statins in pulmonary arterial hypertension in humans, however, the clinical use of statins should be considered investigational.

REFERENCES

1. Fenton JW, 2nd, Brezniak DV, Ofosu FA, Shen GX, Jacobson JR, Garcia JG. Statins and thrombin. Curr Drug Targets Cardiovasc Haematol Disord 2005; 5(2):115–20.

2. Chen Z, Fukutomi T, Zago AC, et al. Simvastatin reduces neointimal thickening in low-density lipoprotein receptor-deficient mice after experimental angioplasty without changing plasma lipids. Circulation 2002; 106(1):20–3.

3. Bea F, Blessing E, Shelley MI, Shultz JM, Rosenfeld ME. Simvastatin inhibits expression of tissue factor in advanced atherosclerotic lesions of apolipoprotein E deficient mice independently of lipid lowering: Potential role of simvastatin-mediated inhibition of Egr-1 expression and activation. Atherosclerosis 2003; 167(2):187–94.

4. Zhu JH, Tao QM, Chen JZ, Wang XX, Shang YP. Statins contribute to enhancement of the number and the function of endothelial progenitor cells from peripheral blood. Sheng Li Xue Bao 2004; 56(3):357–64.

5. Walter DH, Rittig K, Bahlmann FH, et al. Statin therapy accelerates reendothelialization: A novel effect involving mobilization and incorporation of bone marrow-derived endothelial progenitor cells. Circulation 2002; 105(25):3017–24.

6. Llevadot J, Murasawa S, Kureishi Y, et al. HMG-CoA reductase inhibitor mobilizes bone marrow-derived endothelial progenitor cells. J Clin Invest 2001; 108(3):399–405.

7. Szczeklik A, Undas A, Musial J, Gajewski P, Swadzba J, Jankowski M. Antithrombotic actions of statins. Med Sci Monit 2001; 7(6):1381–5.

8. Undas A, Brummel KE, Musial J, Mann KG, Szczeklik A. Simvastatin depresses blood clotting by inhibiting activation of prothrombin, factor V, and factor XIII and by enhancing factor Va inactivation. Circulation 2001; 103(18):2248–53.

9. Gil-Nunez AC, Villanueva JA. Advantages of lipid-lowering therapy in cerebral ischemia: Role of HMG-CoA reductase inhibitors. Cerebrovasc Dis 2001; 11 (Suppl 1):85–95.

10. Mutanen M, Freese R. Fats, lipids and blood coagulation. Curr Opin Lipidol 2001; 12(1):25–9.

11. Mason RP, Walter MF, Jacob RF. Effects of HMG-CoA reductase inhibitors on endothelial function: Role of microdomains and oxidative stress. Circulation 2004; 109(21 Suppl 1):1134–41.

12. Trochu JN, Mital S, Zhang X, et al. Preservation of NO production by statins in the treatment of heart failure. Cardiovasc Res 2003; 60(2):250–8.

13. Ongini E, Impagnatiello F, Bonazzi A, et al. Nitric oxide (NO)-releasing statin derivatives, a class of drugs showing enhanced antiproliferative and antiinflammatory properties. Proc Natl Acad Sci USA 2004; 101(22):8497–502.

14. Bellosta S, Arnaboldi L, Gerosa L, et al. Statins effect on smooth muscle cell proliferation. Sem Vasc Med 2004; 4(4):347–56.

15. Porter KE, Naik J, Turner NA, Dickinson T, Thompson MM, London NJ. Simvastatin inhibits human saphenous vein neointima formation via inhibition of smooth muscle cell proliferation and migration. J Vasc Surg 2002; 36(1):150–7.

16. Jeffery TK, Morrell NW. Molecular and cellular basis of pulmonary vascular remodeling in pulmonary hypertension. Prog Cardiovasc Dis 2002; 45(3):173–202.

17. Sakao S, Taraseviciene-Stewart L, Lee JD, Wood K, Cool CD, Voelkel NF. Initial apoptosis is followed by increased proliferation of apoptosis-resistant endothelial cells. FASEB J 2005; 19(9):1178–80.

18. Dorfmuller P, Humbert M, Capron F, Muller KM. Pathology and aspects of pathogenesis in pulmonary arterial hypertension. Sarcoidosis Vasc Diffuse Lung Dis 2003; 20(1):9–19.

19. Deng Z, Morse JH, Slager SL, et al. Familial primary pulmonary hypertension (gene *PPH1*) is caused by mutations in the bone morphogenetic protein receptor-II gene. Am J Hum Genet 2000; 67(3):737–44.

20. Newman JH, Wheeler L, Lane KB, et al. Mutation in the gene for bone morphogenetic protein receptor II as a cause of primary pulmonary hypertension in a large kindred. N Engl J Med 2001; 345(5):319–24.

21. Trembath RC, Harrison R. Insights into the genetic and molecular basis of primary pulmonary hypertension. Pediatr Res 2003; 53(6):883–8.

22. Machado RD, Pauciulo MW, Thomson JR, et al. BMPR2 haploinsufficiency as the inherited molecular mechanism for primary pulmonary hypertension. Am J Hum Genet 2001; 68(1):92–102.

23. Atkinson C, Stewart S, Upton PD, et al. Primary pulmonary hypertension is associated with reduced pulmonary vascular expression of type II bone morphogenetic protein receptor. Circulation 2002; 105(14):1672–8.

24. Atkinson C, Stewart S, Imamura T, Trembath RC, Morrell NW. Immunolocalisation of BMPR-II and TGF-ss type I and II receptors in primary plexogenic pulmonary hypertension. J Heart Lung Transplant 2001; 20(2):149.

25. Langenfeld EM, Langenfeld J. Bone morphogenetic protein-2 stimulates angiogenesis in developing tumors. Mol Cancer Res 2004; 2(3):141–9.

26. Goumans MJ, Valdimarsdottir G, Itoh S, Rosendahl A, Sideras P, ten Dijke P. Balancing the activation state of the endothelium via two distinct TGF-beta type I receptors. EMBO J 2002; 21(7):1743–53.

27. Pammer J, Reinisch C, Kaun C, Tschachler E, Wojta J. Inhibitors of differentiation/DNA binding proteins Id1 and Id3 are regulated by statins in endothelial cells. Endothelium 2004; 11(3–4):175–80.

28. Fishman AP. Primary pulmonary arterial hypertension: A look back. J Am Coll Cardiol 2004; 43(12 Suppl S):2S–4S.

29. Thompson PD, Moyna NM, White CM, Weber KM, Giri S, Waters DD. The effects of hydroxy-methyl-glutaryl co-enzyme A reductase inhibitors on platelet thrombus formation. Atherosclerosis 2002; 161(2):301–6.

30. Puccetti L, Bruni F, Bova G, et al. Effect of diet and treatment with statins on platelet-dependent thrombin generation in hypercholesterolemic subjects. Nutr Metab Cardiovasc Dis 2001; 11(6):378–87.

31. Notarbartolo A, Davi G, Averna M, et al. Inhibition of thromboxane biosynthesis and platelet function by simvastatin in type IIa hypercholesterolemia. Arterioscler Thromb Vasc Biol 1995; 15(2):247–51.

32. Mraiche F, Cena J, Das D, Vollrath B. Effects of statins on vascular function of endothelin-1. Br J Pharmacol 2005; 144(5):715–26.

33. Hernandez-Perera O, Perez-Sala D, Soria E, Lamas S. Involvement of Rho GTPases in the transcriptional inhibition of preproendothelin-1 gene expression by simvastatin in vascular endothelial cells. Circ Res 2000; 87(7):616–22.

34. Kureishi Y, Luo Z, Shiojima I, et al. The HMG-CoA reductase inhibitor simvastatin activates the protein kinase Akt and promotes angiogenesis in normocholesterolemic animals. Nat Med 2000; 6(9):1004–10.

35. Inoue I, Goto S, Mizotani K, et al. Lipophilic HMG-CoA reductase inhibitor has an anti-inflammatory effect: Reduction of MRNA levels for interleukin-1beta, interleukin-6, cyclooxygenase-2, and p22phox by regulation of peroxisome proliferator-activated receptor alpha (PPARalpha) in primary endothelial cells. Life Sci 2000; 67(8):863–76.

36. Faul JL, Nishimura T, Berry GJ, Benson GV, Pearl RG, Kao PN. Triptolide attenuates pulmonary arterial hypertension and neointimal formation in rats. Am J Respir Crit Care Med 2000; 162(6):2252–8.

37. Nishimura T, Faul JL, Berry GJ, Veve I, Pearl RG, Kao PN. 40-O-(2-hydroxyethyl)-rapamycin attenuates pulmonary arterial hypertension and neointimal formation in rats. Am J Respir Crit Care Med 2001; 163(2):498–502.

38. Nishimura T, Faul JL, Berry GJ, et al. Simvastatin attenuates smooth muscle neointimal proliferation and pulmonary hypertension in rats. Am J Respir Crit Care Med 2002; 166(10):1403–8.

39. Okada K, Bernstein ML, Zhang W, Schuster DP, Botney MD. Angiotensin-converting enzyme inhibition delays pulmonary vascular neointimal formation. Am J Respir Crit Care Med 1998; 158(3):939–50.

40. Nishimura T, Vaszar LT, Faul JL, et al. Simvastatin rescues rats from fatal pulmonary hypertension by inducing apoptosis of neointimal smooth muscle cells. Circulation 2003; 108(13):1640–5.

41. Vaszar LT, Nishimura T, Storey JD, et al. Longitudinal transcriptional analysis of developing neointimal vascular occlusion and pulmonary hypertension in rats. Physiol Genom 2004; 17(2):150–6.

42. Girgis RE, Li D, Zhan X, et al. Attenuation of chronic hypoxic pulmonary hypertension by simvastatin. Am J Physiol Heart Circ Physiol 2003; 285:H938–45.

43. Girgis RE, Ma SF, Ye S, et al. Differential gene expression in chronic hypoxic pulmonary hypertension: Effect of simvastatin treatment. Chest 2005 Dec; 128(6 Suppl):579S.

44. Davidson MH, McGarry T, Bettis R, et al. Ezetimibe coadministered with simvastatin in patients with primary hypercholesterolemia. J Am Coll Cardiol 2002; 40(12):2125–34.

45. Boccuzzi SJ, Bocanegra TS, Walker JF, Shapiro DR, Keegan ME. Long-term safety and efficacy profile of simvastatin. Am J Cardiol 1991; 68(11):1127–31.

46. Pedersen TR, Berg K, Cook TJ, et al. Safety and tolerability of cholesterol lowering with simvastatin during 5 years in the Scandinavian Simvastatin Survival Study. Arch Intern Med 1996; 156(18):2085–92.

47. Thibault A, Samid D, Tompkins AC, et al. Phase I study of lovastatin, an inhibitor of the mevalonate pathway, in patients with cancer. Clin Cancer Res 1996; 2(3):483–91.

48. Kim WS, Kim MM, Choi HJ, et al. Phase II study of high-dose lovastatin in patients with advanced gastric adenocarcinoma. Invest New Drugs 2001; 19(1):81–3.

49. Larner J, Allan G, Kessler C, Reamer P, Gunn R, Huang LC. Phospho-inositol glycan derived mediators and insulin resistance. Prospects for diagnosis and therapy. J Basic Clin Physiol Pharmacol 1998; 9(2–4): 127–37.

50. Kao PN. Simvastatin treatment of pulmonary hypertension: An observational case series. Chest 2005; 127(4):1446–52.

51. Kaye JA, Meier CR, Walker AM, Jick H. Statin use, hyperlipidaemia, and the risk of breast cancer. Br J Cancer 2002; 86(9):1436–9.

52. Hebert PR, Gaziano JM, Chan KS, Hennekens CH. Cholesterol lowering with statin drugs, risk of stroke, and total mortality. An overview of randomized trials. JAMA 1997; 278(4):313–21.

53. Li HY, Appelbaum FR, Willman CL, Zager RA, Banker DE. Cholesterol-modulating agents kill acute myeloid leukemia cells and sensitize them to therapeutics by blocking adaptive cholesterol responses. Blood 2003; 101(9):3628–34.

54. Wong WW, Dimitroulakos J, Minden MD, Penn LZ. HMG-CoA reductase inhibitors and the malignant cell: The statin family of drugs as triggers of tumor-specific apoptosis. Leukemia 2002; 16(4):508–19.

55. Ardati A, Stolley P, Knapp DE, Wolfe SM, Lurie P. Statin-associated rhabdomyolysis. Pharmacoepidemiol Drug Saf 2005; 14(4):287.

56. Ratz Bravo AE, Tchambaz L, Krahenbuhl-Melcher A, Hess L, Schlienger RG, Krahenbuhl S. Prevalence of potentially severe drug-drug interactions in ambulatory patients with dyslipidaemia receiving HMG-CoA reductase inhibitor therapy. Drug Saf 2005; 28(3):263–75.

57. Sochman J, Podzimkova M. Not all statins are alike: Induced rhabdomyolysis on changing from one statin to another one. Int J Cardiol 2005; 99(1):145–6.

58. Baker SK. Molecular clues into the pathogenesis of statin-mediated muscle toxicity. Muscle Nerve 2005; 31(5):572–80.

59. Chu JW, Kao PN, Faul JL, Doyle RL. High prevalence of autoimmune thyroid disease in pulmonary arterial hypertension. Chest 2002; 122(5):1668–73.

16 Transitions and Combination Therapy for Pulmonary Arterial Hypertension

Todd Hirschtritt, M. Kathryn Steiner, and Nicholas S. Hill

Contents

Introduction
Transitions
Combinations
Conclusions
References

Abstract

Pulmonary arterial hypertension (PAH) is a progressive and often fatal disease. Currently available pharmacotherapies are often suboptimal when used singly, due to either a poor clinical response or a complication from the therapy. As a consequence, transitioning patients from one therapy to another or adding a therapy is a frequently encountered clinical conundrum. This chapter examines the rationale and limited data surrounding transitioning patients from one pharmacotherapy to another and combining individual therapies to produce an improvement in clinical outcomes. Much of the research discussed deals with animal models used to test combination therapies, as there are few clinical trials in human subjects, but this is rapidly changing, as a number of controlled trials are currently either in the planning stages or in progress. Transitions clearly have a role in enhancing the convenience and safety of pulmonary hypertension therapy for some patients. Combination therapy looks promising and may well represent the future of PAH pharmacotherapy.

From: *Contemporary Cardiology: Pulmonary Hypertension*
Edited by: N. S. Hill and H. W. Farber © Humana Press, Totowa, NJ

Key Words: pulmonary hypertension therapy; transitions; combination therapy; nitric oxide; endothelin; prostacyclins; phosphodiesterase inhibitors; cyclic guanine monophosphate; cyclic adenine monophosphate; endothelin-receptor antagonists.

1. INTRODUCTION

Prior chapters in this volume have detailed advances in the pharmacotherapy of pulmonary arterial hypertension (PAH), focusing on individual classes of agents. Although these therapies have significantly improved the functional status, quality of life, and, in the case of epoprostenol, survival of PAH patients, responses are usually partial and less than desired. On average, patients with severe pulmonary hypertension experience improvement in pulmonary hemodynamics, but pulmonary arterial pressures remain severely elevated. These agents also have potential adverse side effects and risks, and loss of efficacy may occur after an initial favorable response. This has led investigators to consider switching to an alternative safer or potentially more effective therapy or to ask whether combinations of agents may lead to greater and more durable therapeutic responses than individual agents. An emerging literature in both experimental models and clinical settings is examining these questions. This chapter first discusses the rationale for and information on the transition from one agent to another and then weighs the evidence supporting various combinations of agents. Presently, evidence on many of the possible transitions and combinations is lacking, and our discussion highlights areas where additional study is needed.

2. TRANSITIONS

2.1. Rationale

The presently approved therapies for PAH in the United States have significant limitations. The best established and probably most effective agent, epoprostenol, necessitates intravenous administration and has a half-life of minutes, posing the risks of intravenous catheter-related sepsis and sudden hemodynamic deterioration in the event of abrupt discontinuation. The subcutaneous prostacyclin treprostinil is also effective but causes infusion site pain in virtually all patients, reaching intolerable levels in a minority. The only endothelin-receptor antagonist thus far approved by the Food and Drug Administration, bosentan, causes at least threefold elevations in liver transaminases in approximately 10% of patients *(1)* When these complications occur, transition to an alternative agent should be considered. The following sections examine possible alternative choices and discuss the available evidence.

2.2. From Intravenous Epoprostenol to Subcutaneous or Intravenous Treprostinil

When patients have encountered life-threatening complications from epoprostenol infusion, including catheter-related sepsis (which occurs in up to 0.14 patient-years) (2), catheter-related thrombosis, or abrupt discontinuation due to catheter occlusion, dislodgement, or breakage (3–5), subcutaneous treprostinil offers substantial safety advantages. Catheter-related sepsis is virtually unknown with subcutaneous treprostinil. Furthermore, should the subcutaneous catheter become dislodged, the patient merely replaces it without seeking medical attention, and because of the drug's much longer half-life, there is much less urgency than with epoprostenol. In addition, some patients desire a transition to treprostinil because of the convenience of a much smaller pump and no need for cold packs because of the drug's stability at room temperature. The drug requires no mixing, and the infusion site may be changed as infrequently as every three days or longer. The fact that treprostinil is a prostacyclin is also reassuring to the patient and physician; the likelihood of sustaining the benefit of epoprostenol may be higher than if the switch was to an entirely different drug class.

One study has retrospectively examined the outcomes of eight patients transitioned to subcutaneous treprostinil because they had experienced life-threatening or intolerable complications from intravenous epoprostenol (sepsis in five and cerebral emboli, recurrent syncope, and intractable headache in one each) (6). The patients had all responded favorably to long-term intravenous epoprostenol, with the New York Heart Association class improving from III–IV to I–II in most patients. Patients were transitioned in an intensive care or telemetry unit, with a gradual increase in treprostinil dose (starting with 5 ng/kg/min or half the initial epoprostenol dose, whichever was lower) and continuing such dose increases every 5 hours, while epoprostenol was lowered by 2 ng/kg/min every 2 hours until the transition was complete. No serious complications occurred, but some patients developed signs of prostacyclin excess, necessitating acceleration in the tapering of the epoprostenol dose. At completion of the transition, which took 24 to 96 hours depending on the initial dose, the final treprostinil dose was 83% of the initial epoprostenol dose, and follow-up several months later demonstrated stability of functional status and six-minute walk distance. The main complication of therapy was the infusion site erythema and pain that is also seen with *de novo* initiations of subcutaneous treprostinil. However, despite the much more rapid escalation of dose than is the case with *de novo* starts, the pain appears to be no worse with transitions.

A longer-term study of 17 patients followed for up to 42 months (mean: 16 months) after transitioning from epoprostenol to subcutaneous treprostinil has been reported in preliminary form *(7)*. The 13 patients remained on treprostinil and maintained their functional class and exercise capacity, as evidenced by stability of the six-minute walk distance (6MWD). Two patients died, thought to be related to the progression of the underlying disease, one transitioned to bosentan therapy, and one was lost to follow-up. In a phase IV placebo-controlled trial of the transition from intravenous epoprostenol to subcutaneous treprostinil, 13 of 14 patients randomized to active drug transitioned successfully and 6MWD was well maintained after eight weeks *(8)*. Seven of eight patients randomized to placebo were able to wean entirely from epoprostenol within two weeks but then subsequently deteriorated and resumed epoprostenol. The results unequivocally demonstrate the efficacy of subcutaneous treprostinil for at least the initial eight weeks and underline the need to monitor patients transitioning off infusion to other therapies during transitions, because deteriorations may be delayed.

Recently, the FDA approved intravenous treprostinil for the treatment of pulmonary arterial hypertension. Administered intravenously, treprostinil offers convenience advantages over epoprostenol because it requires no cold packs or mixing, and the drug cassette needs to be changed only every other day rather than daily. A smaller infusion pump is now available as well. However, dose changes are more challenging with the smaller pump due to its narrow range of infusion rates, and the high drug concentration necessary poses a risk of prostacyclin overdose if it enters the circulation too rapidly.

One preliminary report of six PAH patients switched from intravenous epoprostenol to intravenous treprostinil observed a tendency toward an increased pulmonary vascular resistance after the switch, although exercise capacity remained steady. Specific dosing recommendations for intravenous transitions have not been established, but the dose of intravenous treprostinil in the preliminary report *(9)* nearly doubled during the 12 weeks after the transition, from an average of 33 ng/kg/min for epoprostenol prior to the transition to 60 ng/kg/min for treprostinil 12 weeks afterwards. Accordingly, the current recommendation is to transition at a 1:2 dosing ratio, reducing the epoprostenol dose by 2.5–5 ng/kg/min while increasing the treprostinil dose by 5–10 ng/kg/min every few hours (V. Tapson, personal communication). In France, a rapid transition has been used during which patients are transitioned immediately to treprostinil at double the epoprostenol dose while switching from one medication cassette to the next (M. Humbert, personal communication).

Recently, the first clinical study was completed to evaluate the safety and efficacy of transitioning PAH patients from intravenous (IV) epoprostenol to IV treprostinil *(10)*. The 12-week prospective, open-label study transitioned 31 patients over 24 to 48 hours in a monitored setting with a simultaneous reduction of IV epoprostenol and increase in IV treprostinil to a level no lower than the initial dose of IV epoprostenol. Patients were then discharged with titration of IV treprostinil as needed for symptoms throughout the 12-week study period. There was no statistically significant difference in 6MWD between the patients at baseline on IV epoprostenol and at week 12 on IV treprostinil for the 27 patients who completed the study (438 ± 16 m at baseline vs. 439 ± 16 m at week 12). Other parameters including the Naughton–Balke treadmill test and the Borg dyspnea score were similar between the groups as well. Although patients transitioned to roughly the same infusion rate initially, the 12-week treprostinil dose was greater than twice the baseline dose of IV epoprostenol (40 ng/kg/min for IV epoprostenol at baseline vs. 83 ng/kg/min for IV treprostinil at week 12). Several hemodynamic parameters changed after the transition, including an increase in the mean pulmonary artery pressure of 4 ± 1 mm Hg ($p < 0.01$), an increase in the pulmonary vascular resistance of 3 ± 1 Wood units/m^2 ($n = 26$, $p < 0.01$), and a decrease in the cardiac index of 0.4 ± 0.1 L/min/m^2 ($n = 27$, $p = 0.01$). The authors speculated that these differences might have occurred because initial doses of treprostinil after the transition were low. They also noted that the worsening hemodynamics did not correlate with a deterioration in exercise tolerance. Overall, the study demonstrated the safety of transitioning patients from IV epoprostenol to IV treprostinil; however, data are lacking on the long-term efficacy of this transition, including the effect on patient survival.

In summary, most patients in whom IV epoprostenol has caused life-threatening complications or significant inconvenience can be safely switched to subcutaneous treprostinil with the expectation that functional capacity will be maintained. Unfortunately, site pain will often be a problem. The transition from IV epoprostenol to IV treprostinil may improve convenience and safety for patients, but the recommendation that the infusion rate of treprostinil should be at least twice that of epoprostenol must be made with the caveat that it is based on minimal evidence. Furthermore, the relative dosing of subcutaneous versus IV treprostinil has not been fully evaluated, and the best recommendation is to titrate doses to clinical effect.

2.3. From Subcutaneous Treprostinil to Intravenous Epoprostenol

Occasionally, patients transitioned from epoprostenol to treprostinil encounter difficulty tolerating the infusion site pain and must be transitioned back. Also, when pulmonary hypertension progresses despite therapy with treprostinil, some clinicians may attempt intravenous epoprostenol as the therapy of last resort. No description of this transition has been reported, but the authors have transitioned several patients successfully, using the reverse of the process for intravenous epoprostenol to subcutaneous treprostinil outlined above, while patients are monitored in the intensive care unit. One patient, who was receiving 290 ng/kg/min of treprostinil, had the treprostinil dose decreased by 10 ng/kg/min every 6 hours, while the epoprostenol dose was increased by 2 ng/kg/min every 2 hours. After completion of the transition, she was receiving 144 ng/kg/min of epoprostenol. Another patient started on 22 ng/kg/min of treprostinil, which was decreased by 5 ng/kg/min every 5 hours, while epoprostenol was increased by 2 ng/kg/min every 2 hours. Her final infusion rate of epoprostenol was 20 ng/kg/min. Both patients tolerated the transition without difficulty, although both encountered symptoms of prostacyclin excess at times during the process, necessitating reductions in the epoprostenol dose before proceeding with further increases every other hour. The first patient initially improved on the intravenous epoprostenol but then further deteriorated, eventually dying 10 months after the transition. The second patient has remained stable on epoprostenol.

2.4. From Subcutaneous to Intravenous Treprostinil, and Vice Versa

Very little information serves to guide switches from subcutaneous treprostinil to intravenous treprostinil, or vice versa. The two routes of administration have been shown to be bioequivalent, at least during short-term infusions (48 hours) in normal humans at low rates (10 ng/kg/min) (11). Thus, our recommendation would be to perform one-to-one transitions, increasing and lowering doses via the respective routes by perhaps 2–3 ng/kg/min every 2 to 3 hours until the switch is complete.

2.5. From Epoprostenol to Inhaled Iloprost

A small, open-label, uncontrolled trial transitioned three women from intravenous epoprostenol of at least four years' duration to inhaled iloprost. Two had IPAH and the third had progressive PAH after occlusion of an atrial septal defect *(12)*. The patients were given iloprost inhalations (at varying concentrations) every three hours. Central hemodynamics were continuously monitored while epoprostenol was decreased by 1–3 ng/kg/min every 3–10 hours over three days. One patient had temporary reductions in the mean PA pressure in response to inhaled iloprost, but the epoprostenol could only be reduced from 13 to 6 ng/kg/min when symptoms of right heart failure occurred. Another patient was able to completely discontinue epoprostenol but then developed signs of right heart failure and worsening pulmonary hemodynamics during the subsequent several days. The final patient was discharged using inhaled iloprost alone, but right heart failure recurred two weeks later. The authors concluded that iloprost significantly lowers PA pressure in patients with PAH already being treated with epoprostenol, but the effect is not durable. This small case series raises serious questions about the advisability of attempting to transition patients receiving continuous infusion therapy to intermittent inhaled prostacyclin therapy, but the study is too small to draw any firm conclusions. Such attempts should be made very cautiously, with patients undergoing very close follow-up if they are continued on inhalation therapy alone.

2.6. From Intravenous or Subcutaneous Prostacyclins to Oral Therapy

Many patients currently receiving intravenous or subcutaneous therapy are anxious to switch to an oral therapy because of the vastly greater convenience and tolerability. One study transitioned 23 stable (World Health Organization class II or III) patients (stable on their current prostaglandin dose, without evidence of heart failure, and with primary or secondary pulmonary arterial hypertension) from intravenous or subcutaneous prostacyclin therapy to the oral endothelin-receptor antagonist bosentan *(13)*. Initially, patients were excluded if they received more than 50 ng/kg/min of prostacyclin, but that restriction was dropped as experience accrued. The transition occurred over two four-week blocks, with patients admitted to the hospital to begin low-dose bosentan (62.5 mg orally every 12 hours) and to be monitored for signs of prostacyclin excess, leading to reductions in their prostacyclin infusion rate as needed. Four weeks later, the patients were readmitted, started on full-dose bosentan (125 mg orally twice daily), and then discharged and instructed to reduce the prostacyclin infusion rate daily or every other day to taper off the medication within four weeks. Fifteen of the 23 patients (65%) were able to transition to oral bosentan, but four subsequently developed symptoms of worsening pulmonary hypertension after another 7 weeks to 12 months, requiring the resumption of prostacyclin. Furthermore, two patients developed acute liver injury necessitating transition back to prostacyclin. Therefore, 9 of the 23 patients (40%) were able to successfully transition to long-term bosentan therapy. The authors acknowledged that the study was small, nonrandomized, nonblinded, and open-label and had missing data that made statistical analysis unreliable.

In a more recent multicenter trial *(14)*, 10 of 22 patients receiving prostacyclin infusions transitioned to oral bosentan, but 3 of the 10 subsequently deteriorated, two of whom died despite the resumption of intravenous therapy. A lower initial prostacyclin infusion rate and less severe pulmonary hypertension at baseline were associated with successful transitions. The 12 patients who failed transition could not even tolerate lowering of the infusion rate. The authors concluded that although some patients can be transitioned successfully, careful patient selection and close monitoring during the transition are obligatory.

Thus, 30% to 40% of patients currently on parenteral prostacyclin therapy could conceivably be switched to a simpler and potentially safer oral regimen, but further studies are needed to explore the safety of short- and long-term transitional therapy, particularly as newer oral therapies such as specific ETA-receptor blockers and phosphodiesterase-5 inhibitors become available.

3. COMBINATIONS

3.1. Rationale

As detailed in previous chapters, multiple therapies acting via different pathways have now been demonstrated in randomized, controlled trials to improve dyspnea, functional class, exercise capacity, and, in the case of intravenous epoprostenol, survival in patients with PAH. Many investigators have proposed that, similar to the approach with cancer chemotherapy, combining agents that work via different mechanisms might bring about additive benefits. Further, considering that the pathogenesis of PAH is thought to include vasoconstriction as well as vascular remodeling, combining vasodilators with antiproliferative agents has particular appeal. *In situ* thrombosis is also thought to contribute to PAH, so most patients with moderate to severe PAH are placed on anticoagulants as a matter of routine, but this practice has never been subjected to a randomized, controlled trial. Figure 1 illustrates how currently available pharmacotherapies for PAH act via three main therapeutic pathways: prostacyclins, nitric oxide (NO)-cyclic guanylate monophosphate (cGMP), and endothelins. These are by no means the only possible pathways, and agents acting via other pathways are almost certainly to become available as new therapies are developed. However, these three represent the main pathways by which currently available therapies act. In the following, we examine experimental and clinical studies on combinations of PAH therapies that act via different pathways, both in experimental settings and clinically as well as acutely and long-term.

3.2. Combining Prostacyclins-cAMP Pathway with Nitric Oxide-cGMP Pathway

3.2.1. Prostacyclins with Phosphodiesterase Inhibitors

3.2.1.1. Acute Studies. The combination of prostacyclins and phosphodiesterase (PDE) inhibitors is attractive because, as shown in Fig. 1, prostacyclins stimulate cAMP production, causing vasodilating and antiproliferative effects. Inhibitors of phosphodiesterases-3 and -4 potentiate the prostacyclin-induced increase in cAMP by blocking the degradation of cAMP (Fig. 1). Phosphodiesterase-5 inhibitors selectively degrade cGMP, and so inhibitors of PDE5 may potentiate the action of prostacyclins by augmenting intracellular cGMP levels, intensifying the vasodilating and antiproliferative effects. In addition, increases in cGMP may potentiate the prostacyclin-induced increase in cAMP by inhibiting PDE3,4 via a mechanism referred to as "crosstalk."

In initial studies combining prostacyclins with PDE inhibitors by Schermuly et al., subthreshold doses of specific PDE inhibitors including motapizone (PDE3-selective), rolipram (PDE4-selective), and tolafentrine (PDE3/4 dual inhibitor) were administered to isolated rabbit lungs with pulmonary hypertension induced by U46619, the thromboxane A_2 mimetic *(15)*. The combined inhibition of PDE3 and 4 amplified (8 mm Hg vs. 4 mm Hg) and prolonged (>90 min vs. 15 min) the reduction of pulmonary arterial pressure induced by 10 min of aerosolized iloprost. A second similar study by the same investigators used not only the same PDE3 and 4 inhibitors, but also examined the effects of the dual-selective blocker zardaverine and the PDE5 inhibitor zaprinast on pulmonary vasodilator effects

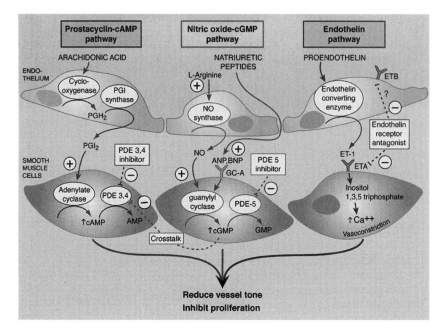

Fig. 1. The three main therapeutic pathways currently targeted in the treatment of PAH are schematized. In the diagram, + signs show where the increased administration of a substance can ameliorate pulmonary hypertension, and − signs show where inhibition might be beneficial. In the prostacyclin-cAMP pathway, prostacyclin agonists (PGI$_2$) act to stimulate cAMP production, and phospho-diesterase (PDE) -3 and -4 inhibitors block the degradation of cAMP, further reducing vasculature tone and inhibiting endothelial remodeling. In the nitric oxide-cGMP pathway, inhaled nitric oxide (iNO) activates soluble guanylate cyclase, stimulating cGMP, while PDE5 inhibitors prevent its degradation. In addition, PDE5 inhibitors act on the cAMP pathway by a "cross-talk" mechanism to inhibit PDE3,4. In the endothelin pathway, endothelin-receptor antagonists either nonselectively block both ET-A and ET-B receptors or selectively block ET-A receptors, inhibiting the vasoconstrictive and mitogenic actions of ET-1. By combining beneficial pharmacological actions in different pathways, a greater therapeutic effect might be achieved. + = increase in the intracellular concentration, activation of an enzyme or a receptor; - = decrease in the intracellular concentration, inhibition of an enzyme, or blockage of a receptor; cGMP= cyclic guanosine monophosphate; cAMP = cyclic adenosine monophosphate; ET-A and ET-B = endothelin-A and -B receptors; ET-1 = endothelin-1; ANP = atrial natriuretic peptide; BNP = brain natriuretic peptide; PGI$_2$ = prostacyclin agonists (i.e., epoprostenol). (To view this figure in color, see insert.)

of inhaled prostacyclin (epoprostenol) on the thromboxane analogue-induced model of pulmonary hypertension in isolated rabbit lungs *(16)*. Once again, although PDE5 inhibition was effective, the greatest potentiation (30–50%) and prolongation (>30 min) of the vasodilator effects were achieved using combined PDE3/4 inhibition.

In a subsequent study using the same experimental model, these investigators observed that currently available nonspecific PDE inhibitors (theophylline, pentoxifylline, and dipyridamole) also potentiated the magnitude and duration of prostacyclin-mediated vasodilating effects on the pulmonary circulation *(17)*. In addition, when both prostacyclin and PDE inhibitors were administered via the inhaled route, the shunt fraction was significantly lowered, indicating that this strategy can have salutary effects not only on pulmonary hemodynamics but also on gas exchange. These investigators also demonstrated that aerosolized iloprost, when combined with the same nonspecific PDE inhibitors, this time given via aerosolization, produced prolonged pulmonary vasodilation, suggesting a potential for the enhancement and prolongation of the effects of iloprost *(18)*. These in vitro acute studies provide a strong rationale for examining the combination of PGI_2 with PDE inhibitors in clinical studies as discussed below.

The dual-selective phosphodiesterase-3/4 inhibitor tolafentrine was tested in combination with iloprost in a study of 11 patients, most with idiopathic PAH *(19)*. In this observational trial, iloprost (1.4 µ g) was given by inhalation. Two hours later, tolafentrine was given intravenously in seven patients and by aerosolization in five patients, followed by a second iloprost inhalation. The combination of agents prolonged (60–120 min) but did not augment the magnitude of the decrease in the pulmonary vascular resistance compared to iloprost alone.

More recent studies have examined the combination of PDE5 inhibition with prostacyclins. Wilkens et al. *(20)* found that the combination of oral sildenafil (25–50 mg) plus inhaled iloprost (8.4–10.5 µ g) lowered the mean pulmonary artery pressure more in five patients with idiopathic PAH than iloprost alone (13.8 ± 1.4 vs. 9.4 ± 1.3, $p < 0.009$). Cardiac output was also increased by the combination, but pulmonary vascular resistance, systemic blood pressure, and heart rates were unchanged. Ghofrani et al. *(21)* examined the same combination of drugs in 30 patients with severe pulmonary hypertension (10 with idiopathic, 6 with connective tissue-related, 13 with chronic thromboembolic, and 1 with aplasia of the left pulmonary artery). They also found that the combination was more potent than either agent alone in lowering the PA pressure and pulmonary vascular resistance and increasing the cardiac output (Fig. 2). In addition, it extended the duration of the effect to more than three hours. These studies show

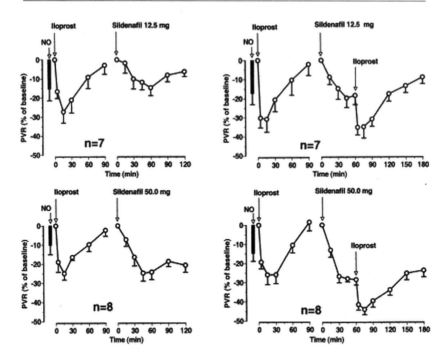

Fig. 2. Effects of inhaled nitric oxide (NO), inhaled iloprost, and increasing doses of oral sildenafil either alone or in combination with inhaled iloprost on pulmonary vascular resistance (PVR) over time. (a) A low dose of sildenafil (12.5 mg) alone is compared with inhaled NO and iloprost. (b) A higher dose of sildenafil (50 mg) is compared with NO and iloprost. (c) Inhaled NO and iloprost are compared to the combination of low-dose sildenafil (12.5 mg) and iloprost. (d) Inhaled NO and iloprost are compared to the combination of high-dose sildenafil (50 mg) and iloprost. Notice the increased and prolonged benefit of combined therapy as well as the improvement with the higher dose of sildenafil. Arrows indicate the administration of therapy. Error bars indicate confidence intervals. [Adapted with permission from *(22)*.]

that combining prostacyclins and PDE inhibitors is a very promising therapeutic strategy to treat PAH, at least acutely.

A Japanese study assessed the acute benefits of the orally active prostacyclin analogue beraprost (40 µg) alone and in combination with sildenafil (25 mg) in six patients with NYHA class II or III PAH *(22)*. The peak reduction in the mean pulmonary artery pressure was 15% lower than baseline in the combination group, with an effect sustained for 4 hours compared to beraprost alone, where the effect persisted for only 2 hours. The mean systemic blood pressure was unchanged. This small, acute study provides further evidence that combination therapy can potentiate and prolong the effects of individual agents on pulmonary hemodynamics.

3.2.1.2. Long-Term Studies. Using the model of monocrotaline-induced pulmonary hypertension in rats, Schermuly et al. *(23)* found that the combination of intravenous iloprost and the dual PDE3/4 blocker tolanfentine, when administered for two weeks during the development of pulmonary hypertension, reduced the right ventricular systolic pressure, right ventricular hypertrophy, and pulmonary vascular remodeling more than either agent alone, approaching normal levels. In addition, when administered for 2 weeks beginning 28 days after monocrotaline administration when the pulmonary hypertension was fully established, hemodynamic, right ventricular, and pulmonary vascular remodeling changes were partially reversed. Another study using the monocrotaline model of pulmonary hypertension in rats found that the combination of the oral PDE5 inhibitor sildenafil and the oral prostacyclin beraprost attenuated the development of pulmonary hypertension more than either agent alone *(24)*. Once again, right ventricular hypertrophy and pulmonary vascular remodeling were attenuated more by combination therapy, in association with greater increases in plasma cAMP and cGMP levels, than with single-agent therapy.

Long-term clinical trials on the combined effects of prostacyclin and PDE inhibitors on pulmonary hypertension include a case series consisting of three patients with severe PAH, with two on both epoprostenol and iloprost and the other on epoprostenol alone *(25)*. Sildenafil was added at doses ranging from 75 mg to 200 mg daily. Five months after the addition of sildenafil, the mean PA pressure had fallen by 14%, 41%, and 22%, the 6MWD improved in all three patients, and in two patients, the pulmonary vascular resistance fell by 52% and 55%, respectively. In another larger observational trial on 73 patients who initially improved on inhaled iloprost, 14 subsequently deteriorated, and sildenafil (25–50 mg tid) was added as rescue therapy *(26)*. In the 14 deteriorating patients, the 6MWD increased from 217 m at baseline to 305 m after the first 3 months of iloprost therapy but then fell by 49 m over the subsequent 15 months. After three months of combined sildenafil and iloprost therapy, the 6MWD had increased to 346 m. Functional class also improved, as did pulmonary vascular resistance (from 2494 to 1950 dyne/s/cm^{-5}) (Fig. 3).

Preliminary results were recently reported of a multicenter, randomized, controlled trial assessing the addition of sildenafil to intravenous epoprostenol, demonstrating a placebo-subtracted improvement of 26 m with add-on therapy *(27)*. These longer-term studies extend

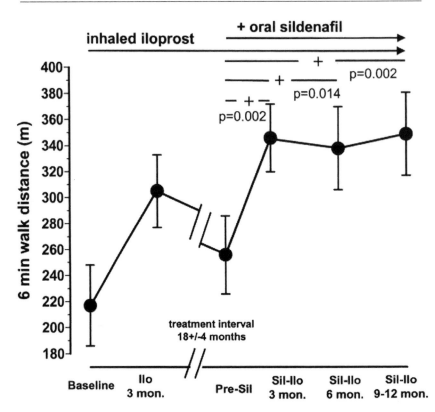

Fig. 3. Improvement in six-minute walk distances in response to iloprost and sildenafil therapy. Results were obtained at baseline, after 3 months of inhaled iloprost (Ilo 3 mo.), following a mean treatment interval of 18 ± 4 months' therapy, and after clinical deterioration occurred, repeat testing occurred (Pre-Sil). After 3, 6, and 9 to 12 months of combination sildenafil and inhaled iloprost (Sil-Ilo) therapy, the 6MWD was measured. Plus signs with horizontal bars adjacent indicate a significant improvement in walk distance with the addition of sildenafil to iloprost (via a Wilcoxon test with two-sided *p* values). [Adapted with permission from *(26)*.]

the findings of the acute studies, suggesting that the addition of sildenafil to prostacyclin is a promising therapeutic approach for PAH and is probably more effective than either agent alone.

3.2.2. Prostacyclins with Nitric Oxide

Another approach to combination therapy is to add an agent that stimulates the production of cAMP (prostacyclin) to one that stimulates the production of cGMP [inhaled nitric oxide (iNO)]. This should intensify the vasodilating and antiproliferative effects of both second messengers and might also further increase cAMP levels via the "cross-talk" phenomenon. Few studies have examined the effect of this combination on pulmonary vascular responses, however. Using intact, anesthetized rats with established pulmonary hypertension four weeks after monocrotaline injection, Hill and Pearl *(28)* found that the combination of iNO and inhaled prostacyclin reduced pulmonary artery pressure more than either agent alone, particularly at lower prostacyclin infusion rates. In a retrospective case-control study on 24 infants and small children with pulmonary hypertension following cardiac surgery, Hermon et al. *(29)* found that patients treated with a prostacyclin infusion (10 ng/kg/min) for 24 hours prior to the withdrawal of iNO were significantly less likely to have rebound ($\geq 5\%$ decrease in SaO_2) after iNO withdrawal. These studies suggest that this combination holds promise, but presently, because both drugs must be administered continuously, this combination is most relevant to the acute setting. As effective NO donors and prostacyclins that require only intermittent administration via inhalational or oral routes are introduced, long-term applications of this combination of agents will become more practical.

3.2.3. NITRIC OXIDE WITH PDE INHIBITORS

Inhaled nitric oxide (iNO) selectively dilates pulmonary vessels by activating soluble guanylate cyclase and stimulating the production of cyclic guanine monophosphate (cGMP). Theoretical advantages of iNO over intravenous vasodilators include improved oxygenation via better ventilation–perfusion matching and its lack of systemic side effects by virtue of its immediate inactivation when combined with hemoglobin. Combining iNO with PDE5 inhibitors has particular appeal because one agent stimulates cGMP production while the other slows its degradation, thus potentially augmenting and prolonging pulmonary vasodilatation (Fig. 1). However, combinations with other PDE inhibitors (3,4 inhibitors) should be efficacious as well, by combining agents that increase cAMP levels by slowing its metabolism with others that stimulate cGMP production.

In one acute study on intact, anesthetized rats, the combination of the PDE5 inhibitor zaprinast and iNO abolished hypoxic pulmonary vasoconstriction, whereas each agent alone caused significantly less blunting *(30)*. In a fetal sheep model, zaprinast had no effect on pulmonary hemodynamic responses to dissolved nitric oxide *(31)*. Based on this finding, the authors surmised that the pulmonary vascular response to NO might involve pathways other than cGMP, but it is important to keep in mind that animals in this study were younger and of a different species than in most other studies; also, zaprinast was combined with an infusion of U46619, which might have influenced the results.

Other studies have examined the combined effects of phosphodiesterase-3 inhibition and iNO on acute pulmonary hemodynamics *(32)*. Intact, anesthetized rabbits, infused with U46619, received incremental doses of the PDE3 inhibitor milrinone, followed by iNO (40 ppm). At each dose of milrinone, iNO had an additive effect on the reductions in the pulmonary vascular resistance but had no effect on the systemic vascular resistance. In an intact, anesthetized piglet model, Foubert et al. combined the nonspecific PDE inhibitor dipyrimadole with iNO (2–10 ppm) *(33)*. Dipyridimole increased plasma cGMP levels, presumably because of the slowing of cGMP degradation. The combination of iNO with dipyridimole had additive effects on reductions in the PVR and blunted the rebound pulmonary hypertension seen after sudden cessation of iNO. In another study by the same authors on intact piglets *(34)*, dipyridimole extended the duration of iNO-induced pulmonary vasodilation from 12 min to 42 min. Overall, these findings suggest that the combination of iNO with PDE inhibition allows the administration of a lower dose of iNO for a similar and prolonged hemodynamic effect and less risk of rebound upon iNO withdrawal.

Few clinical reports are available on the combined effects of iNO and PDE inhibition for the treatment of pulmonary hypertension. Ivy et al. *(35)* exposed children with pulmonary hypertension to iNO (20 ppm), dipyridamole (0.6 mg/kg), and the combination, observing that both treatments lowered the pulmonary vascular resistance similarly, but that iNO was more pulmonary-selective. Nearly half (46%) of the children had more than a 20% additional drop in PVR when iNO was added to dipyridimole than with either agent alone; in a separate group of patients with severe pulmonary hypertension following cardiac surgery, dipyridamole attenuated the rise in PA pressure after the abrupt withdrawal of iNO. In a subsequent case report of an infant with severe pulmonary hypertension following surgical valve replacement for congenital mitral stenosis *(36)*, sildenafil administered for three weeks had additive pulmonary vasodilating effects with iNO. This experience and another case report *(37)* suggest that sildenafil may be useful to facilitate weaning from iNO. These reports are consistent with those on the animal models described above, but too few clinical data are available to draw any firm conclusions.

3.2.4. NATRIURETIC PEPTIDES WITH PDE INHIBITORS

Natriuretic peptides [atrial natriuretic peptide (ANP), brain natriuretic peptide (BNP), and c-type natriuretic peptide (CNP)] activate particulate guanylate cyclase via guanylate cyclase-linked natriuretic peptide receptors (GC-A, B) (Fig. 1), increasing cGMP production. In a recent study on mice with a genetic deficiency of the natriuretic peptide A receptor, sildenafil caused less vasodilation than in wild-type mice, consistent with the idea that greater production of cGMP renders sildenafil more effective *(38)*. In another study on intact anesthetized rats, Preston et al. observed additive blunting effects of ANP and sildenafil on acute hypoxic vasoconstriction as well as on increasing cGMP levels *(39)*. Furthermore, the systemic vascular resistance remained unchanged, indicating pulmonary selectivity. The authors concluded that combinations of agents that stimulate cGMP production with those that inhibit cGMP degradation have additive pulmonary hemodynamic effects and hold promise as therapies for pulmonary hypertension.

Another study on the combination of these two classes of drugs in perfused rabbit lungs found that urodilatin, a renally derived natriuretic peptide that stimulates guanylate cyclase, and a subthreshold dose of dipyridamole reduced the mean PA pressure more than the natriuretic peptide alone, along with significant increases in plasma cGMP *(40)*. However, significant reductions in systemic blood pressure were also seen with both agents, potentially limiting the potential of this combination as a therapy for pulmonary hypertension.

Very few clinical studies have examined the combination of natriuretic peptides with other agents. In a preliminary investigation, Klinger et al. *(41)* infused BNP (2 µg/kg bolus, followed by a 0.01-µg/kg/min infusion for 3 hours) into 13 adult patients with PAH, before and after a 100-mg oral dose of sildenafil. By itself, BNP had nonsignificant hemodynamic effects, but the combination of BNP and sildenafil lowered the PA pressure and pulmonary vascular resistance more than either drug alone. The authors concluded that the combination of BNP and a PDE5 inhibitor has favorable effects on pulmonary hemodynamics and has therapeutic potential, particularly in the acute situation, where the need for intravenous administration would not be a concern, and the lesser effect on systemic hemodynamics as compared to intravenous epoprostenol might be an advantage. As of yet, no reports on the long-term administration of natriuretic peptides to PAH patients have appeared, either alone or in combination with other drugs.

3.3. Combinations of the Prostacyclin-cAMP or the Nitric Oxide-cGMP Pathway with the Endothelin Pathway

3.3.1. PROSTACYCLINS WITH ENDOTHELIN-RECEPTOR ANTAGONISTS

The rationale behind this combination is to correct the imbalance in the production of the vasodilating prostaglandin prostacyclin and of the vasoconstricting prostaglandin thromboxane A_2 in patients with PAH *(42)*, while blocking the effects of endothelin-1. As discussed in Chapter 13, circulating levels and protein expression in plexiform lesions of the potent vasoconstrictor and mitogen endothelin-1 (ET1) are increased in patients with PAH *(43)* and the peptide is thought to contribute to the pathogenesis of the disease. Thus, treating PAH via both pathways could offer a very effective therapeutic approach.

Results from experimental studies support this possibility. Using the monocrotaline model in rats, Ueno et al. *(44)* tested the efficacy of combined therapy with the oral prostacyclin beraprost and an oral ET-A-receptor antagonist (TA-0201). The authors administered the drugs for 20 days starting the day before monocrotaline injection and found that the combination of the two agents was more effective than either drug alone. Rats receiving the two drugs had only a 25% increase in RV pressure at high doses and 53% at moderate doses compared to 60% and 65% in those receiving the ETA inhibitor and 54% and 83% in those receiving beraprost alone, in high and moderate doses, respectively. Furthermore, the combination group had less evidence of pulmonary hypertension by echocardiogram, as evidenced by a greater reduction in the ratio of left ventricular minor to major axis, used as an index of right ventricular systolic pressure. Combination therapy also reduced medial wall thickening of the pulmonary arteries, right ventricular hypertrophy, and the beta/alpha ratio of myosin heavy-chain mRNA (used as an index of the cardiac hypertrophic response) more than either agent alone. This study supports the idea that combination therapy for PAH with a prostacyclin and an endothelin-receptor antagonist may be more effective than single agents alone.

To date, three published studies have reported the effects of this combination of agents in patients with PAH. In an open-label, nonrandomized pilot study, Hoeper et al. *(45)* added the nonspecific endothelin-receptor antagonist bosentan to inhaled iloprost ($n = 9$) or oral beraprost ($n = 11$) in patients who had been on a stable dose of the prostacyclin for at least three months. The maximal oxygen consumption determined by a cardiopulmonary exercise test (from 11.0 ± 2.3 to 13.8 ± 3.6 ml/kg/min), anaerobic threshold, oxygen pulse, peak systolic blood pressure, and minute ventilation/carbon dioxide production slope all increased after three months of bosentan. The 6MWD showed a mean increase of 58 ± 43 m after the initiation of bosentan, but the small sample size precluded an attainment of statistical significance. The combination of medications was well tolerated, with only two patients developing transaminase elevation.

BREATHE-2, a double-blind, placebo-controlled study to examine the efficacy and safety of bosentan combined with intravenous epoprostenol (46), enrolled 33 patients with NYHA class III or IV PAH. Two days after the initiation of intravenous epoprostenol (2 ng/kg/min), patients were randomized to receive bosentan (62.5 mg po twice daily) or placebo (2:1 ratio). Two days later, patients had their epoprostenol dose increased by 2 ng/kg/min, with subsequent two-week increments to a target dose of 12–16 ng/kg/min after 16 weeks. Bosentan was also increased following the initial four weeks to a target dose of 125 mg twice daily. The combination of bosentan and epoprostenol tended to improve the primary endpoint (total pulmonary resistance) and other secondary hemodynamic endpoints, including the mean PA pressure and pulmonary vascular resistance, but the differences were not statistically significant (Fig. 4). Furthermore, there were no significant differences between the two groups in the 6MWD (68 m vs. 74 m median increase in the bosentan/epoprostenol and placebo/epoprostenol groups, respectively) and NYHA functional class. The combination was as well tolerated as placebo/epoprostenol, with leg edema being the only side effect more commonly encountered in the group receiving bosentan (27% vs. 9%). Equal numbers of patients deteriorated and/or died in the two groups. The authors concluded that the combination of bosentan and epoprostenol may be a therapeutic option for PAH, but because the study was underpowered, larger prospective studies are needed.

The double-blind, placebo-controlled STEP (iloprost inhalation solution Safety and pilot efficacy Trial in combination with bosentan for Evaluation in Pulmonary arterial hypertension) trial randomly assigned inhaled iloprost or inhaled placebo to 67 PAH patients already receiving bosentan (47). After 12 weeks, patients in the iloprost plus bosentan group walked 26 m farther in six minutes than patients in the placebo plus bosentan group ($p = 0.51$). Combination therapy was well tolerated and significantly improved other endpoints, including NYHA functional class (34% increased by at least one NYHA class in the combination group vs. 6% in controls), pulmonary arterial pressure, and rate of clinical worsening.

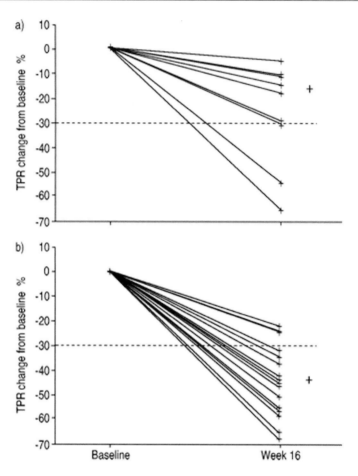

Fig. 4. Results of the BREATHE-2 study. Total pulmonary resistance (TPR) change from baseline are noted (a) comparing placebo plus epoprostenol ($n = 10$) and (b) with bosentan plus epoprostenol ($n = 19$). The isolated + sign indicates median values for each group at the end of the 16-week study period. There was a trend for a greater reduction in mean TPR in the group receiving bosentan plus epoprostenol, but the difference was not statistically significant ($p = 0.08$). [Adapted with permission from *(46)*.]

Another pilot study on 11 patients with symptomatic PAH despite bosentan monotherapy demonstrated significant improvements with inhaled treprostinil at doses of 30 or 45 mcg just four times daily *(48)*. After 12 weeks of therapy, the 6MWD had improved by a mean of 67 m 1 hour after inhalation, NYHA functional class improved from III to II in 9 of 11 patients, and mean PA pressure and pulmonary vascular resistance fell by 10% and 26%, respectively. These data support the idea that combination therapy with prostacyclins and endothelin-receptor antagonists will benefit patients with PAH, but further study is necessary.

3.3.2. ENDOTHELIN-RECEPTOR ANTAGONISTS WITH PDE INHIBITORS

Rats injected with monocrotaline had less mortality and lower PA pressures when treated with a combination of maximally effective doses of bosentan and sildenafil than with either agent alone *(49)*, suggesting that this combination might provide additive benefits in the clinical disease. However, few clinical investigations on the combination of endothelin-receptor antagonists with PDE inhibitors have been reported. Hoeper et al. *(50)* followed a cohort of nine patients with severe idiopathic PAH who were deteriorating on bosentan therapy alone. The six-minute walk distance fell from 403 ± 80 m at initiation to 277 ± 80 m after 11 ± 5 months of bosentan therapy. Three months after the addition of sildenafil (25–50 mg three times daily), the 6MWD increased to 392 ± 62 m ($p = 0.007$), an improvement that was sustained throughout the remainder of the follow-up period (median: 9 months) (see Fig. 5). No adverse events, including liver function abnormalities, were observed. Mathai et al. *(51)* more recently

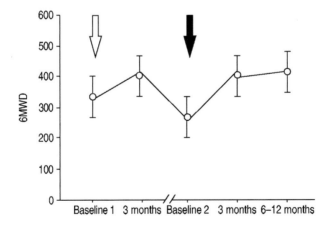

Fig. 5. Graph demonstrating the six-minute walk distances on the nine patients with PAH. The open arrow demonstrates when bosentan therapy was started. Baseline 2 represents the average distance 11 ± 5 months later before the addition of sildenafil, during which time the 6MWD had declined. The closed arrow represents the time when sildenafil was started. The 6MWD was significantly improved at three months, an increase that was sustained for the nine-month follow-up period. [Adapted with permission from *(50)*.]

examined the effect of the addition of sildenafil to patients deteriorating on bosentan monotherapy. They found that patients with idiopathic PAH increased the 6MWD by an average of 47 m, and 5 of 13 such patients improved by at least one NYHA class compared, respectively, to only 7 m and 2 of 12 patients with connective tissue disease-associated PAH. They concluded that although the combination appears to benefit the idiopathic PAH patients, the connective tissue disease patients failed to benefit. These trials show promise for the use of PDE5 inhibitor and endothelin-receptor antagonist combination therapy, but results from adequately powered randomized trials that are currently underway will be necessary before firm conclusions can be drawn.

4. CONCLUSIONS

Despite the introduction of a variety of effective pharmacotherapies for PAH in recent years, the therapeutic options remain suboptimal. Some of the therapies, like intravenous epoprostenol, are cumbersome to administer and entail potentially life-threatening complications. Others, like subcutaneous treprostinil, are painful, while others, like bosentan, incur the risk of liver toxicity. Accordingly, the need to transition from one therapy to another is a common occurrence. Considerable experience has accrued on certain transitions, such as from intravenous epoprostenol to subcutaneous treprostinil or oral bosentan. These transitions can be accomplished safely if carried out with careful monitoring according to guidelines that are continually being refined as experience accrues. Even when therapies are well tolerated and effective, the response is usually partial, so interest in combination therapy is mounting. The idea is to combine therapies with different mechanisms of action that are likely to have additive or synergistic effects. For example, the combination of an agent that increases cAMP (prostacyclin) with one that increases cGMP (phosphodiesterase-5 inhibitor) may have more potent vasodilating and antiproliferative actions than either agent alone. Although studies in animal models show promising results for a variety of combinations, as of yet, relatively few clinical studies have examined the efficacy of combination therapy for PAH. Nonetheless, combination therapy is likely to see increasing use as more agents become available. It is important to assess the various combinations with properly designed controlled trials so that we can determine which combinations are the most beneficial.

REFERENCES

1. Rubin LJ, Badesch DB, Barst RJ, et al. Bosentan therapy for pulmonary arterial hypertension. N Engl J Med 2002; 346(12):896–903.
2. McLaughlin V, Shillington A, Rich S. Survival in primary pulmonary hypertension: The impact of epoprostenol therapy. Circulation 2002; 106(12):1477–82.
3. Barst RJ, Rubin LJ, McGoon MD, Caldwell EJ, Long WA, Levy PS. Survival in primary pulmonary hypertension with long-term continuous intravenous prostacyclin. Ann Intern Med 1994; 121(6):409–15.
4. Badesch DB, Tapson VF, McGoon MD, et al. Continuous intravenous epoprostenol for pulmonary hypertension due to the scleroderma spectrum of disease: A randomized, controlled trial. Ann Intern Med 2000; 132(6):425–34.
5. Falk A, Lookstein RA, Mitty HA. Flolan infusion interruption: A lethal complication during venous access. J Vasc Interv Radiol 2001; 12(5): 667–8.
6. Vachiery JL, Hill N, Zwicke D, Barst R, Blackburn S, Naeije R. Transitioning from IV epoprostenol to subcutaneous treprostinil in pulmonary arterial hypertension*. Chest 2002; 121(5):1561–5.
7. Hill N, Barst R, Vachiery JL, Zwicket D, Naeije R. Long-term follow-up to the effects of transitioning patients with pulmonary arterial hypertension from IV epoprostenol to SC treprostinil. Am J Respir Crit Care Med. A174, 2004.
8. Hill N, Barst RJ, Vachiery J-L, Zwicke D, Naeije R. Long-term follow-up to the effects of transitioning patients with pulmonary arterial hypertension from IV epoprostenol to SC treprostinil. Am J Respir Crit Care Med 2004; 169:A174.
9. Gomberg-Maitland M, Barst RJ, McLaughlin V, et al. Transition from intravenous epoprostenol to intravenous treprostinil for the treatment of pulmonary arterial hypertension (PAH). Proc Am Thorac Soc Abs Issue 2005; 2:A300.
10. Gomberg-Maitland M, Tapson VF, Benza RL, et al. Transition from intravenous epoprostenol to intravenous treprostinil in pulmonary hypertension. Am J Respir Crit Care Med 2005; 172:1586–9.
11. Laliberte K, Arneson C, Jeffs R, Hunt T, Wade M. Pharmacokinetics and steady-state bioequivalence of treprostinil sodium (Remodulin) administered by the intravenous and subcutaneous route to normal volunteers. J Cardiovasc Pharmacol 2004; 44(2):209–14.
12. Schenk P, Petkov V, Madl C, et al. Aerosolized iloprost therapy could not replace long-term IV epoprostenol (prostacyclin) administration in severe pulmonary hypertension. Chest 2001; 119:296–300.
13. Suleman N, Frost A. Transition from epoprostenol and treprostinil to the oral endothelin receptor antagonist bosentan in patients with pulmonary hypertension. Chest 2004; 126(3):808–15.

14. Steiner MK, Preston IR, Klinger JR, et al. Conversion to bosentan from prostacyclin infusion therapy in pulmonary arterial hypertension: A pilot study. Chest. 2006; 130:1471–80.

15. Schermuly R, Roehl A, Weissmann N, et al. Subthreshold doses of specific phosphodiesterase type 3 and 4 inhibitors enhance the pulmonary vasodilatory response to nebulized prostacyclin with improvement in gas exchange. J Pharmacol Exp Ther 2000; 292(2):512–20.

16. Schermuly R, Ghofrani H, Enke B, et al. Low-dose systemic phosphodiesterase inhibitors amplify the pulmonary vasodilatory response to inhaled prostacyclin in experimental pulmonary hypertension. Am J Respir Crit Care Med 1999; 160:1500–6.

17. Schermuly R, Roehl A, Weissmann N, et al. Combination of nonspecific PDE inhibitors with inhaled prostacyclin in experimental pulmonary hypertension. Am J Physiol Lung Cell Mol Physiol 2001; 281(6): L1361–8.

18. Schermuly R, Krupnik E, Tenor H, et al. Coaerosolization of phosphodiesterase inhibitors markedly enhances the pulmonary vasodilatory response to inhaled iloprost in experimental pulmonary hypertension. Maintenance of lung selectivity. Am J Respir Crit Care Med 2001; 164(9):1694–700.

19. Ghofrani H, Rose F, Schermuly R, et al. Amplification of the pulmonary vasodilatory response to inhaled iloprost by subthreshold phosphodiesterase types 3 and 4 inhibition in severe pulmonary hypertension. Crit Care Med 2002; 30(11):2489–92.

20. Wilkens H, Guth A, Konig J, et al. Effect of inhaled iloprost plus oral sildenafil in patients with primary pulmonary hypertension. Circulation 2001; 104(11):1218–22.

21. Ghofrani H, Wiedemann R, Rose F, et al. Combination therapy with oral sildenafil and inhaled iloprost for severe pulmonary hypertension. Ann Intern Med 2002; 136(7):515–22.

22. Ikeda D, Tsujino I, Ohira H, Itoh N, et al. Addition of oral sildenafil to beraprost is a safe and effective therapeutic option for patients with pulmonary hypertension. J Cardiovasc Pharmacol 2005; 45:286–9.

23. Schermuly R, Kreisselmeier K, Ghofrani H, et al. Antiremodeling effects of iloprost and the dual-selective phosphodiesterase 3/4 inhibitor tolafentrine in chronic experimental pulmonary hypertension. Circ Res 2004; 94(8):1101–8.

24. Itoh T, Nagaya N, Fujii T, et al. A combination of oral sildenafil and beraprost ameliorates pulmonary hypertension in rats. Am J Respir Crit Care Med 2004; 169(1):34–8.

25. Stiebellehner L, Petkov V, Vonbank K, et al. Long-term treatment with oral sildenafil in addition to continuous IV epoprostenol in patients with pulmonary arterial hypertension. Chest 2003; 123(4):1293–5.

26. Ghofrani HA, Rose F, Schermuly RT, et al. Oral sildenafil as long-term adjunct therapy to inhaled iloprost in severe pulmonary arterial hypertension. J Am Coll Cardiol 2003; 42(1):158–64.

27. Simmoneau G, Rubin LJ, Galie N, et al. Safety and efficacy of sildenafil-epoprostenol combination therapy in patients with pulmonary arterial hypertension (PAH). Proc Am Thorac Soc 2007; 4:A300.

28. Hill L, Pearl R. Combined inhaled nitric oxide and inhaled prostacyclin during experimental chronic pulmonary hypertension. J Appl Physiol 1999; 86(4):1160–4.

29. Hermon M, Golej J, Burda G, Marx M, Trittenwein G, Pollak A. Intravenous prostacyclin mitigates inhaled nitric oxide rebound effect: A case control study. Artif Organs 1999; 23(11):975–8.

30. Nagamine J, Hill LL, Pearl R. Combined therapy with zaprinast and inhaled nitric oxide abolishes hypoxic pulmonary hypertension. Crit Care Med 2000 Jul; 28(7):2420–4.

31. Skimming J, DeMarco V, Kadowitz P, Cassin S. Effects of zaprinast and dissolved nitric oxide on the pulmonary circulation of fetal sheep. Pediatr Res 1996; 39(2):223–8.

32. Deb B, Bradford K, Pearl R. Additive effects of inhaled nitric oxide and intravenous milrinone in experimental pulmonary hypertension. Crit Care Med 2000; 28(3):795–9.

33. Foubert L, De Wolf D, Mareels K, et al. Intravenous dipyridamole enhances the effects of inhaled nitric oxide and prevents rebound pulmonary hypertension in piglets. Pediatr Res 2002; 52(5):730–6.

34. Foubert L, De Wolf D, Reyntjens K, et al. Intermittent nitric oxide combined with intravenous dipyridamole in a piglet model of acute pulmonary hypertension. Anesth Analg 2003; 97(5):1497–500.

35. Ivy D, Ziegler J, Kinsella J, Wiggins J, Abman S. Hemodynamic effects of dipyridamole and inhaled nitric oxide in pediatric patients with pulmonary hypertension. Chest 1998; 141(1 Suppl):17S.

36. Atz A, Lefler A, Fairbrother D, Uber W, Bradley S. Sildenafil augments the effect of inhaled nitric oxide for postoperative pulmonary hypertensive crises. J Thorac Cardiovasc Surg 2002; 124(3):628–9.

37. Mychaskiw I, George, Sachdev V, Heath BJ. Sildenafil (Viagra) facilitates weaning of inhaled nitric oxide following placement of a biventricular-assist device. J Clin Anesth 2001; 13(3):218–20.

38. Zhao L, Mason NA, Strange JW, Walker H, Wilkins MR. Beneficial effects of phosphodiesterase 5 inhibition in pulmonary hypertension are influenced by natriuretic peptide activity. Circulation 2003; 107(2):234–7.

39. Preston I, Hill N, Gambardella L, Warburton R, Klinger J. Synergistic effects of ANP and sildenafil on cGMP levels and amelioration of acute hypoxic pulmonary hypertension. Exp Biol Med 2004; 229(9):920–5.

40. Schermuly R, Weissmann N, Enke B, et al. Urodilatin, a natriuretic peptide stimulating particulate guanylate cyclase, and the phosphodiesterase 5 inhibitor dipyridamole attenuate experimental pulmonary hypertension: Synergism upon coapplication. Am J Respir Cell Mol Biol 2001; 25(2):219–25.

41. Klinger JR, Thaker S, Houtchens J, Preston IR, Hill NS, Farber HW. Pulmonary hemodynamic responses to brain natriuretic peptide and sildenafil in patients with pulmonary arterial hypertension. Chest 2006; 129:417–25.

42. Christman B, McPherson C, Newman J, et al. An imbalance between the excretion of thromboxane and prostacyclin metabolites in pulmonary hypertension. N Engl J Med 1992; 327(2):70–5.

43. Giaid A, Yanagisawa M, Langleben D, et al. Expression of endothelin-1 in the lungs of patients with pulmonary hypertension. N Engl J Med 1993; 328(24):1732–9.

44. Ueno M, Miyauchi T, Sakai S, Yamauchi-Kohno R, Goto K, Yamaguchi I. A combination of oral endothelin-A receptor antagonist and oral prostacyclin analogue is superior to each drug alone in ameliorating pulmonary hypertension in rats. J Am Coll Cardiol 2002; 40(1):175–81.

45. Hoeper MM, Taha N, Bekjarova A, Gatzke R, Spiekerkoetter E. Bosentan treatment in patients with primary pulmonary hypertension receiving nonparenteral prostanoids. Eur Respir J 2003; 22(2):330–4.

46. Humbert M, Barst RJ, Robbins IM, et al. Combination of bosentan with epoprostenol in pulmonary arterial hypertension: BREATHE-2. Eur Respir J 2004; 24(3):353–9.

47. McLaughlin VV, Oudiz RJ, Frost A, et al. Randomized study of adding inhaled iloprost to existing bosentan in pulmonary arterial hypertension. Am J Respir Crit Care Med 2006; 174:1257–63

48. Channick RN, Olschewski H, Seeger W, Staub T, Voswinckel R, Rubin LJ. Safety and efficacy of inhaled treprostinil as add-on therapy to bosentan in pulmonary arterial hypertension. J Am Coll Cardiol 2006 Oct 3; 48(7):1433–7.

49. Clozel M, Hess P, Rey M, Iglarz M, Binkert C, Qui C. Bosentan, sildenafil, and their combination in the monocrotaline model of pulmonary hypertension in rats. Exp Biol Med 2006; 231:967–73.

50. Hoeper MM, Faulenbach C, Golpon H, Winkler J, Welte T, Niedermeyer J. Combination therapy with bosentan and sildenafil in idiopathic pulmonary arterial hypertension. Eur Respir J 2004; 24(6):1007–10.

51. Mathai SC, Girgis RE, Fisher MR, et al. Addition of sildenafil to bosentan monotherapy in pulmonary arterial hypertension. Eur Respir J 2007;29:469–75.

17 Acute Right Ventricular Dysfunction: Focus on Acute Cor Pulmonale

Antoine Vieillard-Baron and François Jardin

CONTENTS

INTRODUCTION
PHYSIOLOGY AND PATHOPHYSIOLOGY
OF THE RIGHT VENTRICLE
ACUTE COR PULMONALE: DEFINITION,
DIAGNOSIS, AND PATHOPHYSIOLOGY
A FACTOR IN WORSENING OF RV FUNCTION:
MECHANICAL VENTILATION
ACUTE COR PULMONALE IN PULMONARY
EMBOLISM: INCIDENCE, PROGNOSIS,
AND THERAPY
ACUTE COR PULMONALE IN ARDS:
INCIDENCE, PROGNOSIS, AND THERAPEUTIC
IMPACT
ACUTE COR PULMONALE: PRINCIPLES
OF MANAGEMENT
SUMMARY AND CONCLUSIONS
REFERENCES

From: *Contemporary Cardiology: Pulmonary Hypertension*
Edited by: N. S. Hill and H. W. Farber © Humana Press, Totowa, NJ

Abstract

Acute right heart failure related to pulmonary causes (acute cor pulmonale) is caused mainly by acute pulmonary embolism or acute respiratory distress syndrome (ARDS) requiring mechanical ventilatory support. The echocardiogram is even more useful than right heart catheterization in this situation, because the pulmonary arterial pressure correlates poorly with right ventricular function and cardiac output measurements are often unreliable. The echo also gives information not only on the extent of right ventricular dysfunction and dilation, but also on left ventricular filling and function. Acute cor pulmonale due to massive pulmonary embolism occurs in the majority of pulmonary embolism patients admitted to the ICU and may respond rapidly to thrombolytic therapy. Acute cor pulmonale in patients with ARDS is partly related to positive pressure ventilation and its effect on increasing the impedance of the pulmonary vasculature. Lung-protective ventilatory strategies using limited tidal volumes and plateau pressures can greatly lower the occurrence of acute cor pulmonale in ARDS patients. The therapy for acute cor pulmonale aims at minimizing the pulmonary vascular resistance and optimizing fluid volume. Vasopressor agents should be used in hypotensive patients to maintain coronary perfusion, but inhaled vasodilator agents like inhaled nitric oxide and prostacyclin are seeing increasing use in critical care settings to selectively dilate the pulmonary arterial bed.

Key Words: cor pulmonale; echocardiography; acute right heart syndrome; lung-protective ventilator strategy; ARDS; inhaled nitric oxide; inhaled prostacyclin; vasopressors.

1. INTRODUCTION

Acute right ventricular dysfunction refers to the acute deterioration of right ventricular function as a consequence of pump failure related to the loss of contractility or the inability to handle an increase in afterload, or some combination of the two. Several clinical scenarios are associated with acute right ventricular failure: right ventricular infarction *(1)*, myocarditis *(2)*, severe sepsis *(3)*, and sudden pulmonary hypertension as in massive pulmonary embolism or acute respiratory distress syndrome (ARDS), leading to acute cor pulmonale *(4)*. Because the focus of this book is on pulmonary hypertension, only the last scenario is detailed below.

2. PHYSIOLOGY AND PATHOPHYSIOLOGY OF THE RIGHT VENTRICLE

Whereas the left ventricle (LV) is a thick-walled pump, the right ventricle (RV) has a thin free wall, adapted to handling large shifts in volume, but not pressure. Under physiological conditions, the RV acts against a low-resistance, high-compliance circuit, i.e., the pulmonary circulation. Consequently, the RV ejects blood quasi-continuously into the pulmonary bed, acting partly as a passive conduit *(5)*. Redington et al. have characterized the normal RV pressure-volume relation as a triangular shape with short isovolemic contraction and relaxation times and a prolonged ejection long after the RV pressure has decreased *(6)*. For these reasons, the RV systolic function is sensitive to even slight increases in pulmonary vascular resistance that can overload the RV and impair its systolic function. To compensate, the RV is able to dilate acutely unlike the left ventricle, because of a significantly lower diastolic elastance *(7)*; its diastolic function is tolerant.

RV perfusion has a great impact on RV function, particularly when the RV fails. Under physiological conditions, RV perfusion persists throughout the cardiac cycle. Because of its thin free wall, the systolic intramyocardial pressure developed by the RV is much lower than the systemic, leading to a relatively constant RV perfusion pressure, not only in diastole but also in systole *(8)*. With RV failure, the RV dilates, end-diastolic and end-systolic pressures increase, and the systemic arterial pressure decreases. Together, these lead to an increase in RV oxygen demand while the coronary driving pressure decreases, thus causing RV ischemia, which leads to a downward spiral that further aggravates the RV failure. This process was well documented by Vlahakes et al. in an experimental model of RV failure induced by increased RV afterload *(9)*. In this model, a phenylephrine infusion raised RV perfusion pressure, thereby significantly improving RV function *(9)*. Guyton et al. demonstrated that optimal RV adaptation to an acute increase in pulmonary vascular resistance can only be achieved if the systemic arterial pressure is maintained *(10)*. Using echocardiography, we noted a marked functional improvement of the failing RV following infusion of a low dose of norepinephrine, thus restoring a normal systemic pressure and, presumably, adequate RV perfusion *(11)*. Maintenance of adequate systemic perfusion pressure is an extremely important aspect of the management of acute RV failure and is illustrated below.

3. ACUTE COR PULMONALE: DEFINITION, DIAGNOSIS, AND PATHOPHYSIOLOGY

In 1831, Testa was the first to use the term "cor pulmonale" to describe the concept of cardiopulmonary interaction *(12)*. In 1935, McGinn and White described the clinical features of acute cor pulmonale resulting from pulmonary embolism *(13)*. Acute cor pulmonale may be defined as the consequences on the RV of a sudden and excessive increase in afterload, leading to systolic and diastolic overload. In the most severe cases, acute cor pulmonale may induce shock, requiring prompt and physiologically adapted treatment. Massive pulmonary embolism is the most frequent cause of acute cor pulmonale *(14)*, where the obstruction of the pulmonary circulation is proximal. The second most common cause is severe ARDS *(15)*, where the obstruction is more distal. These situations are described in more detail below.

Echocardiography, by a transthoracic or transesophageal approach, is the best tool to diagnose and characterize acute cor pulmonale. Echocardiography allows a direct and simple visualization of the kinetics and size of cardiac cavities, especially of the RV. In acute cor pulmonale, paradoxical septal motion reflects the RV systolic overload and is associated with RV enlargement, indicating diastolic overload of the ventricle *(4)*. Elzinga et al. have demonstrated in cats that the progressive constriction of the pulmonary artery prolongs RV isovolemic contraction and ejection times compared to the left ventricle *(16)*. This reverses the normal transseptal pressure gradient at end systole when the LV is relaxed but the RV is still ejecting blood. The persistence of elevated RV pressure into early LV diastole causes bowing (or paradoxical motion) of the septum toward the LV. We have reported the same phenomenon in humans by applying a high positive end-expiratory pressure (PEEP) in patients with ARDS on mechanical ventilation (Fig. 1) *(17)*.

A   **B**

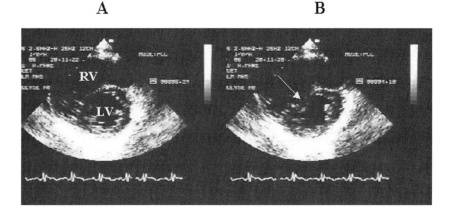

Fig. 1. Short-axis view of the left ventricle by a transthoracic approach in a patient who presented acute cor pulmonale related to massive pulmonary embolism. Paradoxical septal motion consists of a movement of the interventricular septum toward the left ventricular cavity, as noted by the arrow. A = end diastole; B = end systole; RV = right ventricle; LV = left ventricle.

In acute cor pulmonale, echocardiography also demonstrates the effects of RV dilation on LV diastolic function. Because the two ventricles are enclosed within a stiff pericardium, any acute RV dilation is responsible, via septal displacement, for a decrease in LV diastolic dimensions and an impairment in LV relaxation *(18)*. This is illustrated by alterations in Doppler mitral flow, shown in Fig. 2. Using echocardiography, acute cor pulmonale is classically separated from chronic cor pulmonale by the absence of thickening of the RV free wall and by less of an increase in the pulmonary artery pressure. Whereas the pulmonary artery pressure is indeed lower in acute than in chronic cor pulmonale, because the RV is unable to sustain a mean pressure gradient > 30 cm H_2O in acute conditions, we have previously reported early RV thickening in acute cor pulmonale *(15)*, reflecting the ability of the RV to adapt quickly to the new hemodynamic conditions. However, this thickening is only slight; it is less than 6 mm when the normal value is less than 3 mm. Finally, we never use the RV fractional area contraction, a parameter proposed for evaluating the RV systolic function, since we have observed a large range of values in normal volunteers and a marked overlap in patients with or without acute cor pulmonale (Fig. 3).

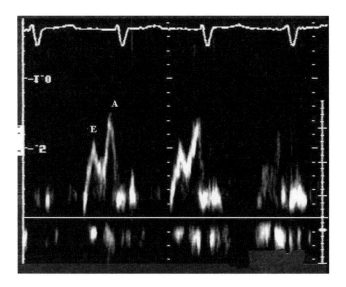

Fig. 2. Typical pattern of mitral flow by Doppler with an inverted E/A ratio in a patient with acute cor pulmonale. This reflects left ventricular relaxation impairment. The E wave represents the passive filling of the left ventricle, while the A wave represents the active filling at end diastole induced by atrial contraction.

RVFAC (%)

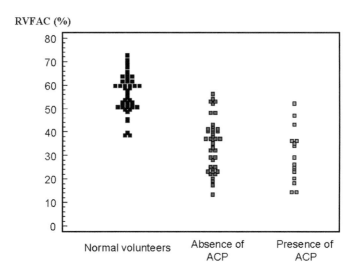

Fig. 3. Right ventricular fractional area contraction (RVFAC) measured by echocardiography in a long-axis view in normal volunteers and in patients with ARDS complicated or not by acute cor pulmonale (ACP). Note the large range of the values in the normal volunteers, between 38% and 74%, and the large overlap among the three groups.

Two echocardiographic examples of acute cor pulmonale are given in Fig. 4. Narrated videos are also available online in the supplementary material of our previously published clinical commentary regarding acute cor pulmonale in the intensive care unit *(19)*.

Pulmonary artery catheterization has difficulty accurately diagnosing acute cor pulmonale. The severity of pulmonary hypertension is not the primary determinant of the tolerance of the RV to increased afterload. This depends primarily on the intrinsic properties of the RV and secondly on associated factors that can increase the pulmonary vascular impedance, such as mechanical ventilation *(20)*. In other words, although higher PA pressures predispose to the development of acute cor pulmonale, for the same abnormal pulmonary artery pressures, acute cor pulmonale may or may not develop, as illustrated in Fig. 5. Moreover, cardiac output measurement by thermodilution may be inaccurate in marked pulmonary hypertension because of the high incidence of significant tricuspid regurgitation and its well-known negative effect on the validity of measurements *(21)*. Finally, some authors have suggested that acute cor pulmonale may be present when the central venous pressure is greater than the pulmonary capillary wedge pressure *(22)*, but this has never been confirmed.

Long axis view   **Short axis view**

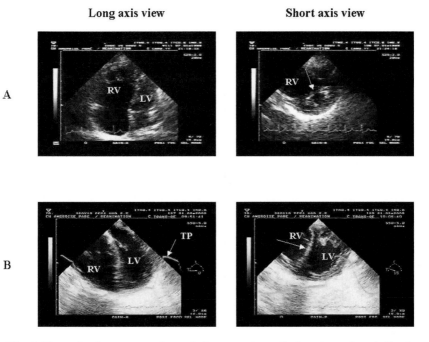

Fig. 4. Example of acute cor pulmonale in two patients. Patient A was hospitalized for massive pulmonary embolism and patient B for ARDS requiring mechanical ventilation. The long-axis view of the left ventricle, by a transthoracic approach in patient A and a transesophageal approach in patient B, demonstrated marked RV dilation. The short-axis view, by a transthoracic approach in A and a transgastric approach in B, demonstrated a paradoxical septal motion (arrows). Note also that the left ventricle appeared severely restricted. RV = right ventricle; LV = left ventricle; TP = tracheal pressure.

4. A FACTOR IN WORSENING OF RV FUNCTION: MECHANICAL VENTILATION

Mechanical ventilation, well known to be the usual treatment of respiratory failure and some cases of shock, is also well known to induce significant hemodynamic alterations and lower cardiac output *(23,24)*. Mechanical ventilation, particularly when administered using high inflation pressures, compresses pulmonary vessels, increases RV afterload *(25)*, and decreases RV stroke volume. By increasing the transpulmonary pressure, i.e., the distending pressure of the lung, high tidal volumes or PEEP may further increase the resistance to flow in the intra-alveolar vessels. This has been known since 1962 when Permutt et al. applied the concept of the Starling resistor to the pulmonary circulation *(26)*. Our unit has previously found a strong relationship

SPAP (mmHg)

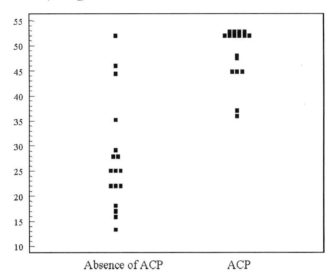

Fig. 5. Systolic pulmonary artery pressure (SPAP) evaluated by Doppler measurement on the third day of mechanical ventilation in patients hospitalized for ARDS. Note the overlap of SPAP whether or not acute cor pulmonale (ACP) was present.

between the increase in transpulmonary pressure and increased RV afterload, using either right heart catheterization *(27)* or, more recently, echocardiography *(28)*. In septic states, which depress intrinsic RV systolic function *(3,29)*, the imposition of positive pressure during mechanical ventilation may in itself be sufficient to induce acute cor pulmonale, as illustrated in Fig. 6.

5. ACUTE COR PULMONALE IN PULMONARY EMBOLISM: INCIDENCE, PROGNOSIS, AND THERAPY

Pulmonary embolism causes acute cor pulmonale when the obstruction of the pulmonary circulation is substantial, usually involving at least two lobar arteries. Kasper et al. were the first to report a significant correlation between an angiographic score of pulmonary obstruction and the severity of RV dilation *(30)*, and our group has since confirmed these results in 57 patients *(31)*. We have also reported a 61% incidence of acute cor pulmonale in a population of 161 patients hospitalized in our ICU for proven pulmonary embolism involving at least two lobar arteries *(14)*. In this study, greater RV dilation was associated with LV restriction, a smaller LV stroke volume, and shock

A   B

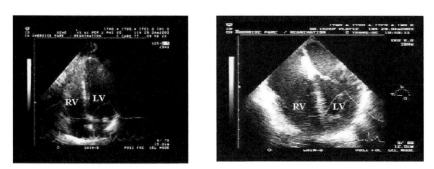

Fig. 6. Patient hospitalized in intensive care unit for septic shock. (a) Initially, the patient was breathing spontaneously and transthoracic echocardiography demonstrated a right ventricle in the normal size range. (b) Because of severe hypoxia, mechanical ventilation was started and transesophageal echocardiography demonstrated marked RV dilation associated with paradoxical septal motion (not shown). RV = right ventricle; LV = left ventricle.

that were observed in only 67% of the patients with acute cor pulmonale *(14)*. We also found that acute cor pulmonale is associated with a typical pattern of pulmonary artery flow: a biphasic pattern of the Doppler profile associated with a markedly reduced maximal velocity (Fig. 7).

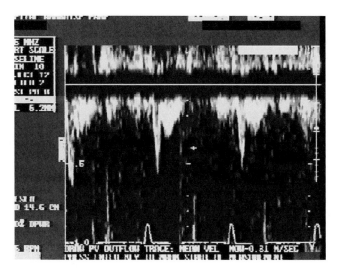

Fig. 7. Typical pattern of pulmonary artery flow by Doppler in a patient with massive pulmonary embolism. Note the biphasic pattern of the flow with two velocity peaks.

In 11 patients with acute cor pulmonale related to massive pulmonary embolism, we used echocardiography to follow the evolution of the RV function during anticoagulation therapy *(32)*. We found that parameters of RV function were nearly corrected after seven days (Fig. 8) and completely corrected after 31 days of treatment *(32)*. When thrombolysis is used soon after an acute pulmonary embolism, acute cor pulmonale resolves within a few hours.

Because it is so often associated with massive pulmonary embolism, acute cor pulmonale determined by echocardiogram increases the likelihood of pulmonary embolism sufficiently to begin anticoagulation therapy without awaiting a definitive radiological diagnosis *(33)*. If deemed necessary, definitive radiological procedures can be obtained later, once the patient has stabilized. Echocardiography therefore appears especially useful for the management of shock in the intensive care unit; the visualization of acute cor pulmonale quickly raises the possibility of pulmonary embolism, thus guiding acute therapy and subsequent diagnostic procedures.

The prognostic impact of acute cor pulmonale complicating pulmonary embolism is currently a matter of debate. Some authors argue that RV dysfunction is an independent predictor of mortality *(34,35)* and serves as an indication for thrombolytic therapy, regardless of the clinical presentation. However, in our study of 161 cases of pulmonary embolism, the only independent factor of mortality was the presence of metabolic acidosis, reflecting inadequate tissue perfusion *(14)*.

D1   D7

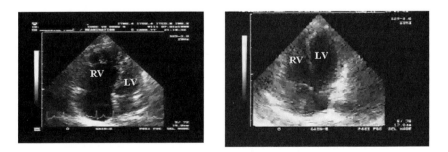

Fig. 8. Echocardiographic evolution in a patient with massive pulmonary embolism. Transthoracic echocardiography was initiated (D1) and then repeated after seven days of anticoagulant treatment (D7). RV = right ventricle; LV = left ventricle.

6. ACUTE COR PULMONALE IN ARDS: INCIDENCE, PROGNOSIS, AND THERAPEUTIC IMPACT

In 1977, Zapol and Snider first described the presence of pulmonary hypertension in ARDS leading to RV overload *(36)*. Contributing factors to the pulmonary hypertension included pulmonary vasoconstriction, obstruction of distal arteries by clumped platelets, inflammatory cells and fibrin microthrombi, and pulmonary vascular remodeling *(37)*. As discussed above, mechanical ventilation also has an important effect on RV function. As is well known, lung compliance is markedly reduced in ARDS, thus necessitating high transpulmonary pressures for a given tidal volume. The enormous impact of mechanical ventilation on RV function in ARDS is demonstrated by comparing two echocardiographic studies from our unit, consisting, respectively, of 23 *(38)* and 75 *(15)* mechanically ventilated ARDS patients. In the first study, performed before 1990, patients were ventilated with large tidal volumes (13 ml/kg) to maintain normocapnia, airway pressures were therefore excessive *(38)*, and the incidence of acute cor pulmonale was 61% *(38)*. In the second study, performed after 1996, patients were ventilated with relatively low tidal volumes (8 ml/kg), plateau pressure was below 30 cm H_2O in all cases, PEEP was limited, and the incidence of acute cor pulmonale was only 25% *(15)*. In this second study, echocardiography was performed by a transesophageal approach on the third day of mechanical ventilation and was repeated periodically until the patient recovered *(15)*. We observed that acute cor pulmonale was associated with marked hemodynamic alterations, including a significant decrease in LV dimensions and stroke index, associated with a significant increase in heart rate *(15)*. Acute cor pulmonale was reversible in all patients who recovered (Fig. 9) *(15)*. The level of hypercapnia and of plateau pressure were strongly associated with acute cor pulmonale *(15)*; the more pronounced the hypercapnia, the more frequent the acute cor pulmonale. This suggests the need to limit hypercapnia, a condition well known to induce pulmonary vasoconstriction *(39,40)*. However, the hypercapnia may also merely be a marker of more severe disease. Hypercapnia should never be controlled by increasing the plateau pressure, but rather by other means *(41)*.

Evidence regarding the prognostic impact of acute cor pulmonale complicating ARDS is conflicting. In our first study, when patients were ventilated with high tidal volumes, acute cor pulmonale was markedly and significantly associated with a poor prognosis: Mortality was 57% in cases, compared to 33% in those without acute cor

Long axis view   Short axis view

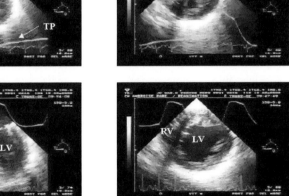

D3

D14

Fig. 9. Transesophageal echocardiography in a patient on mechanical ventilation for ARDS related to extensive pneumonia. After three days (D3), the patient was severely hypoxic and shock was present. The long-axis view of the left ventricle demonstrated RV dilation and the short-axis view indicated paradoxical septal motion (arrow). The patient recovered after 14 days (D14). Echocardiography thus demonstrated normalization of RV function. RV = right ventricle; LV = left ventricle; TP = tracheal pressure.

pulmonale *(38)*. In our second study, which used lower tidal volumes, acute cor pulmonale had no influence on mortality, which was 25% in patients with and without acute cor pulmonale *(15)*. However, in the latter study, acute cor pulmonale was managed with more stringent limitations on plateau pressure and more frequent use of prone positioning rather than increases in PEEP. This suggests that when mechanical ventilator strategies are used that limit the impact on RV overload, the RV is able to successfully adapt.

7. ACUTE COR PULMONALE: PRINCIPLES OF MANAGEMENT

The main goal, of course, is to treat the cause of RV overload: anticoagulation or thrombolysis in massive pulmonary embolism, and antibiotics or other specific medications in ARDS. But pending reversal of the cause, acute cor pulmonale requires specific management, including adaptation of mechanical ventilation, judicious fluid administration, choice of the right vasoactive drug, and sometimes use of inhaled nitrite oxide or prostacyclin.

7.1. Mechanical Ventilation

Whereas some investigators have proposed combining mechanical ventilation with transesophageal echocardiography in critically ill patients to easily visualize thrombi in the pulmonary arteries at the bedside *(42)*, we strongly discourage this practice and instead recommend transthoracic echocardiography with avoidance of mechanical ventilation in massive pulmonary embolism if at all possible. In ARDS, the situation is very different because mechanical ventilation is virtually always required. As discussed above, the institution of a so-called lung-protective ventilatory strategy in recent years has accompanied a substantial reduction (from 61% to 25%) in the occurrence of acute cor pulmonale in mechanically ventilated patients with ARDS. Therefore, we advocate the limitation of plateau pressure to <30 cm H_2O and tidal volume to ≤8 ml/kg, levels that were associated with the marked decrease in acute cor pulmonale in our earlier studies *(43)*. The association we found between more severe hypercapnia and acute cor pulmonale suggests that limitation of the level of hypercapnia may be advantageous, but not at the expense of excessive inflation pressures or tidal volumes.

7.2. Fluid Administration

RV dysfunction and especially acute cor pulmonale necessitate judicious fluid management. Schneider et al. have demonstrated that RV dysfunction is the main factor explaining the absence of fluid responsiveness in septic patients *(44)*. In acute cor pulmonale complicating ARDS or massive pulmonary embolism, the inferior vena cava diameter is markedly increased *(14,15)*, associated with volume overload of the RV. In this situation, fluid infusion is not only useless but may be dangerous because it may further dilate the RV and compress the LV. Acute cor pulmonale may also alter the effectiveness of pulse pressure variation in predicting fluid responsiveness. We have reported that pulse pressure variation, a parameter of LV preload deficiency, may be present in severe acute cor pulmonale. This deficiency is related to the marked dilation of the RV and interference with LV filling due to ventricular interdependence. Infusing more fluid in this situation further dilates the RV and may aggravate the problem with LV filling. The failure of cardiac output to respond to a bolus fluid challenge in a patient with clinical features of acute cor pulmonale should serve as a signal to forego further attempts at fluid resuscitation and adopt alternative strategies such as those discussed below *(45)*.

7.3. Vasoactive Agents

Acute cor pulmonale often induces circulatory failure, thus necessitating the infusion of vasoactive drugs. In our experience and in that of other investigators *(46,47)*, isolated RV dysfunction with normal LV function responds to norepinephrine infusion. By normalizing the systemic arterial pressure, norepinephrine restores RV perfusion, leading to improved RV function (Fig. 10). However, if LV failure is associated with acute cor pulmonale, the infusion of an inotropic drug such as dobutamine is preferred, considering the fact that norepinephrine infusion may aggravate LV failure *(11)*, although tolerance to dobutamine can develop rapidly *(48)*. Infusion of the phosphodiesterase-3 inhibitor milrinone would be an alternative consideration, but data are lacking on its efficacy for acute right heart failure.

7.4. Vasodilators

Various intravenous vasodilators have been used to treat acute right heart failure, including prostaglandin E1, nitroglycerin, nitroprusside, and prostacyclin *(47)*. If these lower pressures in the right side of the

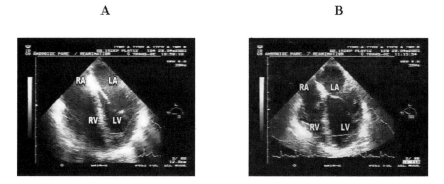

A   B

Fig. 10. Patient mechanically ventilated for septic shock related to pneumonia. (a) At baseline, transesophageal echocardiography demonstrated acute cor pulmonale with marked right ventricular dilatation. (b) Low-dose norepinephrine infusion restored systemic arterial pressure and corrected RV function. RV = right ventricle; LV = left ventricle; RA = right atrium; LA = left atrium.

heart are more than on the left, they can improve coronary perfusion of the right heart and help to restore hemodynamic stability. Unfortunately, this is often not the case, and the inhibition by these agents of hypoxic pulmonary vasoconstriction can disrupt ventilation–perfusion relationships and aggravate hypoxemia. Therefore, enthusiasm has been decreasing for the use of intravenous vasodilators and increasing for inhaled vasodilators to treat acute cor pulmonale.

Because these must be delivered to ventilated regions of the lung, inhaled agents usually improve oxygenation. Furthermore, agents like inhaled nitric oxide (iNO), which is inactivated by combining with hemoglobin circulating in the pulmonary vessels), and inhaled prostacyclin are pulmonary-selective by virtue of their short half-lives that minimize any systemic hemodynamic effects. Bhorade et al. *(49)* reported the effects of iNO (average concentration: 35 ppm) in 26 patients with various causes for their right heart failure. Although the mean pulmonary arterial pressure did not fall from an average of 73 mm Hg, the pulmonary vascular resistance dropped significantly and cardiac output, stroke volume, and oxygen saturation improved significantly. Approximately half of the patients had at least a 20% drop in pulmonary vascular resistance or a 20% increase in cardiac output, which permitted a reduction in the dose of vasoactive drugs in half of these "responders." However, mortality was still very high, approaching 80% in the responders, and in a separate study, these investigators also demonstrated that approximately one-quarter of patients become hemodynamically unstable when withdrawn from long-term iNO *(50)*. Partially in response to this limitation, some investigators have begun combining agents that enhance inotropy (dobutamine) *(51)* or inhibit the degradation of cGMP with iNO, but clinical data on these approaches are lacking.

Inhaled prostacyclin has seen increasing use to treat acute right heart syndrome in recent years, because it combines the pulmonary selectivity and favorable effects on oxygenation of iNO *(52)* and a substantially lower cost for acute administration. Inhaled iloprost, available in some European countries but not yet in the United States, has also been reported to improve right ventricular hemodynamics in a patient with acute right heart failure *(53)*. Nesiritide (synthetic BNP) and an investigational agent that improves cardiac output, lowers systemic and pulmonary vascular resistances, and selectively enhances right ventricular efficiency, levosimendan *(54)*, have been proposed as agents that might be advantageous to treat acute right heart failure, but once again, clinical data are lacking.

8. SUMMARY AND CONCLUSIONS

Acute right heart failure related to pulmonary causes (acute cor pulmonale) is caused mainly by acute pulmonary embolism or ARDS requiring mechanical ventilatory support. The echocardiogram is even more useful than right heart catheterization in this situation, because pulmonary arterial pressure correlates poorly with right ventricular function and cardiac output measurements are often unreliable. The echo also gives information not only on the extent of right ventricular dysfunction and dilation but also on left ventricular filling and function. Acute cor pulmonale due to massive pulmonary embolism occurs in the majority of pulmonary embolism patients admitted to the ICU and may respond rapidly to thrombolytic therapy. Acute cor pulmonale in patients with ARDS is partly related to positive pressure ventilation and its effect on increasing the impedance of the pulmonary vasculature. Lung-protective ventilatory strategies using limited tidal volumes and plateau pressures can greatly lower the occurrence of acute cor pulmonale in ARDS patients. The therapy of acute cor pulmonale aims at minimizing the pulmonary vascular resistance and optimizing fluid volume. Vasopressor agents should be used in hypotensive patients to maintain coronary perfusion, but inhaled vasodilator agents like inhaled nitric oxide and prostacyclin are seeing increasing use in critical care settings to selectively dilate the pulmonary arterial bed.

REFERENCES

1. Cohn JN, Guiha NH, Broder MI, Limas CJ. Right ventricular infarction. Clinical and hemodynamic features. Am J Cardiol 1974; 33:209–14.
2. McFalls EO, Jan van Suylen R. Myocarditis as a cause of primary right ventricular failure. Chest 1993; 103:1607–8.
3. Kimchi A, Ellrodt GA, Berman DS, Riedinger M, Riedinger MS, Swan HJC, Murata GH. Right ventricular performance in septic shock: A combined radionuclide and hemodynamic study. J Am Coll Cardiol 1984; 4:945–51.
4. Jardin F, Dubourg O, Bourdarias JP. Echocardiographic pattern of acute cor pulmonale. Chest 1997; 111:209–17.
5. Brooks H, Kirk E, Vokonas P, Urschel C, Sonnenblick E. Performance of the right ventricle under stress: Relation to right coronary flow. J Clin Invest 1971; 50:2176–83.
6. Redington AN, Gray JJ, Hodson ME, Rigby ML, Oldershaw PJ. Characterization of the normal right ventricular pressure-volume relation by biplane angiography and simultaneous micromanometer pressure measurements. Br Heart J 1988; 59:23–30.

7. Laks M, Gardner D, Swan JHC. Volumes and compliance measured simultaneously in the right and left ventricle of the dogs. Circ Res 1967; 66:612.

8. Hess DS, Bache RJ. Transmural right ventricular myocardial blood flow during systole in the awake dog. Circ Res 1979; 45:88–94.

9. Vlahakes GJ, Turley K, Hoffman J. The pathophysiology of failure in acute right ventricular hypertension: Hemodynamic and biochemical correlations. Circulation 1981; 63:87–95.

10. Guyton A, Lindsey A, Gilluly J. The limits of right ventricular compensation following acute increase in pulmonary circulatory resistance. Circ Res 1954; 11:326–32.

11. Vieillard-Baron A, Prin S, Chergui K, Dubourg O, Jardin F. Hemodynamic instability in sepsis. Bedside assessment by Doppler echocardiography. Am J Respir Crit Care Med 2003; 168:1270–6.

12. Testa AG. Delle Malattie del Cuore. Milano, 1831.

13. McGinn S, White P. Acute cor pulmonale resulting from pulmonary embolism. JAMA 1935; 104:1473–8.

14. Vieillard-Baron A, Page B, Augarde R, Prin S, Qanadli S, Beauchet A, Dubourg O, Jardin F. Acute cor pulmonale in massive pulmonary embolism: Incidence, echocardiographic pattern, clinical implications and recovery rate. Intens Care Med 2001; 27:1481–6.

15. Vieillard-Baron A, Schmitt JM, Augarde R, Fellahi JL, Prin S, Page B, Beauchet A, Jardin F. Acute cor pulmonale in acute respiratory distress syndrome submitted to protective ventilation: Incidence, clinical implications, and prognosis. Crit Care Med 2001; 29:1551–5.

16. Elzinga G, Pienne H, De Jong J. Left and right ventricular pump function and consequences of having two pumps in one heart. A study on isolated cat heart. Circ Res 1980; 46:564–74.

17. Jardin F, Farcot JC, Boisante L, Curien N, Margairaz A, Bourdarias JP. Influence of positive end-expiratory pressure on left ventricular performance. N Engl J Med 1981; 304:387–92.

18. Jardin F, Dubourg O, Gueret P, Delorme G, Bourdarias JP. Quantitative two-dimensional echocardiography in massive pulmonary embolism: Emphasis on ventricular interdependence and leftward septal displacement. J Am Coll Cardiol 1987; 10:1201–6.

19. Vieillard-Baron A, Prin S, Chergui K, Dubourg O, Jardin F. Echo-Doppler demonstration of acute cor pulmonale at the bedside in the medical intensive care unit. Am J Respir Crit Care Med 2002; 166: 1310–9.

20. Jardin F, Vieillard-Baron A. Right ventricular function and positive pressure ventilation in clinical practice: From hemodynamic subsets to respirator settings. Intens Care Med 2003; 29:1426–34.

21. Cigarroa R, Lange R, Williams R, et al. Underestimation of cardiac output by thermodilution in patients with tricuspid regurgitation. Am J Med 1989; 86:417–20.

22. Monchi M, Bellenfant F, Cariou A, Joly LM, Thebert D, Laurent I, Dhainaut JF, Brunet F. Early predictive factors of survival in the acute

respiratory distress syndrome. A multivariate analysis. Am J Respir Crit Care Med 1998; 158:1076–81.

23. Cournand A, Motley M, Werko L, Richard D. Physiological studies on the effects of intermittent positive pressure breathing on cardiac output in man. Am J Physiol 1948; 152:162.

24. Scharf S, Brown R, Saunders N, Green L. Hemodynamic effects of positive pressure inflation. J Appl Physiol 1980; 49:124.

25. Whittenberger J, McGregor M, Berglund E, Borst H. Influence of state of inflation of the lung on pulmonary vascular resistance. J Appl Physiol 1960; 15:878–82.

26. Permutt S, Bromberger-Barnea B, Bane HN. Alveolar pressure, pulmonary venous pressure, and the vascular waterfall. Med Thorac 1962; 19:239–60.

27. Jardin F, Brun-Ney D, Cazaux P, Dubourg O, Hardy A, Bourdarias JP. Relation between transpulmonary pressure and right ventricular isovolumetric pressure change during respiratory support. Cathet Cardiovasc Diag 1989; 16:215–20.

28. Vieillard-Baron A, Loubières Y, Schmitt JM, Page B, Dubourg O, Jardin F. Cyclic changes in right ventricular output impedance during mechanical ventilation. J Appl Physiol 1999; 87:1644–50.

29. Parker M, McCarty K, Ognibene F, Parillo J. Right ventricular dysfunction, similar to left ventricular changes, characterizes the cardiac depression of septic shock in humans. Chest 1990; 97:126–31.

30. Kasper W, Meinertz T, Kersting F, Lollgen H, Limbourg P, Just H. Echocardiography in assessing acute pulmonary hypertension due to pulmonary embolism. Am J Cardiol 1980; 45:567–72.

31. Mansencal N, Joseph T, Vieillard-Baron A, Qanadli S, Jondeau G, Lacombe P, Jardin F, Dubourg O. Comparison of different echocardiographic indexes secondary to right ventricular obstruction in acute pulmonary embolism. Am J Cardiol 2003; 92:116–9.

32. Valtier B, Dubourg O, Jondeau G, De Lassence A, Loubières Y, Dib JC, et al. Left and right intracardiac Doppler blood flow analysis in patients with severe acute pulmonary embolism. Eur Heart J 1993; 13 (Suppl):12.

33. Vieillard-Baron A, Qanadli S, Antakly Y, Fourme T, Loubières Y, Jardin F, Dubourg O. Transesophageal echocardiography for the diagnosis of pulmonary embolism with acute cor pulmonale: A comparison with radiological procedures. Intens Care Med 1998; 24:429–33.

34. Goldhaber SZ, Visani L, De Rosa M. Acute pulmonary embolism: Clinical outcomes in the International Cooperative Pulmonary Embolism Registry (ICOPER). Lancet 1999; 353:1386–9.

35. Konstantinides S, Geibel A, Olschewski M, Heinrich F, Grosser K, Rauber K, Iversen S, Redecker M, Kienast J, Just H, Kasper W. Association between thrombolytic treatment and the prognosis of hemodynamically stable patients with major pulmonary embolism: Results of a multi-center registry. Circulation 1997; 96:882–8.

36. Zapol W, Snider M. Pulmonary hypertension in severe acute respiratory failure. N Engl J Med 1977; 296:476–80.
37. Moloney ED, Evans TW. Pathophysiology and pharmacological treatment of pulmonary hypertension in acute respiratory distress syndrome. Eur Respir J 2003; 21:720–7.
38. Jardin F, Gueret P, Dubourg O, Farcot JC, Margairaz A, Bourdarias JP. Two-dimensional echocardiographic evaluation of right ventricular size and contractility in acute respiratory failure. Crit Care Med 1985; 13: 952–6.
39. Viitanen A, Salmenpera M, Heinonen J. Right ventricular response to hypercarbia after cardiac surgery. Anesthesiology 1990; 73:393–400.
40. Carvalho C, Barbas C, Medeiros D, Magaldi RB, Lorenzi Filho G, Kairalla RA, Deheinzelin D, Munhoz C, Kaufmann M, Ferreira M, Takagaki TY, Amato MB. Temporal hemodynamic effects of permissive hypercapnia associated with ideal PEEP in ARDS. Am J Respir Crit Care Med 1997; 156:1458–66.
41. Prin S, Chergui K, Augarde, R, Page B, Jardin F. Ability and safety of a heated humidifier to control hypercapnic acidosis in severe ARDS. Intens Care Med 2002; 28:1756–60.
42. Pruszczyk P, Torbicki A, Kuch-Wocial A, Chlebus M, Miskiewicz C, Jedrusik P. Transesophageal echocardiography for definition diagnosis of hemodynamically significant pulmonary embolism. Eur Heart J 1995; 16:534–8.
43. Vieillard-Baron A, Jardin F. Why protect the right ventricle in patients with acute respiratory distress syndrome? Curr Opin Crit Care 2003; 9:15–21.
44. Schneider A, Teule G, Groeneveld A, Nauta J, Heidendal G, Thijs L. Biventricular performance during volume loading in patients with early septic shock, with emphasis on the right ventricle: A combined hemodynamic and radionuclide study. Am Heart J 1988; 116:103–12.
45. Vieillard-Baron A, Chergui K, Rabiller A, Peyrouset O, Page B, Beauchet A, Jardin F. Superior vena caval collapsibility as a gauge of volume status in ventilated septic patients. Intens Care Med 2004 Sep; 30(9):1734–9.
46. Angle MR, Molloy DW, Penner B, Jones D, Prewitt RM. The cardiopulmonary and renal effects of norepinephrine in cnine pulmonary embolism. Chest 1989; 95:1333–7.
47. Mebazza A, Karpati P, Renaud E, Algotsson L. Acute right ventricular failure—From pathophysiology to new treatments. Intens Care Med 2003; 30:185–96.
48. Unverferth DA, Blanford M, Kates RE, Leier CV. Tolerance to dobutamine after a 72 hour continuous infusion. Am J Med 1980; 69: 262–6.
49. Bhorade S, Christenson J, O'Connor M, Lavoie A, Pohlman A, Hall JB. Response to inhaled nitric oxide in patients with acute right heart syndrome. Am J Respir Crit Care Med 1999; 159:571–9.

50. Christenson J, Lavoie A, O'Connor M, Bhorade S, Pohlman A, Hall JB. The incidence and pathogenesis of cardiopulmonary deterioration after abrupt withdrawal of inhaled nitric oxide. Am J Respir Crit Care Med 2000; 161:1443–9.

51. Bradford KK, Deb B, Pearl RG. Combination therapy with inhaled nitric oxide and intravenous dobutamine during pulmonary hypertension in the rabbit. J Cardiovasc Pharmacol 2000; 36:146–51.

52. Lowson SM, Doctor A, Walsh BK, Doorley PA. Inhaled prostacyclin for the treatment of pulmonary hypertension after cardiac surgery. Crit Care Med 2002; 30:2762–4.

53. Langer F, Wendler O, Wilhelm W, Tscholl D, Schafers HJ. Treatment of a case of acute right heart failure by inhalation of iloprost, a long-acting prostacyclin analogue. Eur J Anaesthesiol 2001; 18:770–3.

54. Ukkonen H, Saraste M, Akkila J, et al. Myocardial efficiency during levosimendan infusion in congestive heart failure. Clin Pharmacol Ther 2000; 68:522–31.

18 Lung Transplantation and Atrial Septostomy for Pulmonary Arterial Hypertension

E. P. Trulock

CONTENTS

INTRODUCTION
LUNG TRANSPLANTATION
ATRIAL SEPTOSTOMY
SUMMARY
REFERENCES

Abstract

Improvements in medical therapy for PAH patients have led to dramatic changes in the way PAH is managed, with much less emphasis on surgical techniques than in the past. Nevertheless, the current drug regimens are still ineffective or lose effectiveness in many patients, related to the progression of the underlying disease. For these patients, lung transplantation and atrial septostomy offer the hope of improved function, prolonged survival, and, most important to some patients, enhanced quality of life. However, both procedures are risky, with the potential for substantial morbidity and mortality, and patients must be selected carefully. Most lung transplant recipients now undergo double-lung transplants and experience higher perioperative mortality rates than those undergoing transplants for other diagnoses. Infection and acute rejection are early causes of morbidity, and most patients later suffer from bronchiolitis obliterans, thought to be related to chronic rejection. This is the main reason for a survival rate that approaches only 50% at five years' posttransplant. Septostomies are reserved for patients with high-rate atrial pressures who are

From: *Contemporary Cardiology: Pulmonary Hypertension*
Edited by: N. S. Hill and H. W. Farber © Humana Press, Totowa, NJ

suffering from low cardiac output syndromes or syncope. They have been associated with mortality rates of 16% in the past, but more recent studies using graded balloon septostomy report rates approaching 5%.

Key Words: septostomy; lung transplantation; pulmonary hypertension; surgery; right atrial pressure; graded septostomy; idiopathic pulmonary arterial hypertension; Eisenmenger's syndrome.

1. INTRODUCTION

Lung transplantation and atrial septostomy are the final options in the management of pulmonary arterial hypertension (PAH). With the advent of effective drug treatments, selecting patients for these procedures and timing the interventions have become more complex. Schemes for integrating atrial septostomy and transplantation into a sequential management strategy have been proposed (1–5), and evidence-based clinical practice guidelines have recently been published for both medical therapy and other interventions (5,6).

Prostaglandins, endothelin-receptor antagonists, phosphodiesterase inhibitors, and nitric oxide improve symptoms, exercise tolerance, and hemodynamic parameters not only in patients with idiopathic pulmonary arterial hypertension (IPAH) but also in patients with other forms of PAH (3,4). Furthermore, intravenous epoprostenol has conferred a significant survival advantage in patients with IPAH (7,8). Thus, medical management can delay the need for surgical intervention in many patients, sometimes indefinitely.

However, drug treatment has limitations. Although it can alter the clinical course of IPAH in many patients, the impact on the underlying pathobiology is less certain. Most patients already have moderate to severe PAH when the diagnosis is made, and some do not improve with drug treatment. Only a small minority of patients with IPAH respond to a calcium channel antagonist (9). Moreover, approximately 25% of patients with IPAH fail to respond to epoprostenol treatment, and those who remain in functional class III or IV with epoprostenol treatment have three-year survival rates in the range of 30% to 60% (7,8). Hence, unless future drug regimens are more effective, transplantation will ultimately be the only option in a significant proportion of cases. Unfortunately, because of the limited supply of donor organs, transplantation cannot be done on demand if a patient's status deteriorates while on the waiting list. Moreover, some patients will not be acceptable candidates for transplantation, and transplantation will not be accessible to patients in some countries. If medical therapy fails, atrial septostomy has a role in appropriately selected patients either as a bridge to transplantation or as an alternative procedure if transplantation is not an option.

2. LUNG TRANSPLANTATION

2.1. Pretransplantation Assessment

Overall, the purpose of the pretransplantation assessment is to identify patients whose prognosis will be improved by transplantation and whose cardiopulmonary status or other medical problems will not overly jeopardize the success of transplantation, i.e., to choose the right patient and time for transplantation. The major specific goals of the evaluation for transplantation are to *(1)* confirm the diagnosis, *(2)* assess the severity of the disease, *(3)* optimize medical management, *(4)* determine the potential role of transplantation and select suitable candidates, and *(5)* choose a transplant procedure.

Consensus guidelines for selecting patients for transplantation have been promulgated by the major societies *(10)*, and most transplant centers use similar criteria. In general, patients referred for transplantation should have physiologically severe pulmonary hypertension with right ventricular dysfunction despite the use of optimal medical therapy, but no significant secondary effects of chronic right ventricular failure on other organs, such as cardiac cirrhosis or renal insufficiency. In addition, any other medical problems should be fully characterized to ascertain their potential impact on the outcome of transplantation, and all health maintenance testing that is appropriate for the patient should be completed.

2.2. Choice of Transplant Operation

Heart-lung transplantation should be reserved for patients who are not candidates for lung transplantation alone. Most forms of PAH except complex congenital heart disease do not require heart-lung transplantation unless there is a significant cardiac problem other than cor pulmonale. The threshold of unrecoverable right ventricular dysfunction is unknown, if such a boundary even exists. Severe right ventricular dysfunction has been reversible after isolated lung transplantation *(11–16)*. Thus, cor pulmonale is not a contraindication to lung transplantation. However, right ventricular function does not revert to normal immediately after lung transplantation even though afterload is promptly reduced or normalized, and hemodynamic instability is a common problem during the early postoperative period.

Both single- and double-lung transplantation have been performed for IPAH and some other types of PAH *(11,14–17)*. These operations have been combined with repair of some cardiovascular anomalies for Eisenmenger's syndrome *(14,16,18)*. Single-lung transplantation creates a ventilation–perfusion imbalance with perfusion going predominantly to the allograft because of its low vascular resistance, but ventilation is usually evenly split between the allograft and the remaining native lung. Although this is a physiologically workable situation, any complication in the allograft can cause severe hypoxemia. Probably because of this tenuous physiology with single-lung transplantation, approximately 85% of lung transplants for IPAH have been bilateral procedures *(19)*. Nevertheless, recipient survival rates are similar between single and bilateral transplantation for IPAH, and either of these operations is an acceptable choice. However, in patients with certain cardiac defects and Eisenmenger's syndrome, heart-lung transplantation may be preferable. In an analysis of transplantation for Eisenmenger's syndrome, survival rates were significantly better after heart-lung transplantation than after lung transplantation, a difference that was not apparent for recipients with IPAH *(18)*. The survival advantage of heart-lung transplantation was most pronounced for patients with a ventricular septal defect *(18)*, and heart-lung transplantation should be strongly considered for this subgroup. Unfortunately, donor organs for heart-lung transplantation are relatively scarce because of the competition for donor hearts for cardiac transplantation, and this disadvantage has to be weighed when the procedure is being selected.

2.3. Timing of Transplantation

Ideally, transplantation should be postponed until it offers a survival advantage over continuing medical therapy. Practically, however, this strategy is not straightforward. The survival statistics for transplantation are well known, but reliable prognostic indices to forecast survival with various medical therapies are not available, and many relevant clinical gauges of an individual patient's condition are more qualitative than quantitative. Moreover, transplantation cannot be done on demand or even timed with any precision, because the availability of donor organs is not predictable.

Hence, clinical judgment plays a major role in the decision about the right time to move toward transplantation. The waiting time for transplantation depends on the organ allocation system, and organ distribution systems vary significantly in countries around the world. In the United States, the organ allocation system for lung transplantation was changed in 2005. In the new system, priority on the waiting list is determined by medical urgency (the likelihood of dying without transplantation) and transplant benefit (the probability of surviving after transplantation). Time on the waiting list, which was the primary determinant under the previous system, is no longer a factor in the allocation scheme.

Regardless of the allocation system, a long wait before transplantation should be anticipated, and during the waiting period both medical management and transplantation strategy must be adjusted to changing clinical circumstances. Patients should have regular evaluations with noninvasive tests plus periodic right heart catheterizations to monitor their cardiopulmonary status and regulate their therapy.

Patients with IPAH who have not responded either functionally or hemodynamically to intravenous epoprostenol have a guarded prognosis (7,8), and proceeding toward transplantation may be advisable in many of these cases. Repeatable, noninvasive tests with prognostic value are needed to complement clinical judgment about the trend in the patient's disease and the timing of transplantation. As drug treatment for PAH has improved, it is being extended to its limit, and perhaps beyond, in many patients before transplantation. If refractory right heart failure develops on such maximal medical therapy, little can be done to restore cardiopulmonary status, and other organs deteriorate, especially the liver and kidney. In this scenario, a patient can quickly be transformed into a high-risk or totally unacceptable candidate for transplantation, and the opportunity for transplantation may be forfeited.

Some noninvasive tests may be helpful in timing transplantation. Both the six-minute walk distance and cardiopulmonary exercise testing have shown prognostic implications (20,21). The predictive value of these tests deserves further study. The six-minute walk distance (6MWD) correlated well with peak oxygen uptake in one study of IPAH patients, and a 6MWD less than 332 m portended a poor prognosis, with a one-year mortality rate of approximately 40% (20). In a study of cardiopulmonary exercise testing in patients with IPAH, both peak oxygen uptake and peak systolic blood pressure were prognostically important (21). A peak oxygen uptake lower than 10.4 ml/kg/min and a peak exercise systolic blood pressure less than 120 mm Hg were associated with one-year mortality rates of approximately 50% and 70%, respectively. Among patients with both of these risk factors, only 23% survived for one year (21). Thus, transplantation would offer a survival advantage to patients with these profiles, and these thresholds might be useful in timing transplantation.

Plasma brain natriuretic peptide (BNP) is a potentially useful biomarker that increases in proportion to the degree of right ventricular dysfunction in PAH *(22)*, and it can be easily measured serially. In one study of patients with IPAH, BNP was an independent predictor of mortality *(23)*, and an increase in BNP during follow-up was strongly and independently associated with mortality. Therefore, BNP may be a bellwether for the course of IPAH, and a persistently high or a rising BNP in spite of intensive medical therapy is probably a signal that drug treatment is failing and transplantation is indicated.

2.4. Transplant Activity

Table 1 summarizes the indications for lung and heart-lung transplantation *(24)*. Heart-lung transplantation was initially performed for pulmonary vascular disease *(25)*, and it was the transplant operation of choice for IPAH and Eisenmenger's syndrome throughout the 1980s.

Table 1
Indications for Adult Lung (1995–2003) and Heart-Lung (1996–2003) Transplantation

	Single Lung	*Bilateral Lung*	*Heart-Lung*
Diagnosis	$n = 5793$	$n = 5166$	$n = 750$
Chronic obstructive pulmonary disease	3091 53.0%	1201 23.0%	25 3.3%
Idiopathic pulmonary fibrosis	1369 24.0%	503 9.7%	14 1.9%
Cystic fibrosis	131 2.3%	1615 31.0%	124 16.5%
α1-Antitrypsin deficiency emphysema	493 8.5%	491 9.5%	25 3.3%
Primary pulmonary hypertension	66 1.1%	391 7.6%	144 19.2%
Sarcoidosis	143 2.5%	144 2.8%	NA
Bronchiectasis	21 0.4%	254 4.9%	NA
Eisenmenger's syndrome/CHD	13 0.2%	107 2.1%	273 36.4%
Lymphangioleiomyomatosis	50 0.9%	72 1.4%	NA
Retransplantation	116 2.0%	90 1.7%	6 0.8%
Others	300 5.2%	281 5.4%	139 18.5%

Source: Data from the Registry of the International Society for Heart and Lung Transplantation *(24)*.

As lung transplantation became more successful in the 1990s, the preferred operation shifted away from heart-lung transplantation. Now bilateral lung transplantation is the procedure that is usually performed for IPAH and Eisenmenger's syndrome with a simple, surgically correctable defect, and heart-lung transplantation is usually reserved for more complex congenital heart disease with pulmonary hypertension. Recently, annual worldwide transplant activity has been in the range of 75 cases per year for IPAH and 65 cases per year for Eisenmenger's syndrome/congenital heart disease *(19)*.

2.5. Outcomes of Lung Transplantation

2.5.1. SURVIVAL

Survival, physiological function, quality of life, and cost-effectiveness are key outcome measures for lung transplantation. Actuarial survival is well known from the U.S. Scientific Registry *(26)*, the ISHLT Registry *(19)*, and reports from individual centers *(15,16,27–30)*. Survival rates from the ISHLT Registry are presented for IPAH and Eisenmenger's syndrome in Fig. 1 and 2. Both IPAH and Eisenmenger's syndrome/congenital heart disease have been associated with a significantly higher risk of death than other diagnoses in the first year after lung transplantation *(19)*. Attributable to the complexity of the transplant surgery for pulmonary vascular disease, the increased mortality has been concentrated in the perioperative period; thereafter, the attrition rates for recipients with IPAH and Eisenmenger's syndrome parallel those for recipients with other diagnoses since later complications are not strongly influenced by the pretransplantation diagnosis. Causes of death for all recipients are compiled in the ISHLT Registry *(19)*. Primary graft dysfunction, usually related to

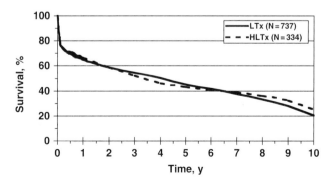

Fig. 1. Survival after lung (LTx) and heart-lung (HLTx) transplantation for PPH. [Data from *(24)*.]

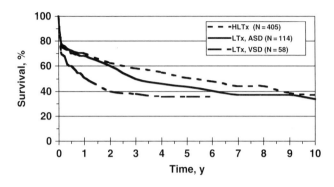

Fig. 2. Survival after lung (LTx) and heart-lung (HLTx) for Eisenmeger's syndrome. [Data from *(24)*.]

ischemia-reperfusion injury, and infection have been the major sources of mortality within the first 30 days. Thereafter, infection and chronic rejection have been the main causes of death.

2.5.2. Physiological Function

Lung and heart-lung transplantation alleviate pulmonary hypertension and right ventricular dysfunction *(11–16,29,31,32)*, and these responses are sustained if recipients avoid complications. Pulmonary hemodynamics can normalize after heart-lung and bilateral lung transplantation *(14,16,29,32,33)*. Likewise, the hemodynamic pattern has improved dramatically after single-lung transplantation *(15,16)*. Performance status returns to New York Heart Association functional class I or II in practically all recipients who avoid complications. A stereotypical pattern of maximal exercise limitation, which is probably related to peripheral oxygen utilization, has been detected by cardiopulmonary exercise testing in all lung and heart-lung transplant recipients regardless of their pretransplantation diagnosis *(34)*, but most survivors report no activity limitations *(19)*.

2.5.3. Quality of Life

Quality of life is at least as important to transplant recipients as survival or physiological function. Although psychiatric comorbidity has been identified in a significant portion of patients awaiting lung transplantation and has been associated with a poorer quality of life and other adverse effects on symptoms and health habits before transplantation *(35)*, several studies have observed significant posttransplant improvements in both overall and health-related quality of life among heart-lung and lung transplant recipients *(36–41)*. With multidimensional profiles, the improvement in quality of life has extended across most domains, and it is sustained unless complications such as chronic rejection arise *(37,41)*. Despite these improvements, the psychological and emotional health of recipients has been below par when compared to population norms *(39)*. Nevertheless, even if the survival advantage of transplantation is marginal, many patients would sacrifice some longevity for a better quality of life *(42)*. Almost 90% of surviving recipients have expressed satisfaction with their decision to have a transplant and would encourage a friend with a similar problem to seek transplantation *(37)*.

2.5.4. Cost and Cost-Effectiveness

The cost of transplantation depends on the health-care system, health-care policies, and socioeconomic factors, which vary substantially from one country to another. At two U.S. centers from 1993 to 1994, the average cost for lung transplantation and the associated postoperative inpatient care was in the range of $154,000 to $165,000 *(42,43)*. At one of the centers, the average charges for posttransplantation care were $16,628 per month during the first six months, $5,440 per month during the second six months, and $4,525 per month after the first year *(42)*. During the same period, the average monthly charge for patients on the transplant waiting list was $3,395. Cost estimates have also been reported from the U.K. and the Netherlands, where the national health-care systems differ substantially from that in the United States *(44–46)*. The average cost for lung transplantation in the Dutch system (1990–1995) and inpatient follow-up care was G138,323 ($82,994) *(44)*. In the U.K. (1995–2000), the cost for donor acquisition, transplantation, and inpatient follow-up care was estimated at £29,000–£30,000 ($48,000–$49,000) for bilateral lung, single-lung, or heart-lung transplantation *(46)*. The costs for posttransplantation care were highest in the first year (£12,500–£15,000). Thereafter, the annual cost estimations were much lower, approximately £5,500 ($9,020) in years 2 and 3, £3,500 ($5,740) in years 4 to 10, and £1,800 ($2,952) in years 11 to 15.

The costs of routine posttransplantation care and common clinical events were assessed by the program at U.K.'s Papworth Hospital (1984–1997) *(45)*. In the first five years after transplantation, the distribution of costs was 57% for routine care (including maintenance immunosuppression, infection prophylaxis, clinic visits, and tests), 16.5% for rejection episodes, 3.1% for cytomegalovirus (CMV) infection, and 23.5% for other infectious complications. Typical costs per event were £1,850 ($2,750) for rejection, £3,380 ($5,000) for CMV infection, and £2,790 ($4,200) for other infections.

Determining the cost-effectiveness of lung transplantation is difficult. Analyses of cost-effectiveness often rely on some assumptions and extrapolations that are reasonable, but debatable, and results must be interpreted cautiously. In the United States, the incremental cost per quality-adjusted life-year (QALY) gained through lung transplantation at one center was calculated to be $176,817. In the Dutch program, the cost per QALY gained was G167,000 ($100,200), and in the U.K. it was £29,415 ($48,241) for single-lung, £20,002 ($32,803) for double-lung, and £17,856 ($29,285) for heart-lung transplantation.

2.5.5. COMPLICATIONS

Most posttransplantation complications are similar regardless of the pretransplantation diagnosis (Table 2), and the occurrences of some of these are shown in Table 3. A detailed review of these complications is beyond the scope of this chapter; however, primary graft dysfunction and rejection are briefly summarized.

Table 2
Complications of Lung Transplantation and Posttransplantation Immunosuppressive Therapy

Primary graft dysfunction (ischemia-reperfusion injury)
Diaphragmatic dysfunction/paralysis
Vocal cord paresis/paralysis
Chylothorax
Airway
  Anastomotic dehiscence or stricture
  Bronchomalacia
Rejection
  Hyperacute
  Acute
  Chronic (bronchiolitis obliterans syndrome, BOS)
Infection
  Bacterial (especially *Staphylococcus aureus*, *Pseudomonas aeruginosa*)
  Viral (especially CMV; other respiratory viruses)
  Fungal (especially *Aspergillus* species)
Neoplasms
  Lymphoproliferative disorders/lymphoma
  Skin
  Other organs
Cardiovascular
  Air embolism
  Dysrhythmias (mainly supraventricular)

Systemic hypertension
Gastrointestinal
    Gastroparesis
    Gastroesophageal reflux
Renal
    Calcineurin inhibitor (cyclosporine, tacrolimus) nephropathy
Neurological
    Reversible posterior leukoencephalopathy
    Seizures
Musculoskeletal
    Steroid myopathy
    Rhabdomyolosis (cyclosporine + statin therapy)
    Osteopenia/osteoporosis
    Avascular necrosis (hip; shoulder)
Metabolic
    Obesity
    Diabetes mellitus
    Hypercholesterolemia/hypertriglyceridemia
    Idiopathic hyperammonemia
Hematologic
    Anemia, leukopenia, thrombocytopenia
    Thrombotic microangiopathy

Table 3
Cumulative Morbidities for Survivors of Lung Transplantation

	Cumulative Incidence Among Survivors	
Condition	Within 1 Year	Within 5 Years
Systemic hypertension	50.4%	86.4%
Renal dysfunction	25.8%	38.4%
Abnormal creatinine		
<2.5 mg/dl	(15.7%)	(21.3%)
>2.5 mg/dl	(8.1%)	(12.9%)
Chronic dialysis	(1.9%)	(3.4%)
Renal transplant	(0.0%)	(0.7%)
Hyperlipidemia	16.3%	45.4%
Diabetes mellitus	20.1%	29.4%
Malignancy	3.8%	13.0%
Lymphoid	(2.0%)	(2.8%)
Skin	(0.7%)	(6.6%)
Others	(1.1%)	(3.6%)

Source: Modified from (19).

2.5.5.1. Primary Graft Dysfunction. Primary graft dysfunction is a nonspecific acute lung injury with diffuse alveolar damage and increased vascular permeability. It is the consequence of insults that are inherent in the transplantation process (brain death in the donor; harvest and preservation; implantation and reperfusion in the recipient), and it has been called reperfusion edema, reimplantation response, and ischemia-reperfusion injury. The definition, grading scheme, risk factors, management, and outcome have been thoroughly reviewed *(47–51).*

Primary graft dysfunction is characterized primarily by hypoxemia and diffuse pulmonary infiltrates that appear within 72 hours of transplantation, but the clinical presentation can be mimicked by hyperacute rejection, pulmonary venous obstruction, pulmonary edema, and pneumonia. Overall, up to 50% of recipients may have some degree of primary graft dysfunction. The severity is variable, but approximately 10% to 20% of recipients may have severe graft dysfunction (grade 3–$pO_2/F_IO_2 < 200$, with diffuse infiltrates). In one analysis, recipients with IPAH were more prone to this complication than recipients with other diagnoses *(52).*

Primary graft dysfunction is associated with longer postoperative ventilator support, longer intensive care unit and hospital stays, higher costs, and excess mortality. The short-term mortality rate for recipients with grade 3 primary graft dysfunction has been in the range of 40% to 60%. For survivors of primary graft dysfunction, the impact on long-term outcomes remains uncertain, but there is particular concern that primary graft dysfunction may be a risk factor for chronic rejection.

Management follows the general paradigm for acute lung injury and uses fluid management and protective ventilation strategies similar to those for acute respiratory distress syndrome. In severe cases, nebulized epoprostenol or inhaled nitric oxide may be helpful, and extracorporeal membrane oxygenation has been utilized for refractory cases. Lastly, retransplantation may be an option for selected recipients without other end-organ failure.

2.5.5.2. Acute Rejection. Acute rejection is an immunological response to direct or indirect alloantigen recognition and is manifested by arteriolar and bronchiolar lymphocytic inflammation. Although it is rarely fatal, acute rejection is a significant problem for several reasons. First, the incidence is high. In most series, 50% or more of recipients have at least one episode during the first year after transplantation. Second, clinical diagnosis is unreliable because the signs and symptoms are nonspecific and overlap with other complications, especially CMV and other viral infections. Third, silent acute rejection has been detected in about 20% of surveillance biopsies in asymptomatic, clinically and physiologically stable recipients; therefore, pathological evidence of rejection can evade clinical detection. Finally, acute rejection is the primary risk factor for the subsequent development of chronic rejection. The diagnosis of acute rejection is best confirmed by transbronchial lung biopsy. Treatment of acute rejection typically includes a short course of high-dose corticosteroid therapy and adjustment of the maintenance immunosuppressive regimen. Therapy is usually effective, but persistent or recurrent acute rejection is not rare.

2.5.5.3. Chronic Rejection (Bronchiolitis Obliterans Syndrome). Chronic rejection is the main impediment to better medium-term survival rates and is the cause of considerable morbidity because of its impact on lung function and quality of life. The pathogenesis remains a mystery, but both alloimmune and non-alloimmune mechanisms are probably involved *(53,54)*. Clinically, chronic rejection is a form of graft dysfunction synonymous with bronchiolitis obliterans syndrome (BOS) *(55,56)*. BOS is characterized physiologically by airflow obstruction and pathologically by bronchiolitis obliterans. The sensitivity of transbronchial biopsy for detecting the definitive lesion is low, and pathological confirmation is not necessary. However, bronchoscopy with biopsies and bronchoalveolar lavage are important to exclude other causes of graft dysfunction. A formal diagnosis of BOS is made when there is a sustained decrement of 20% or more in the FEV1 without an alternative explanation.

Physiological changes are far downstream from the primary immunological events, but currently there are no clinically applicable tests to monitor the adequacy of immunosuppression after transplantation. There is ongoing interest and research in various biomarkers, but none is ready for routine clinical implementation. Abnormalities in some physiological tests precede the decrement in FEV1 seen with BOS. Perhaps the most useful is the FEF25-75%, which usually declines before the FEV1 and may presage BOS, but after single-lung transplantation this parameter is influenced by the native lung and is more difficult to interpret than after double-lung or heart-lung transplants.

The prevalence of BOS approaches 50% by five years after transplantation *(19)*. Both antecedent acute rejection and lymphocytic bronchitis/bronchiolitis have been recognized as risk factors, and CMV pneumonia has been implicated, albeit inconsistently *(57)*. Neither the

pretransplantation diagnosis nor other recipient and donor characteristics have been risk factors in most studies, but IPAH was identified
as a risk factor in one analysis *(58)*.

BOS is usually treated with augmented immunosuppression, but
there is no consensus on therapy. While immunosuppressive protocols
may stabilize lung function in some cases, the overall results have
been disappointing. Although the course of BOS may be prolonged,
the median survival after onset has been approximately three years.
Retransplantation is the last resort, but its role is controversial, and it
has been performed infrequently. Overall, the results of retransplantation have been poor in comparison to first transplants; however, the
outcomes have been acceptable if the recipient had survived more
than two years with the first transplant, was ambulatory, and was not
ventilator-dependent *(59)*. Survival rates have been similar between
recipients undergoing retransplantation for BOS and those having a
second transplant for other reasons, and BOS has not seemed to recur
at an accelerated pace.

3. ATRIAL SEPTOSTOMY

Right ventricular failure in pulmonary hypertension is associated
with a poor prognosis and is often unresponsive to drug therapy.
Creating an interatrial communication can decompress the failing right
ventricle and improve cardiac output at the cost of decreased arterial
oxygen content because of the right-to-left shunt. The net benefit of
atrial septostomy hinges on maintaining or improving systemic oxygen
transport while partially unloading the right heart, and the procedure
must be approached with attention to this balance.

Although atrial septostomy has been performed as a palliative
procedure for IPAH for more than 20 years, its precise role in
management is still uncertain *(60)*. The mortality rate associated with
the procedure has been high in some series, but it can be performed
safely in appropriately selected patients, and sustained clinical and
hemodynamic improvement can result *(61–63)*.

3.1. Indications and Patient Selection

The principal indication for atrial septostomy is persistent right
heart failure or recurrent syncope despite maximal medical treatment.
The procedure can be a bridge to transplantation if the patient is a
suitable candidate, or it can be a palliative technique if transplantation
is not an option. However, septostomy is not a rescue procedure for
moribund patients. Candidates for the procedure should, of course,

have an intact atrial septum, and their hemodynamic status should be optimized as much as possible with medical therapy before the procedure. If significant hypoxemia is present, the integrity of the septum should be interrogated by bubble-contrast echocardiography to exclude a patent foramen ovale or other interatrial communication. Baseline oxygenation should be satisfactory (SpO_2 > 90%) on room air or relatively little supplemental oxygen so that oxygenation can be adequately maintained with supplemental oxygen after opening the right-to-left shunt. Moreover, a hematocrit > 35% is recommended to assure sufficient oxygen-carrying capacity. Lastly, the left ventricular function must be preserved to avoid left ventricular overload when the shunt is created (63). Preprocedure hemodynamic factors associated with death within one month after septostomy were reported in an analysis of 64 cases collected from the literature through 1998 (62). The significant variables associated with death versus survival in the univariate comparison included a higher mean right atrial pressure (22 vs. 11 mm Hg), a lower cardiac index (1.60 vs. 2.19 L/min/m^2), a pulmonary vascular resistance index > 55 units/m^2, and a lower one-year survival probability (64% vs. 38%) among the fatalities (64). Based upon these findings, the predictors of procedure-related failure or death in the Executive Summary of the World Symposium—Primary Pulmonary Hypertension 1998 were as follows: mean right atrial pressure > 20 mm Hg; pulmonary vascular resistance index > 55 units/m^2; and a predicted one-year survival < 40% (65). Patients with any of these risk factors should be instrumented with caution.

3.2. Techniques

Two techniques have been used: blade balloon atrial septostomy and graded balloon dilation atrial septostomy (62,63). The latter approach gives more control over the size of the septostomy. Baseline hemodynamics are measured during simultaneous right and left heart catheterizations. There should be a pressure gradient from the right to left atrium, and the left ventricular diastolic pressure should be less than 12 mm Hg to minimize the risk of pulmonary edema when the septostomy is created (63).

After puncture of the interatrial septum with a Brockenbrough needle, the septostomy is created by stepwise transseptal balloon dilation, usually beginning in the range of 4 mm. The size is increased until any of the following endpoints is reached: left ventricular end-diastolic pressure reaches 18 mm Hg; SaO_2 or SpO_2 nears 80% (on room air) or decreases 10% from baseline; or a 16-mm dilation is achieved. These guidelines are designed to minimize the possibility of pulmonary edema related to left ventricular volume overload and to avoid severe hypoxemia.

3.3. Outcomes

Because of the very tenuous clinical and hemodynamic status of patients undergoing septostomy, some mortality related to the procedure is inevitable. In the original compilation of the worldwide experience, the mortality rate within the first month after septostomy was 16% *(62)*. However, the publication and adoption of the afore-mentioned guidelines along with increasing experience seem to have had an impact, because the first-month mortality rate decreased to only 5.4% in 74 cases that have been reported since 1998 *(60)*.

The immediate effects of septostomy on resting pulmonary hemody-namics have been modest but vary among patients *(62)*. Typically, the mean right atrial pressure declines by 3 mm Hg, the cardiac index increases by 0.7 L/min/m², and systemic oxygen transport rises despite a decrement in arterial oxygenation saturation. The baseline mean right atrial pressure is the best indicator of the hemodynamic response (Table 4). A baseline mean right atrial pressure lower than 10 mm Hg changes very little after the procedure. On the other hand, a baseline mean right atrial pressure between 10 and 20 mm Hg improves moderately after the procedure, and these patients appear to have the most favorable benefit-risk ratio. A baseline mean right atrial pressure greater than 20 mm Hg changes the most after the procedure, but the risk of mortality is also the highest.

The long-term hemodynamic effects of septostomy have not been studied extensively, but a favorable immediate response to the procedure is a good sign. In one comparison, patients who had a

Table 4
Hemodynamic Effects of Atrial Septostomy Stratified by Baseline Mean Right Atrial Pressure

RAP, mm Hg	N	Change After Septostomy			
		ΔRAP, %	ΔCI, %	ΔSaO_2, %	ΔSOT, %
<10	15	−5.5 ± 47	13 ± 14	−4.4 ± 4.3	8 ± 13
10–20	18	−31 ± 22	39 ± 27	−14 ± 7	19 ± 22
>20	6	−32 ± 20	69 ± 49	−17 ± 15	34 ± 22

RAP = right atrial pressure; N = number of patients; CI = cardiac index; SaO_2 = arterial oxygen saturation; SOT = systemic oxygen transport; Δ, change in.
Source: From *(62)*.

significantly greater increment in cardiac index (52% vs. 15%) and systemic oxygen transport (37% vs. 4%) shortly after the procedure also had a better sustained clinical response *(66)*. In another series with late follow-up in 8 of 15 patients, the mean right atrial pressure was lower and both the cardiac index and systemic oxygen transport were higher 16 to 27 months after the procedure compared to soon after the procedure *(61)*.

The influence of atrial septostomy on survival is difficult to ascertain because no prospective, controlled study has been done. As mentioned previously, the mortality rate in the first month after septostomy has ranged from 16% in a compilation of 64 cases through 1998 to 5.4% in a more recent cohort *(60,62)*. Long-term survival estimates were generated for 54 patients who lived more than one month after septostomy *(62)*. The median survival for the group was 19.5 months. Most deaths were related to progression of the underlying pulmonary vascular disease.

4. SUMMARY

Medical therapy for PAH has improved dramatically in the last decade and has changed the course of the disease in many patients. Nevertheless, the current drug regimens are still ineffective or lose effectiveness in many patients, related to the progression of the underlying disease. For these patients, lung transplantation and atrial septostomy offer the hope of improved function, prolonged survival, and, most important to some patients, enhanced quality of life.

REFERENCES

1. Rubin LJ. Primary pulmonary hypertension. N Engl J Med 1997; 336: 111–7.
2. Barst RJ. Role of atrial septostomy in the treatment of pulmonary vascular disease. Thorax 2000; 55:95–6.
3. Hoeper MM, Galiè N, Simonneau G, Rubin LJ. New treatments for pulmonary arterial hypertension. Am J Respir Crit Care Med 2002; 165:1209–16.
4. Galiè N, Seeger W, Naeije R, Simonneau G, Rubin LJ. Comparative analysis of clinical trials and evidence-based treatment algorithm in pulmonary arterial hypertension. J Am Coll Cardiol 2004; 43 (Suppl):81S–88S.
5. Badesch DB, Abman SH, Ahearn GS, et al. Medical therapy for pulmonary arterial hypertension. ACCP evidence-based guidelines. Chest 2004; 126:35S–62S.

6. Doyle RL, McCrory D, Channick RN, Simonneau G, Conte J. Surgical treatments/interventions for pulmonary arterial hypertension. ACCP evidence-based clinical practice guidelines. Chest 2004; 26:63S–71S.

7. McLaughlin VV, Shillington A, Rich S. Survival in primary pulmonary hypertension. The impact of epoprostenol therapy. Circulation 2002; 106:1477–82.

8. Sitbon O, Humbert M, Nunes H, et al. Long-term intravenous epoprostenol infusion in primary pulmonary hypertension. Prognostic factors and survival. J Am Coll Cardiol 2002; 40:780–8.

9. Rich S, Kaufman E, Levy PS. The effect of high doses of calcium channel blockers on survival in primary pulmonary hypertension. N Engl J Med 1992; 327:76–81.

10. International guidelines for the selection of lung transplant candidates. Joint statement of the American Society for Transplant Physicians (ASTP)/American Thoracic Society (ATS)/European Respiratory Society (ERS)/International Society for Heart and Lung Transplantation (ISHLT). Am J Respir Crit Care Med 1998; 158:335–9.

11. Pasque MK, Trulock EP, Kaiser LR, Cooper JD. Single-lung transplantation for pulmonary hypertension: Three-month hemodynamic follow-up. Circulation 1991; 84:2275–9.

12. Ritchie M, Waggoner AD, Dávila-Román VG, Barzilai B, Trulock EP, Eisenberg PR. Echocardiographic characterization of the improvement in right ventricular function in patients with severe pulmonary hypertension after single-lung transplantation. J Am Coll Cardiol 1993; 22:1170–4.

13. Kramer MR, Valantine HA, Marshall SE, Starnes VA, Theodore J. Recovery of the right ventricle after single-lung transplantation in pulmonary hypertension. Am J Cardiol 1994; 73:494–500.

14. Bando K, Armitage JM, Paradis IL, et al. Indications for and results of single, bilateral, and heart-lung transplantation for pulmonary hypertension. J Thorac Cardiovasc Surg 1994; 108:1056–65.

15. Pasque MK, Trulock EP, Cooper JD, et al. Single lung transplantation for pulmonary hypertension: Single institution experience in 34 patients. Circulation 1995; 92:2252–8.

16. Gammie JS, Keenan RJ, Pham SM, et al. Single- versus double-lung transplantation for pulmonary hypertension. J Thorac Cardiovasc Surg 1998; 115:397–403.

17. Mendeloff EN, Meyers BF, Sundt TM, et al. Lung transplantation for pulmonary vascular disease. Ann Thorac Surg 2002; 73:209–19.

18. Waddell TK, Bennett L, Kennedy R, Todd TRJ, Keshavjee SH. Heart-lung or lung transplantation for Eisenmenger syndrome. J Heart Lung Transplant 2002; 21:731–7.

19. Trulock EP, Edwards LB, Taylor DO, Boucek MM, Keck BM, Hertz MI. The Registry of the International Society for Heart and Lung Transplantation: Twenty-first official adult lung and heart-lung transplant report—2004. J Heart Lung Transplant 2004; 23:804–15.

20. Miyamoto S, Nagaya N, Satoh T, et al. Clinical correlates and prognostic significance of six-minute walk test in patients with primary pulmonary hypertension. Am J Respir Crit Care Med 2000; 161:487–92.

21. Wensel R, Opitz CF, Anker SD, et al. Assessment of survival in patients with primary pulmonary hypertension. Importance of cardiopulmonary exercise testing. Circulation 2002; 106:319–24.

22. Nagaya N, Nishikimi T, Okano Y, et al. Plasma brain natriuretic peptide levels increase in proportion to the extent of right ventricular dysfunction in pulmonary hypertension. J Am Coll Cardiol 1998; 31:202–8.

23. Nagaya N, Nishikimi T, Uematsu M, et al. Plasma brain natriuretic peptide as a prognostic indicator in patients with primary pulmonary hypertension. Circulation 2000; 102:865–70.

24. Registry of the International Society for Heart and Lung Transplantation, http://www.ishlt.org/registries/slides.asp; accessed July 18, 2004.

25. Reitz BA, Wallwork JL, Hunt SA, et al. Heart-lung transplantation. Successful therapy for patients with pulmonary vascular disease. N Engl J Med 1982; 306:557–64.

26. 2003 Annual Report of the U.S. Organ Procurement and Transplantation Network and the Scientific Registry of Transplant Recipients: Transplant Data 1993–2002. Department of Health and Human Services, Health Resources and Services Administration, Office of Special Programs, Division of Transplantation, Rockville, MD; United Network for Organ Sharing, Richmond, VA; University Renal Research and Education Association, Ann Arbor, MI.

27. Whyte RI, Robbins RC, Atlinger J, et al. Heart-lung transplantation for primary pulmonary hypertension. Ann Thorac Surg 1999; 67:937–42.

28. Ueno T, Smith JA, Snell GI, et al. Bilateral sequential single lung transplantation for pulmonary hypertension and Eisenmenger's syndrome. Ann Thorac Surg 2000; 69:381–7.

29. Franke U, Wiebe K, Harringer W, et al. Ten years experience with lung and heart-lung transplantation in primary and secondary pulmonary hypertension. Eur J Cardiothorac Surg 2000; 18:447–52.

30. Stoica SC, McNeil KD, Perreas K, et al. Heart-lung transplantation for Eisenmenger syndrome: Early and long-term results. Ann Thorac Surg 2001; 72:1887–91.

31. Levine SM, Gibbons WJ, Bryan CL, et al. Single lung transplantation for primary pulmonary hypertension. Chest 1990; 98:1107–15.

32. Conte JV, Borja MJ, Patgel CB, Yang SC, Jhaveri RM, Orens JB. Lung transplantation for primary and secondary pulmonary hypertension. Ann Thorac Surg 2001; 72:1673–80.

33. Dawkins KD, Jamieson SW, Hunt SA, et al. Long-term results, hemodynamics, and complications after combined heart and lung transplantation. Circulation 1985; 71:919–26.

34. Howard DA, Iademarco E, Trulock EP. The role of cardiopulmonary exercise testing in lung and heart-lung transplantation. Clin Chest Med 1994; 15:405–20.

35. Parekh PI, Blumenthal JA, Babyak MA, et al. Psychiatric disorder and quality of life in patients awaiting lung transplantation. Chest 2003; 124:1682–8.

36. Ramsey SD, Patrick DL, Lewis S, Albert RK, Raghu G. Improvement in quality of life after lung transplantation: A preliminary study. J Heart Lung Transplant 1995; 14:870–7.

37. Gross C, Savik K, Bolman RM, Hertz MI. Long-term health status and quality of life outcomes of lung transplant recipients. Chest 1995; 108:1587–93.

38. TenVergert EM, Essink-Bot M-L, Geertsma A, van Enckevort PJ, de Boer WJ, van der Bij W. The effect of lung transplantation on health-related quality of life: A longitudinal study. Chest 1998; 113:358–64.

39. Limbos MM, Joyce DP, Chan CKN, Kesten S. Psychological functioning and quality of life in lung transplant candidates and recipients. Chest 2000; 118:408–16.

40. Lanuza DM, Lefavier C, McCabe M, Farcas GA, Garrity E, Jr. Prospective study of functional status and quality of life before and after lung transplantation. Chest 2000; 118:115–22.

41. Vermeulen KM, Ouwens J-P, van der Bij W, de Boer WJ, Koëter GH, TenVergert EM. Long-term quality of life in patients surviving at least 55 months after lung transplantation. Gen Hosp Psychiatry 2003; 25:95–102.

42. Ramsey SD, Patrick DL, Albert RK, et al. The cost-effectiveness of lung transplantation: A pilot study. Chest 1995; 108:1594–601.

43. Gartner SH, Sevick MA, Keenan RJ, Chen GJ. Cost-utility of lung transplantation: A pilot study. J Heart Lung Transplant 1997; 16:1129–34.

44. Maiwenn J. AI, Koopmanschap MA, van Enckevort PJ, et al. Cost-effectiveness of lung transplantation in the Netherlands. Chest 1998; 113:124–30.

45. Sharples LD, Taylor GJ, Karnon J, et al. A model for analyzing the cost of the main clinical events after lung transplantation. J Heart Lung Transplant 2001; 20:474–82.

46. Anyanwu AC, McGuire A, Rogers CA, Murday AJ. An economic evaluation of lung transplantation. J Thorac Cardiovasc Surg 2002; 123:411–20.

47. Christie JD, Carby M, Bag R, et al. Report of the ISHLT Working Group on primary lung graft dysfunction, Part II: Definition. A consensus statement of the International Society for Heart and Lung Transplantation. J Heart Lung Transplant 2005; 24:1454–9.

48. de Perrot M, Bonser RS, Dark J, et al. Report of the ISHLT Working Group on primary lung graft dysfunction, Part III: Donor-related risk factors and markers. J Heart Lung Transplant 2005; 24:1460–7.

49. Barr ML, Kawut SM, Whelan TP, et al. Report of the ISHLT Working Group on primary lung graft dysfunction, Part IV: Recipient-related risk factors and markers. J Heart Lung Transplant 2005; 24:1468–82.

50. Arcasoy SM, Fisher A, Hachem RR, et al. Report of the ISHLT Working Group on primary lung graft dysfunction, Part V: Predictors and outcomes. J Heart Lung Transplant 2005; 24:1483–8.

51. Shargall Y, Guenther G, Ahya VN, et al. Report of the ISHLT Working Group on primary lung graft dysfunction, Part VI: Treatment. J Heart Lung Transplant 2005; 24:1489–500.

52. Christie JD, Kotloff RM, Pochettino A, et al. Clinical risk factors for primary graft failure following lung transplantation. Chest 2003; 124:1232–41.

53. Boehler A, Kesten S, Weder W, Speich R. Bronchiolitis obliterans after lung transplantation. A review. Chest 1998; 114:1411–26.

54. Estenne M, Hertz MI. Bronchiolitis obliterans after human lung transplantation. Am J Respir Crit Care Med 2002; 166:440–4.

55. Cooper JD, Billingham M, Egan T, et al. A working formulation for the standardization of nomenclature and for clinical staging of chronic dysfunction in lung allografts. J Heart Lung Transplant 1993; 12:713–6.

56. Estenne M, Maurer JR, Boehler A, et al. Bronchiolitis obliterans syndrome 2001: An update of the diagnostic criteria. J Heart Lung Transplant 2002; 21:297–310.

57. Sharples LD, McNeil K, Stewart S, Wallwork J. Risk factors for bronchiolitis obliterans: A systematic review of recent publications. J Heart Lung Transplant 2002; 21:271–81.

58. Kroshus TJ, Kshettry VR, Savik K, John R, Hertz MI, Bolman RM III. Risk factors for the development of bronchiolitis obliterans syndrome after lung transplantation. J Thorac Cardiovasc Surg 1997; 114:195–202.

59. Novick RJ, Stitt LW, Al-Kattan K, et al. Pulmonary retransplantation: Predictors of graft function and survival in 230 patients. Ann Thorac Surg 1998; 65:227–34.

60. Klepetko W, Mayer E, Sandoval J, et al. Interventional and surgical modalities of treatment for pulmonary arterial hypertension. J Am Coll Cardiol 2004; 43 (Suppl):73S–80S.

61. Kerstein D, Levy PS, Hsu DT, Hordof AJ, Gersony WM, Barst RJ. Blade balloon atrial septostomy in patients with severe primary pulmonary hypertension. Circulation 1995; 91:2028–35.

62. Sandoval J, Rothman A, Pulido T. Atrial septostomy for pulmonary hypertension. Clin Chest Med 2001; 22:547–60.

63. Sandoval J, Pepke Zaba J, Vachiery JL. Atrial septostomy for primary pulmonary hypertension. Task force paper for Third World Symposium on Pulmonary Arterial Hypertension; Venice; June 23–25, 2003.

64. D'Alonzo GE, Barst RJ, Ayres SM, et al. Survival in patients with primary pulmonary hypertension: Results from a national prospective registry. Ann Intern Med 1991; 115:343–9.

65. Sandoval J, Barst RJ, Rich S, Rothman A. Atrial septostomy for pulmonary hypertension, World Symposium on Primary Pulmonary Hypertension 1998, Evian, France, 1998. Vol. Executive summary. World Health Organization, 1998.

66. Rothman A, Sklansky MS, Lucas VW, et al. Atrial septostomy as a bridge to lung transplantation in patients with severe pulmonary hypertension. Am J Cardiol 1999; 84:682–6.

19 New Directions in Pulmonary Hypertension Therapy

Christopher M. Carlin
and Andrew J. Peacock

CONTENTS

INTRODUCTION
GENERAL MEASURES
TARGETS: IN SEARCH OF THE MAGIC BULLET
AMMUNITION: HOW BEST TO HIT THE
    TARGET?
ARMOR: RECOGNIZING AND PROTECTING
    THE SUSCEPTIBLE
CLINICAL TRIALS AND ENDPOINTS
CONCLUSIONS
REFERENCES

Abstract

Great progress in the understanding of the pathogenesis of as well as the therapy for pulmonary hypertension has been made in the last 20 years, but many challenges remain. Combinations of prostanoids, endothelin antagonists, and phosphodiesterase inhibitors are seeing increasing use, and clinical trials currently underway should identify which combinations work best. Nebulized treprostinil, selective endothelin-A antagonists, and newer phosphodiesterase inhibitors may offer advantages and expand our therapeutic armamentarium in the near future. Clinical trials of statins, SSRIs, VIP, potassium channel activators, or antiplatelets are also ongoing or are likely to commence in the near future. Agents that interrupt signaling pathways such as Rho kinases and tyrosine kinases also show promise. The biological plausibility, availability,

From: *Contemporary Cardiology: Pulmonary Hypertension*
Edited by: N. S. Hill and H. W. Farber © Humana Press, Totowa, NJ

and relative safety of these newer agents make it tempting to prescribe them now, particularly when faced with gravely ill patients. However, these and all future therapies require proof of efficacy and safety from properly conducted clinical trials before widespread use can be advocated. Too many patients are still severely limited by and dying of pulmonary arterial hypertension to warrant therapeutic complacency at this time. While we await proof of safety and efficacy, we must continue to enroll patients in clinical trials.

Key Words: future directions of pulmonary hypertension; Rho kinase inhibitors; tyrosine kinase inhibitors; potassium channels; growth factors; serotonin; serotonin transporter; apoptosis.

1. INTRODUCTION

This is an exciting time for the pulmonary hypertension community. The "holy grails" in the management of pulmonary arterial hypertension—early recognition, side effect-free targeted treatment, robust tools for noninvasive follow-up—are being actively and successfully pursued. Preceding chapters have reviewed the progress made in our understanding of the pathobiology of pulmonary arterial hypertension (PAH) and the targeted therapeutic options that are currently available. Progress in the management of lung transplantation, the role of atrial septostomy, and also the intriguing promise shown by statin drugs and nitric oxide donors has also been outlined. Here we propose to outline the progress that we anticipate will continue to improve clinical outcomes for patients with PAH.

Progress in our understanding of the abnormal pathophysiological processes that lead to pulmonary arterial hypertension, and the mechanisms by which we may influence these, has led to the recognition and application of the currently available targeted therapies for PAH. Pursuing this further by completely dissecting the abnormal cellular and molecular pathways at the heart of PAH, recognizing therapeutic targets within these, and exploring these therapies in model systems is an obvious direction for pursuing new therapies. Recent developments have identified a number of possible targets. It seems timely to review these and suggest the ones we consider most promising. Progress in the development of novel therapeutic modalities (e.g., gene transfer, cardiac pacing strategies) and new drugs for other diseases that may be applicable to the management of PAH are also discussed.

Impediments to the exploration of new PAH therapies are inevitable. The worldwide patient pool is limited and has been extensively utilized in recent clinical trials. Placebo-based trials may soon be inappropriate in the face of validated, effective therapy. If we are to fully exploit progress in the laboratory, then robust trials utilizing validated endpoints are required. All of the recent placebo-controlled trials have been brief (12–16 weeks) and primarily used exercise capacity and pulmonary hemodynamics to assess the response to therapy. This approach becomes problematic when assessing agents that influence pulmonary vascular remodeling; agents acting over a longer period will require a different trial approach. Targeted therapy has improved the prognosis of PAH in the short to mid-term. We will need to shift our focus and either undertake prolonged clinical trials (with the expense and long-term uncertainty) or identify and validate relevant surrogate endpoints that reflect the disease aspects being explored and allow long-term conclusions about efficacy.

Our understanding of the genetic influences underlying PAH and the early pathobiological events that initiate pulmonary vascular remodeling is evolving. We are also acquiring new techniques that may aid in early diagnosis and assessment. Recognition of risk factors and the ability to detect early disease may allow us to develop preventive strategies for PAH. We acknowledge, however, that the prospect of genetic testing and presymptomatic investigations raises significant ethical issues.

New drugs and investigation techniques potentially place a considerable financial burden on health-care services. Clinical trials to assess the efficacy of new agents should also assess effects on quality of life; this information may help in deciding which therapies should be supported in the face of limited resources. We recognize that rationing of resources is not ideal but is an essential and sometimes hidden feature of all health-care systems. While we do not discuss ethical or financial issues further, these should be borne in mind when considering the implementation of new developments.

Figure 1a illustrates the processes by which symptomatic disease in PAH develops. We can potentially assess and influence these processes at various stages, as illustrated in Fig. 1b. The focus of most current work is on agents targeting pulmonary vascular remodeling. The use of combination agents, targeting multiple steps in the pathogenesis of the disease, is a promising approach. Progress in the management of diseases of the systemic circulation such as atherosclerosis, systemic hypertension, and left heart failure may be relevant to the management of PAH and may offer new therapeutic directions. The principal future developments that we anticipate for the therapy of PAH include

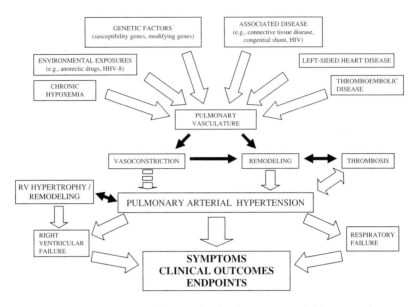

Fig. 1a. Etiology and pathogenesis of pulmonary arterial hypertension.

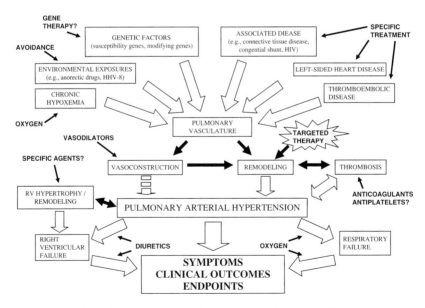

Fig. 1b. Therapy for pulmonary arterial hypertension.

- the utilization of new agents for the ancillary management of PAH,
- the new use of currently available targeted agents—expanding indications and use of combinations,
- the recognition and development of new classes of agents for targeted therapy.

We speculate on these approaches as well as on new techniques for drug delivery and for nonpharmacological management. In a rapidly evolving field, it is recognized that any speculation may soon be rendered irrelevant by events. We hope that this proves to be the case; positive developments are urgently needed for the patients still suffering and dying from these devastating diseases.

2. GENERAL MEASURES

General management of PAH consists of treating concomitant disease aggressively, managing respiratory and cardiac failure, and administering anticoagulants in the absence of contraindications. Better measures to prevent and treat hypoxic lung disease, liver disease, connective tissue disease, thromboembolic disease, and HIV will hopefully prevent or significantly delay the development of PAH in these patient groups. Improvements in our understanding of how and why PAH develops in these conditions should give us insight into how best to manage the underlying disorder once PAH has developed. Progress with these ancillary measures has been made and may be relevant for PAH management.

2.1. Oxygen Therapy

Many patients with PAH have hypoxemia at rest or on exertion. Long-term oxygen therapy is traditionally provided via an oxygen concentrator to those with significant hypoxemia. Previously, difficulties with portable oxygen systems limited the utility of these systems. Improved portable cylinders and liquid oxygen systems are increasingly available, facilitating the provision of supplementary oxygen. Aggressive attempts to maintain normoxemia, both in patients with established respiratory failure and in those with purely exertional hypoxemia, would theoretically be of benefit for all patients with PAH. This point could be explored in a clinical trial. At present, the increased portability and convenience of oxygen delivery systems permit an enhancement of the patient's quality of life. Newer developments, such as truly portable concentrators and more compact, longer-acting portable systems, should sustain this progress.

2.2. Diuretics

Right heart failure and intractable edema are common manifestations of advanced PAH. Diuretics are used judiciously to alleviate symptomatic edema and reduce right ventricular preload. Care, however, has to be taken to avoid overzealousness, which can reduce left ventricular filling pressure and lead to systemic hypotension. Loop diuretics are widely used with potassium-sparing diuretics added as required. Of the potassium-sparing diuretics, spironolactone tends to be favored: Patients in heart failure typically have significant secondary hyperaldosteronism.

Diuretics have traditionally been regarded as palliative therapy for patients with heart failure. Symptomatic relief can be dramatic if fluid overload is adequately controlled. However, diuretics have not been shown to improve outcomes like survival, and more effective approaches would be welcome. One possible approach is to alter the renin-angiotensin system, the importance of which in PAH is unclear. The addition of low-dose aldosterone antagonists to "maximal" heart failure therapy improves mortality and symptomatic outcome in patients with severe left ventricular systolic dysfunction (1,2), but ACE inhibitors are unhelpful in PAH (3,4). Possible beneficial effects of aldosterone antagonists that are relevant to the pulmonary circulation include increased serum potassium, reduction in the incidence of arrhythmias (1,2), improved endothelial function (5–7), enhanced nitric oxide synthesis (8), and altered ventricular remodeling (9). Furthermore, loop diuretics are theoretically detrimental, as they can lead to increased activation of the renin-angiotensin system. It is conceivable that diuretic regimens favoring aldosterone antagonists rather than loop diuretics would benefit PAH patients. Aldosterone antagonists could be studied in PAH experimental models, and placebo-controlled studies to explore the effects of small doses of an aldosterone antagonist compared to best standard care could be undertaken in PAH patients. The new aldosterone antagonist eplerenone may benefit patients who develop side effects with spironolactone but require this class of diuretic.

2.3. Neurohormonal Agents

Several neurohormonal agents are undergoing phase II and phase III clinical studies to explore their role in the management of acute and chronic left-sided cardiac failure. Of these, nesiritide (a recombinant brain natriuretic peptide analogue, administered parenterally) and tolvaptan (a V2 vasopressin receptor analogue, administered orally) have recently reported positive outcomes *(10–12)*. The application of these agents as therapies for PAH is biologically plausible *(13,14)*. The key benefit of these agents is an effective reduction in systemic congestion with reduced incidence of electrolyte disturbance, renal dysfunction, and arrhythmia compared with standard heart failure regimens. These agents may be useful in managing right heart failure in PAH and may also have disease-modifying effects. Experimental work and clinical studies of these agents are merited.

2.4. Anticoagulants and Antiplatelets

Thrombosis may contribute to disease progression in PAH *(15,16)*. Local (pulmonary vascular) and systemic coagulation, fibrinolytic, and antithrombotic mechanisms are disordered in PAH, favoring thrombosis *(17,18)*. No robust trial evidence favors the use of anticoagulation, but reported case series are supportive *(19,20)*. The benefits of anticoagulation seem to be additive to other therapies, with an independent benefit on survival *(19)*. The dramatic effect seen in these studies, combined with the pathological observations, has led to the adoption of routine anticoagulation as the standard of care for most PAH patients. The difficulties with warfarin therapy (requirement for monitoring, diet and drug interactions, bleeding risk, inconsistency) are well recognized and newer, safer agents are needed.

The oral direct thrombin inhibitor ximelagatran has efficacy in various settings *(21–26)*. A fixed dosage regimen has a predictable anticoagulant effect without the need for blood monitoring. It is likely to lead to improved stability of anticoagulation compared with warfarin. Ximelagatran also has few significant drug interactions, but liver function monitoring is likely to be required. Despite this, ximelagatran offers the likelihood of warfarin equivalency, improved physician and patient convenience, and cost-effectiveness and is likely to enter clinical use in the near future.

New anticoagulants (e.g., fondaparinux and idraparinux) offer additional options for parenteral anticoagulation *(27)*. Further agents are in preclinical and early clinical development. All of these new agents target different clotting factors compared with vitamin K antagonists and would potentially have different effects on PAH pathophysiology.

The role of antiplatelet agents in PAH is unclear but is being reappraised. Single or combination antiplatelet regimens may offer comparable or additive antithrombotic efficacy compared to warfarin. Platelets release 5HT, thromboxane, and PDGF. Antiplatelet agents, particularly aspirin, would potentially be of benefit in modifying pulmonary vascular remodeling, in addition to affecting pulmonary vascular thrombosis. Antiplatelet agents or anticoagulants targeting non-vitamin K-dependent clotting factors may thus have different effects on PAH progression than warfarin. Nonwarfarin regimens may also have fewer side effects, be easier to manage, and be less expensive. Experimental work should explore the potential antiremodeling effects of anticoagulant and antiplatelet drugs, and clinical studies should be considered.

3. TARGETS: IN SEARCH OF THE MAGIC BULLET

The significant progress in our understanding of the pathophysiology of PAH has been reviewed earlier in this book (see Chapter 4). One of the key observations made is that the central pathophysiological process in PAH is not vasoconstriction but rather pulmonary vascular remodeling, typified by a proliferative/fibrotic arteriopathy *(28)*. As a consequence, the focus of speculation about, and research into, novel agents has shifted from agents acting as vasodilators to agents that halt or reverse the remodeling progress.

Prostanoids, endothelin antagonists, and phosphodiesterase-5 inhibitors were identified as promising agents for PAH primarily via observations regarding their potential for selective pulmonary arterial vasodilation. While vasodilator effects are demonstrable in a subgroup of patients with PAH *(19)*, even patients who do not demonstrate a vasodilator response may benefit *(29)*. In addition to their vasodilator effect, these agents seem likely to have a clinically relevant antiproliferative and antiremodeling effect *(30–36)*. Translation of this effect into improved long-term outcomes, especially survival, has thus far only been demonstrated for intravenous epoprostenol *(37)*, although data are accumulating for bosentan *(38,39)*.

There appears to be no single, central process leading to PAH that is common to all disease types. PAH develops in only a minority of patients harboring the key *BMPR2* mutation or suffering from PAH-associated diseases *(40)*. Therefore, it is unlikely that there is a single therapeutic "magic bullet" for PAH. If, however, we could halt the remodeling process, reverse the obstructive vascular pathology, and enhance the function of the right ventricle, we would, in effect, provide a cure. The pathology seen in PAH appears to be at least partially reversible, so we suspect that a multiple "bullet" approach consisting of several agents with complementary actions may be the ultimate solution for our patients.

Recent work has highlighted key cellular and molecular processes that appear to be central to the initiation and progression of PAH (Fig. 2a). Figure 2b illustrates potential avenues to influence these processes. Some of these breakthroughs have already been successfully exploited (endothelin-receptor antagonists, phosphodiesterase-5 inhibitors) and have been discussed in previous chapters. Here we consider those pathways that seem to hold the most promise for novel therapies.

3.1. TGF-β Superfamily

The recognition that mutations of the *BMPR2* gene are found in a large proportion of cases of familial PAH was a key breakthrough *(41)*. This gene is a member of the TGF-β superfamily of genes; as a consequence of this discovery, much research is now focused on related signaling proteins, inhibitors, receptors, and downstream intracellular pathways. Work thus far reported suggests that reduced BMPR2 activity and abnormal downstream signaling are common factors in the development of not only familial, but also sporadic, idiopathic

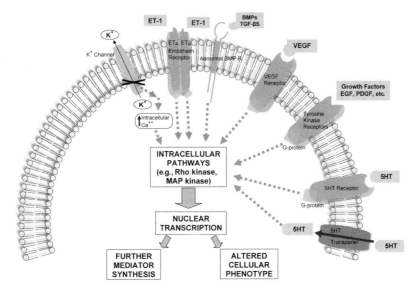

Fig. 2a. Selected cellular/molecular processes implicated in pulmonary arterial hypertension. See text and Chapter 4 for details. Dotted arrows indicate intermediate processes. Each process is restricted and variable in the different cell type (endothelial, smooth muscle or fibroblast) within the pulmonary vasculature. To provide an overview of the molecular processes, we illustrate a generic cell.

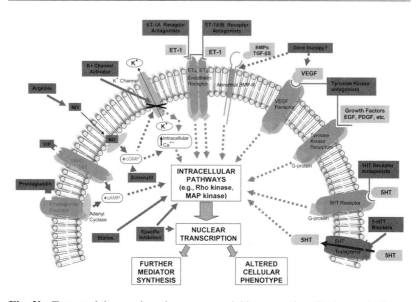

Fig. 2b. Targetted therapy in pulmonary arterial hypertension. Dark gray indicates processes or therapies that may inhibit remodeling.

PAH and may influence the development of PAH secondary to other processes *(42)*. Work is in progress to clarify this and determine which pulmonary artery cell populations are influenced by the BMP/BMPR signaling system.

The effects of TGF- β molecules on cellular processes are diverse and difficult to predict. Different effects are seen for the same ligand at different locations in the body, and in similar locations at different stages of development. Tissue specificity seems to relate to variations in receptor structure and variable expression of downstream mediators (e.g., SMAD proteins).

Bone morphogenetic proteins (ligands for BMPR) have shown safety and therapeutic benefit when administered locally via collagen matrices, enhancing skeletal growth *(43)*. Whether these could be delivered to and benefit the pulmonary circulation requires assessment. Whether simply overcoming abnormal signaling by providing large amounts of ligand will be successful is doubtful and, in the presence of an abnormal receptor complex with dysfunctional downstream signaling, could even be harmful. However, the diversity and tissue specificity of this system may allow us to target PAH selectively. Statin drugs have many intriguing effects including upregulation of BMP-2 expression in human osteoblasts *(44)* and systemic vascular smooth muscle cells *(45)*. Whether there is any such effect in the pulmonary vasculature is unknown. Considering the complexity of the TGF-β system, this effect could be harmful or helpful, emphasizing the importance of cautious optimism regarding statins for PAH. The TGF-β system is clearly important in PAH, and ongoing efforts to fully characterize this will almost certainly lead to new therapies.

3.2. Serotonin (5HT): Receptors and Transporter

The influence of serotonin on PAH pathophysiology is well known; serotoninergic drugs can induce disease (46), the LL polymorphism of the serotonin transporter gene promoter (which leads to increased 5HTT expression) seems to confer susceptibility to the disease (47,48), and platelet and serum levels of serotonin are deranged in PAH patients (49). The combination of increased intracellular 5HT (via the transporter) and increased cell surface 5HT-receptor signals seems to have additive effects leading to adverse cellular responses (vasoconstriction and proliferation) in pulmonary artery smooth muscle cells and fibroblasts (49,50). Blockade of the 5HT transporter and receptors has been beneficial in experimental models of pulmonary hypertension (51–55), and clinical studies of SSRI drugs (transporter blockers) and/or receptor antagonists (e.g., ketanserin) seem likely to follow. On the basis of current evidence, excessive activation of serotonin systems does not appear to initiate disease; few patients with carcinoid syndrome (with massively elevated serum serotonin levels) develop PAH. Rather, the serotonin receptor/transporter systems appear to enhance and accelerate the disease process, suggesting that antagonists could retard pulmonary vascular remodeling and ameliorate pulmonary hypertension.

3.3. Vasodilators: Vasoactive Intestinal Peptide (VIP) and Potassium Channel Blockers

VIP is a potent pulmonary and systemic vasodilator. An acute vasodilator response has been observed following the inhalation of VIP in patients with idiopathic PAH (56). It also has antiproliferative effects on vascular smooth muscle cells (56,57), inhibits monocrotaline-induced PAH in rabbits (58), and has the potential to inhibit human pulmonary vascular remodeling. A single small study of VIP administered four times daily (by inhalation) to patients with idiopathic PAH has reported favorable changes in hemodynamics (at 3 months) and the six-minute walk distance (at 12 and 24 weeks), without significant adverse side effects (56). Clearly, further study of this agent is indicated.

Voltage-gated potassium (Kv) channels are downregulated in pulmonary artery smooth muscle cells from patients with idiopathic PAH (though not secondary PAH) *(59)*. DNA microarray analysis performed on lungs from patients with IPAH demonstrates the downregulation of Kv channel genes *(60)*. The consequence of this combination is decreased intracellular potassium, release of intracellular calcium from stores, and vasoconstriction. These electrolyte changes also facilitate cell proliferation and escape from apoptosis *(61)*. Acquired Kv channel abnormalities may be a disease-initiating process or contribute to ongoing pulmonary vascular remodeling. Agents such as dichloroacetate may augment Kv channel function and have positive effects in PAH; whether this benefit is limited to the subgroup of patients with idiopathic disease remains to be determined.

3.4. Growth Factors

Experimental work suggests that a variety of growth factors [e.g., PDGF *(62,63)*, EGF *(64)*, and bFGF *(65)*] may influence PASMC proliferation in PAH. Various small molecule tyrosine kinase antagonists (which antagonize the ligand effect on these receptors) have been studied in other diseases. Toxicity has been problematic, reflecting the importance of these pathways throughout the body. Nevertheless, these pathways merit further exploration because some potentially useful antagonists that may retard pulmonary vascular remodeling are in development. Local delivery to the lungs may be possible to minimize systemic effects.

Recent studies have highlighted two important endothelial growth factor systems: vascular endothelial growth factor (VEGF)/VEGF-receptor (VEGF-R) and angiopoietin-1/TIE2. VEGF is abundantly expressed in lung tissue, but its physiological role and downstream signaling mechanisms remain unclear. Experimental models of pulmonary hypertension suggest that the VEGF-A isoform may be protective while the B isoform may be harmful *(66)*. VEGF receptors are differentially increased in human PAH lesions *(67)*. Antagonism of the VEGF-2 receptor contributes to the development of PAH in a rat model *(68)*, but cell-based VEGF gene transfer has been shown to prevent the development of PAH in monocrotaline-exposed rats *(69)*. Thus, in PAH, VEGF has theoretical potential for harm as well as benefit, and its complex role in PAH must be better understood before we can confidently predict effective treatment strategies. However, augmentation of VEGF activity could be beneficial in PAH by stabilizing vessel status or inducing healthy neovascularization.

The role angiopoietin-1 plays and its demonstrated interactions with 5HT and BMPR appear to be a key in the pathogenesis of PAH, although studies are continuing and current data are conflicting. Nonetheless, these interactions may prove to be an important target for therapeutic intervention.

3.5. Intracellular Pathways: Rho/Rho-Kinase and p38 MAPK

Evidence is accruing to support the view that a restricted number of intracellular pathways transduce signals via the abnormal extracellular molecule/membrane receptor systems that have been discussed above. Certain intracellular pathways seem to play a key role in directing the abnormal cellular behavior seen in pulmonary vascular remodeling. Targeting these pathways offers the potential to block the effects of multiple harmful signals with single agents.

Rho-A is a small GTP-binding protein that acts via its downstream effector Rho kinase. This pathway couples membrane receptor/G-protein signaling with phosphorylation of intracellular proteins. Rho/Rho-kinase signaling seems important in pulmonary arterial vasoconstriction and proliferation and has been linked to various key upstream mediators (e.g., thromboxane, endothelin, and serotonin) *(70)*. Isoprenylation of Rho is an essential activation step, providing its membrane anchor *(71)*. Statins reduce isoprenyl synthesis and consequently inhibit Rho pathways. Many of the pleiotropic effects of statins are thought to be mediated via this mechanism *(72)*. The intriguing effects of statins on experimental PAH are discussed in Chapter 15.

Selective rho-kinase inhibitors have antiproliferative effects in cell culture and in animal models of PAH *(73–75)*. One such inhibitor, fasudil, has been studied in clinical trials as an antianginal *(76)* and for treatment of cerebral vasospasm *(77)* with successful outcomes and apparent safety. The positive experimental work and familiarity with statins and rho-kinase inhibitors suggest the need for clinical trials.

Various intracellular kinases have been explored in pulmonary vascular cells and implicated in processes relevant to pulmonary vascular remodeling. p38 mitogen-activated protein kinase (MAPK) seems to be a key intracellular effector of various upstream mechanisms, with resultant cellular proliferation. A key feature of BMPR mutations is that the abnormal protein signals via p38 to induce proliferation, rather than via "healthy" SMAD pathways *(42)*. Experimental work suggests that p38-MAPK antagonism can block the fibroblast proliferation that results from abnormal stimuli *(50,78,79)*. The relative importance of the four p38 isoforms *(80)* is unknown, but targeting of the relevant isoform (when confirmed) may improve the therapeutic efficacy and minimize systemic effects. Further work should clarify this and determine the importance of p38 in other cells and as an effector of other signaling systems. Nonselective antagonists of p38-MAPK are available, and phase I studies have been conducted on this promising therapeutic target *(81)*.

3.6. Matrix Proteins

Alteration in the structure of the extracellular matrix within the arterial wall seems important in pulmonary vascular remodeling. Intimal migration of fibroblasts is an early step that requires matrix degradation. Increased elastase activity is an early change seen in the pulmonary arteries of rats exposed to hypoxia or monocrotaline *(82)*. Elastase inhibitors significantly attenuate monocrotaline-induced pulmonary hypertension, leading to animal survival with regression of structural pulmonary artery changes. Elastase effects matrix changes by activating matrix metalloproteinases (MMPs), which modify the matrix structure *(83,84)*. Matrix degradation facilitates cellular migration and proliferation. It also leads to release of biologically active growth factors from the matrix. Thus, the inhibition of matrix degradation may slow or halt pulmonary vascular remodeling.

Inhibitors of MMPs have been assessed in cancer trials. Toxicity was a problem early on, but newer agents have shown promise and merit further study *(85,86)*. However, in a hypoxic PAH model, MMP inhibition led to increased fibroproliferation, and the effects of proteases in human PAH need to be better understood before considering clinical studies.

3.7. Apoptosis and Gene Transfer

Vascular cell proliferation accounts for much of the increase in the pulmonary arterial wall thickness seen in PAH. Thus, attempting to retard the fibroproliferative process is an attractive therapeutic approach. However, we acknowledge that many patients present with advanced disease with profound, fixed pulmonary vascular resistance. It may not be enough for these (or indeed any) patients to simply inhibit further disease progression: We may also need to reverse the obstructive pathology. One approach to consider is to enhance apoptosis and reduce the vascular cell population directly. Small molecules that induce apoptosis are currently under investigation and may prove to be useful for the therapy of PAH.

Transfection of apoptosis-promoting genes is another attractive concept. In order to debulk the pulmonary vasculature, triggering apoptosis in only a portion of the smooth muscle cell population may be adequate. However, sustaining gene expression has long been an obstacle for effective gene therapy *(87)*. Short-term expression of apoptosis genes may be effective at removing cells, and intermittent treatment may overcome the problem of temporary effect.

The pulmonary circulation is an ideal site in which to attempt gene therapy. Inhaled adenoviral vectors may be effective, without systemic effects. In addition to transfecting apoptosis genes, we may be able to overcome inherited genetic defects (e.g., *BMPR2*) or provide an intermittent boost of "helpful" protein (e.g., VEGF, Kv channels) by the regular inhalation of vectors containing relevant genetic material.

3.8. Mechanics: Supporting the Right Ventricle

Patients with PAH die predominantly of right heart failure. The thin-walled right ventricle is put under great strain by the increased afterload posed by pulmonary hypertension and progressively dilates, remodels, and fails. The damaged right ventricle can recover [e.g., following lung transplantation or pulmonary thromboendarterectomy *(88)*], and so supporting or enhancing right ventricular function is a rational avenue to explore for useful PAH therapy.

In advanced PAH, the right ventricular (RV) pressures may exceed the left ventricular (LV) pressures during late RV systole and early LV diastole. As a consequence, the intraventricular septum "bows" into the left ventricle, impairing left ventricular filling and further compromising cardiac output. This may be the mechanism under-lying exertional syncope in advanced PAH. Atrial septostomy can successfully improve this unhealthy situation in carefully selected patients. Careful cardiac resynchronization (or desynchronization) with multichamber pacing may help to normalize intracardiac pressure relationships. Though theoretical, this strategy may lead to some mechanical improvement in advanced PAH.

Right ventricular failure develops less frequently in patients with congenital heart disease-related PAH than with idiopathic PAH *(89)*. This may be related to a phenotypic change in RV myocytes in early childhood, rendering them better able to adapt to high pressures and thus behave more like LV myocytes. In patients with RV pressure overload later in life, this phenotypic switch may not occur. If we could identify the mechanisms underlying the phenotypic difference between adult LV and RV myocytes, we may be able to alter RV myocyte behavior and render them better able to cope with pulmonary arterial hypertension.

Another approach would be to augment the myocyte population. Skeletal myocytes have been administered into areas of infarcted left ventricle, with resultant reductions in remodeling and improved function *(90)*. Areas of RV damage can be demonstrated in severe PAH *(91)*, and it may be possible to improve RV function by augmenting the RV myocyte population in a similar fashion.

4. AMMUNITION: HOW BEST TO HIT THE TARGET?

Prostanoid therapy is effective but suffers primarily through cumbersome delivery systems and systemic side effects. Key qualities required of new therapies for PAH are selectivity, simple administration, and lack of side effects.

Selectivity for the pulmonary circulation can be achieved either by targeting a pathophysiological system that is restricted to the lung (e.g., phosphodiesterase-5) or by administering the drug locally, thus minimizing systemic exposure (e.g., nitric oxide). Some of the molecular pathways outlined above, e.g., abnormal TGF-β system signaling or p38 MAPK, may be selective or semiselective for the pulmonary circulation *(79)*. Experimental work comparing molecular pathways in systemic and pulmonary arterial systems and assessing the differential effects of mediators should continue.

The design of drugs and delivery systems is an advanced science. The pulmonary circulation, preferentially exposed to inhaled agents, offers unique opportunities for selective drug targeting. Systemic effects can be minimized if we can provide the drug via a delivery system limiting it to the lungs. This has been shown to be effective for nitric oxide and iloprost. Continuous nitric oxide therapy is, however, logistically unfeasible. Furthermore, the requirement for a specialized device and the inconvenience of the number of daily inhalations required with nebulized iloprost limit the use of this agent. Agents with a long half-life are preferable. Nebulized treprostinil shows some promise and may require many fewer daily doses *(92)*. It is conceivable that we could design effective therapies for PAH, administered via a simple inhalation device.

Regardless of the mechanisms by which we achieve it, it is clear that we require not only effective agents, but also safe and convenient agents, if we are to improve our patients' quality of life.

5. ARMOR: RECOGNIZING AND PROTECTING THE SUSCEPTIBLE

Previous sections have highlighted risk factors for the development of PAH including *BMPR2* mutations, connective tissue diseases, and hypoxic lung disease. The recognition of PAH as a disease of progressive vascular remodeling has led to the suggestion that treatment should be initiated early. Identification of at-risk patients at a presymptomatic stage allows for intervention with effective agents to halt the remodeling process and potentially prevent the disease.

Screening poses problems when dealing with unusual diseases. Screening techniques should be robust, noninvasive, sensitive, and specific, and limiting the population to be screened by identifying those with risk factors is helpful. Patients at high risk for pulmonary hypertension are currently screened using resting transthoracic echocardiograms, but these and other routine investigations (ECG, chest X-ray) are insensitive for early disease. New imaging techniques [e.g., amplification of the signals by exercise *(93–95)*] and biomarkers offer the tantalizing potential for earlier disease detection with greater sensitivity and specificity.

At present, we lack the sophisticated techniques necessary to accurately detect early disease or predict future disease development. Without these, it is difficult to envisage clinical trials of targeted therapies for these at-risk patients. Screening, treating, and preventing disease thus remain goals for the future. Achieving these will potentially be achieved as new assessment tools become available and validated. In the meantime, we should continue to consider targets by which we might treat early disease and also maintain our epidemiological data to aid future investigation.

6. CLINICAL TRIALS AND ENDPOINTS

The time from a basic scientific breakthrough to validated, commercially available therapy is slow (20 years for prostacyclin, 10 years for bosentan) and increasingly costly. The development of effective new therapies requires not just recognition and synthesis of novel agents but also robust clinical studies utilizing appropriate, validated endpoints. We must continue to direct resources toward improved trial design and validation of new endpoints if progress in the clinical arena is to match that at the bench.

Clinical assessment, six-minute walk distance (6MWD), echocardiography, and measurement of resting hemodynamics at cardiac catheterization are the workhorses of routine clinical follow-up. Quality-of-life data and time to clinical worsening have been used along with these (in various combinations) as the primary endpoints in recent clinical studies. Each endpoint has various deficiencies: Clinical assessment is a subjective tool; echocardiography is unreliable in a proportion of patients; cardiac catheterization is generally safe but is time-consuming and unattractive to patients if repeated frequently; and resting hemody-namics may not fully reflect disease burden. The 6MWD has been widely used, is reproducible, is easy to conduct, provides an easily communicable endpoint, and has been accepted by the pulmonary vascular community and regulatory authorities. Unfortunately, the 6MWD becomes an insensitive tool when used to monitor patients with early disease, because exercise limitation in this subgroup is usually minimal. As we move toward earlier treatment and disease prevention, we need endpoints that reflect disease progress in this patient group.

Another deficiency of most studies to date is that they have been relatively short-term. Currently available therapies have been approved on the basis of results from 12- to 16-week trials, but we lack understanding about the relationship between short-term changes and medium- to long-term clinical outcome or endpoints that are suitable for long-term studies in patients with minimal disease. Recent symposia in Scotland and Venice considered these issues and attempted to refine clinical endpoints. New quality-of-life question-naires have been developed and are in the process of being validated. Newer echocardiography techniques may provide additional diagnostic and prognostic information. Although cardiopulmonary MRI provides detailed, reproducible images and shows promise, it is not yet widely available and cannot be used in claustrophobic patients as a useful technique, or in those with metallic implants or permanent pacemakers. Certain biomarkers [BNP/NT-proBNP *(96,97)*, troponin T *(98)*, and uric acid *(99–101)*] correlate with hemodynamic status and disease prognosis, and the search for other serum markers continues. Changes in levels of these over time or following intervention may reflect disease progression. These newer potential endpoints still require validation and long-term study.

7. CONCLUSIONS

Great progress in the understanding of the pathogenesis of as well as the therapy for pulmonary hypertension has been made in the last 20 years, but many challenges remain. We have outlined the foundations of currently available therapies and the directions we think therapies for pulmonary arterial hypertension will take. The next few years seem likely to bring increasing use of combinations of prostanoids, endothelin antagonists, and phosphodiesterase inhibitors. Nebulized treprostinil, selective endothelin-A antagonists, and newer phosphodi-esterase inhibitors may offer advantages and expand our therapeutic armamentarium in the near future. Clinical trials of statins, SSRIs,

VIP, potassium channel activators, or antiplatelets are ongoing or are likely to commence in the near future.

The biological plausibility, availability, and relative safety of these newer agents make it tempting to prescribe them now, particularly when faced with gravely ill patients. However, we urge caution. These and all future therapies require proof of efficacy and safety from properly conducted clinical trials before widespread use can be advocated. The gratifying progress we have made in the past decade will come to a halt if we fail to design and conduct trials of the most promising new agents. Even of more concern, these trials cannot be done if clinicians place patients on untested but promising new agents without entering them in trials. Too many patients are still severely limited by and dying of pulmonary arterial hypertension to warrant therapeutic complacency at this time. While we await proof of safety and efficacy, we must continue to enroll patients in clinical trials.

REFERENCES

1. Pitt B, Zannad F, Remme WJ, et al. The effect of spironolactone on morbidity and mortality in patients with severe heart failure. N Engl J Med 1999; 341:709–17.
2. Pitt B, Remme WJ, Zannad F, et al. Eplerenone, a selective aldosterone blocker, in patients with left ventricular dysfunction after myocardial infarction. N Engl J Med 2003; 348:1309–21.
3. Ikram H, Maslowski AH, Nicholls GM, et al. Haemodynamic and hormonal effects of captopril in primary pulmonary hypertension. Br Heart J 1982; 48:541–5.
4. Leier CV, Bambach D, Nelson S, et al. Captopril and primary pulmonary hypertension. Circulation 1983; 67:155–61.
5. Schafer A, Fraccarollo D, Hildemann SK, Tas P, Ertl G, Bauersachs J. Addition of the selective aldosterone receptor antagonist eplerenone to ACE inhibition in heart failure: Effect on endothelial dysfunction. Cardiovasc Res 2003; 58(3):655–62.
6. Macdonald JE, Kennedy N, Struthers AD. Effects of spironolactone on endothelial function, vascular angiotensin converting enzyme activity, and other prognostic markers in patients with mild heart failure already taking optimal treatment. Heart 2004; 90(7):765–70.
7. Abiose AK, Mansoor GA, Barry M, Soucier R, Nair CK, Hager D. Effect of spironolactone on endothelial function in patients with congestive heart failure on conventional medical therapy. Am J Cardiol 2004; 93(12):1564–6.
8. Mitchell BM, Smith AD, Webb RC, Dorrance AM. Aldosterone decreases endothelium-dependent relaxation by down-regulating GYP cyclohydrolase. Hypertension. 2003; 42:435(P161). Abstract.

9. Fraccarollo D, Galuppo P, Hildemann S, Christ M, Ertl G, Bauersachs J. Additive improvement of left ventricular remodeling and neurohormonal activation by aldosterone receptor blockade with eplerenone and ACE inhibition in rats with myocardial infarction. J Am Coll Cardiol 2003; 42(9):1666–73.

10. Yancy CW, Saltzberg MT, Berkowitz RL, et al. Safety and feasibility of using serial infusions of nesiritide for heart failure in an outpatient setting (from the FUSION 1 trial). Am J Cardiol 2004; 94:595–601.

11. Kurian DC, Wagner IJ, Klapholz M. Nesiritide in pulmonary hypertension. Chest 2004; 126(1):302–5.

12. Gheorghiade M, Gattis WA, O'Connor CM, et al. Effects of tolvaptan, a vasopressin antagonist, in patients hospitalized with worsening heart failure. JAMA 2004; 291:1963–71.

13. Klinger JR, Warburton RR, Pietras L, Hill NS. Brain natriuretic peptide inhibits hypoxic pulmonary hypertension in rats. J Appl Physiol 1998; 84(5):1646–52.

14. Lok BL, Ashrafian H, Mukerjee D, Coghlan JG, Timms PM. The natriuretic peptides and their role in disorders of right heart dysfunction and pulmonary hypertension. Clin Biochem 2004; 37:847–56.

15. Wagenvoort CA, Mulder PG. Thrombotic lesions in primary plexogenic arteriopathy. Similar pathogenesis or complication? Chest 1993; 103:844–9.

16. Fuster V, Steele PM, Edwards WD, et al. Primary pulmonary hypertension: Natural history and the importance of thrombosis. Circulation 1984; 70:580–7.

17. Welsh CH, Hassell KL, Badesch DB, Kressin DC, Marlar RA. Coagulation and fibrinolytic profiles in patients with severe pulmonary hypertension. Chest 1996; 110:710–7.

18. Eisenberg PR, Lucore C, Kaufman L, et al. Fibrinopeptide A levels indicative of pulmonary vascular thrombosis in patients with primary pulmonary hypertension. Circulation 1990; 82:841–7.

19. Rich S, Kaufmann E, Levy PS. The effects of high doses of calcium-channel blockers on survival in primary pulmonary hypertension. N Engl J Med 1992; 327:76–81.

20. Frank H, Mlczoch J, Huber K, et al. The effect of anticoagulant therapy in anorectic induced pulmonary hypertension. Chest 1997; 112:714–21.

21. Eriksson BI, Agnelli G, Cohen AT, et al. Direct thrombin inhibitor melagatran followed by oral ximelagatran in comparison with enoxaparin for prevention of venous thromboembolism after total hip or knee replacement. Thromb Haemost 2003; 89:288–96.

22. Francis CW, Davidson BL, Berkowitz SD, et al. Ximelagatran versus warfarin for the prevention of venous thromboembolism after total knee arthroplasty. A randomized, double-blind trial. Ann Intern Med 2002; 137:648–55.

23. Francis CW, Berkowitz SD, Comp PC, et al. Comparison of ximelagatran with warfarin for the prevention of venous thromboembolism after total knee replacement. N Engl J Med 2003; 349:1703–12.

24. Schulman S, Wåhlander K, Lundström T, et al. Secondary prevention of venous thromboembolism with the oral direct thrombin inhibitor ximelagatran. N Engl J Med 2003; 349:1713–21.

25. Olsson SB; Executive Steering Committee on behalf of the SPORTIF III Investigators. Stroke prevention with the oral direct thrombin inhibitor ximelagatran compared with warfarin in patients with non-valvular atrial fibrillation (SPORTIF III): Randomised controlled trial. Lancet 2003; 362(22):1691–8.

26. Halperin JL, Executive Steering Committee, SPORTIF III and V Study Investigators. Ximelagatran compared with warfarin for prevention of thromboembolism in patients with nonvalvular atrial fibrillation: Rationale, objectives, and design of a pair of clinical studies and baseline patient characteristics (SPORTIF III and V). Am Heart J 2003; 146(3):431–8.

27. Koopman MM, Buller HR. Short- and long-acting synthetic pentasaccharides. J Intern Med 2003; 254(4):335–42.

28. Jeffery TK, Morrell NW. Molecular and cellular basis of pulmonary vascular remodelling in pulmonary hypertension. Prog Cardiovasc Dis 2002; 45:173–202.

29. McLaughlin VV, Genthner DE, Panella MM, Rich S. Reduction in pulmonary vascular resistance with long-term epoprostenol (prostacyclin) therapy in primary pulmonary hypertension. N Engl J Med 1998; 338(5):273–7.

30. Jasmin JF, Lucas M, Cernacek P, Dupuis J. Effectiveness of a nonselective ETA/B and a selective ETA antagonist in rats with monocrotaline-induced pulmonary hypertension. Circulation 2001; 103:314–8.

31. Wong J, Reddy VM, Hendricks-Munoz K, et al. Endothelin-1 vasoactive responses in lambs with pulmonary hypertension and increased pulmonary blood flow. Am J Physiol 1995; 269:H1965– H1972.

32. Rondelet B, Kerbaul F, Motte S, et al. Bosentan for the prevention of overcirculation-induced experimental pulmonary arterial hypertension. Circulation 2003; 107:1329–35.

33. Prie S, Leung TK, Cernacek P, Ryan JW, Dupuis J. The orally active ET(A) receptor antagonist (+)-(S)-2-(4,6-dimethoxy-pyrimidin-2-yloxy)-3-methoxy-3,3-diphenyl-propionic acid (LU 135252) prevents the development of pulmonary hypertension and endothelial metabolic dysfunction in monocrotaline-treated rats. J Pharmacol Exp Ther 1997; 282:1312–8.

34. Prie S, Stewart DJ, Dupuis J. Endothelin-A receptor blockade improves nitric oxide-mediated vasodilation in monocrotaline-induced pulmonary hypertension. Circulation 1998; 97:2169–74.

35. Hill NS, Warburton RR, Pietras L, Klinger JR. Nonspecific endothelin-receptor antagonist blunts monocrotaline-induced pulmonary hypertension in rats. J Appl Physiol 1997; 83(4):1209–15.

36. Zhao L, Mason NA, Morrell NW, et al. Sildenafil inhibits hypoxia induced pulmonary hypertension. Circulation 2001; 104:424–8.

37. McLaughlin VV, Shillington A, Rich S. Survival in primary pulmonary hypertension: The impact of epoprostenol therapy. Circulation 2002; 106:1477–82.

38. Sitbon O, Badesch DB, Channick RN, et al. Effects of the dual endothelin antagonist bosentan in patients with pulmonary arterial hypertension: A 1-year follow-up study. Chest 2003; 124:247–54.

39. McLaughlin V, Sitbon O, Rubin LJ, et al. The effect of first-line bosentan on survival of patients with primary pulmonary hypertension (Abstract). Am J Respir Crit Care Med 2003; 167:A442.

40. Newman JH, Wheeler L, Lane KB, et al. Mutations in the gene for bone morphogenetic protein receptor 2 as a cause of primary pulmonary hypertension in a large kindred. N Engl J Med 2001; 345:319–24.

41. Lane KB, Machado RD, Pauciulo JR, et al. Heterozygous germline mutations in BMPR2, encoding a TGF-beta receptor, cause familial primary pulmonary hypertension. The International PPH Consortium. Nat Genet 2000; 26:81–4.

42. Humbert M, Morrell NW, Archer SL, et al. Cellular and molecular pathobiology of pulmonary arterial hypertension. J Am Coll Cardiol 2004; 43:13S–24S.

43. Khan SN, Lane JM. The use of recombinant human bone morphogenetic protein-2 (rhBMP-2) in orthopaedic applications. Exp Opin Biol Ther 2004; 4(5):741–8.

44. Ohnaka K, Shimoda S, Nawata H, et al. Pitavastatin enhanced BMP-2 and osteocalcin expression by inhibition of Rho-associated kinase in human osteoblasts. Biochem Biophys Res Commun 2001; 287(2):337–42.

45. Emmanuele L, Ortmann J, Doerflinger T, Traupe T, Barton M. Lovastatin stimulates human vascular smooth muscle cell expression of bone morphogenetic protein-2, a potent inhibitor of low-density lipoprotein-stimulated cell growth. Biochem Biophys Res Commun 2003; 302(1): 67–72.

46. Abenhaim L, Moride Y, Brenot F, et al. Appetite-suppressant drugs and the risk of primary pulmonary hypertension. International Primary Pulmonary Hypertension Study Group. N Engl J Med 1996; 335:609–16.

47. Marcos E, Fadel E, Sanchez O, et al. Serotonin-induced smooth muscle hyperplasia in various forms of human pulmonary hypertension. Circ Res 2004; 94:1263–70.

48. Eddahibi S, Chaouat A, Morrell N, et al. Polymorphism of the serotonin transporter gene and pulmonary hypertension in chronic obstructive pulmonary disease. Circulation 2003; 108:1839–44.

49. Herve P, Launay JM, Scrobohaci ML, et al. Increased plasma serotonin in primary pulmonary hypertension. Am J Med 1995; 99:249–54.

50. Welsh DJ, Harnett M, MacLean M, Peacock AJ. Proliferation and signalling in fibroblasts: Role of 5-hydroxytryptamine2A receptor and transporter. Am J Respir Crit Care Med 2004; 170:252–9.

51. Eddahibi S, Fabre V, Boni C, Martres MP, Raffestin B, Hamon M, Adnot S. Induction of serotonin transporter by hypoxia in pulmonary

vascular smooth muscle cells: Relationship with the mitogenic action of serotonin. Circ Res 1999; 84:329–36.

52. Eddahibi S, Hanoun N, Lanfumey L, Lesch K, Raffestin B, Hamon M, Adnot S. Attenuated hypoxic pulmonary hypertension in mice lacking the 5-hydroxytryptamine transporter gene. J Clin Invest 2000; 105:1555–62.

53. Keegan A, Morecroft I, Smillie D, Hicks MN, MacLean MR. Contribution of the 5-HT1B receptor to hypoxia-induced pulmonary hypertension: Converging evidence using 5-HT1B-receptor knockout mice and the 5-HT1B/1D-receptor antagonist GR127935. Circ Res 2001; 89:1231–9.

54. Launay JM, Herve P, Peoc'h K, et al. Function of the serotonin 5-hydroxytryptamine 2B receptor in pulmonary hypertension. Nat Med 2002; 8:1129–35.

55. MacLean MR, Deuchar GA, Hicks MN, et al. Overexpression of the 5-hydroxytryptamine transporter gene: Effect on pulmonary hemody-namics and hypoxia induced pulmonary hypertension. Circulation 2004; 109(17):2150–5.

56. Petkov V, Mosgoeller W, Ziesche R, Raderer M, Stiebellehner L, Vonbank K, Funk GC, Hamilton G, Novotny C, Burian B, Block LH. Vasoactive intestinal peptide as a new drug for treatment of primary pulmonary hypertension. J Clin Invest. May 2003; 111(9):1339–46.

57. Maruno K, Absood A, Said SI. VIP inhibits basal and histamine-stimulated proliferation of human airway smooth muscle cells. Am J Physiol 1995; 268:L1047–L1051.

58. Gunayadin S, Imai Y, Takanashi Y, et al. The effects of vasoactive intestinal polypeptide on monocrotaline induced pulmonary hypertensive rabbits following cardiopulmonary bypsass: A comparative study with isoproternol and nitroglycerine. Cardiovasc Surg 2002; 10:138–45.

59. Yuan JX, Wang J, Juhaszova M, Gaine SP, Rubin LJ. Attenuated K^+ channel gene transcription in primary pulmonary hypertension. Lancet 1998; 351:726–7.

60. Geraci MW, Moore M, Gesell T, et al. Gene expression patterns in the lungs of patients with primary pulmonary hypertension: A gene microarray analysis. Circ Res 2001; 88:555–62.

61. Krick S, Platoshyn O, McDaniel SS, et al. Augmented K^+ currents and mitochondrial membrane depolarization in pulmonary artery myocyte apoptosis. Am J Physiol Lung Cell Mol Physiol 2001; 281:L887–L894.

62. Katayose D, Ohe M, Yamauchi K, et al. Increased expression of PDGF A- and B-chain genes in rat lungs with hypoxic pulmonary hypertension. Am J Physiol 1993; 264:L100–L106.

63. Berg JT, Breen EC, Fu Z, et al. Alveolar hypoxia increases gene expression of extracellular matrix proteins and platelet-derived growth factor-B in lung parenchyma. Am J Respir Crit Care Med 1998; 157:1920–8.

64. Powell PP, Klagsbrun M, Abraham JA, et al. Eosinophils expressing heparin-binding EGF-like growth factor mRNA localize around lung microvessels in pulmonary hypertension. Am J Pathol 1993; 143: 784–93.

65. Arcot SS, Fagerland JA, Lipke DW, et al. Basic fibroblast growth factor alterations during development of monocrotaline-induced pulmonary hypertension in rats. Growth Factors 1995; 12:121–30.

66. Wanstall JC, Gambino A, Jeffery TK, et al. Vascular endothelial growth factor-B–deficient mice show impaired development of hypoxic pulmonary hypertension. Cardiovasc Res 2002; 55:361–8.

67. Hirose S, Hosoda Y, Furuya S, Otsuki T, Ikeda E. Expression of vascular endothelial growth factor and its receptors correlates closely with formation of the plexiform lesion in human pulmonary hypertension. Pathol Int 2000; 50:472–9.

68. Taraseviciene-Stewart T, Kasahara Y, Alger L, et al. Inhibition of the VEGF receptor-2 combined with chronic hypoxia causes cell death dependent pulmonary endothelial cell proliferation and severe pulmonary hypertension. FASEB J 2001; 15:427–38.

69. Campbell AI, Zhao Y, Sandhu R, Stewart DJ. Cell-based gene transfer of vascular endothelial growth factor attenuates monocrotaline-induced pulmonary hypertension. Circulation 2001; 104:2242–8.

70. Nagoaka T, Morio Y, Casanova N, et al. Rho/Rho-kinase signalling mediates increased basal pulmonary vascular tone in chronically hypoxic rats. Am J Physiol Lung Cel Mol Physiol 2004; 287(4):L665–72.

71. Takemoto M, Liao JK. Pleiotropic effects of 3-hydroxy-3-methylglutaryl coenzyme A reductase inhibitors. Arterioscler Thromb Vasc Biol 2001; 21:1712–9.

72. Kwak BR, Mulhaupt F, Mach F. Atherosclerosis: Anti-inflammatory and immunomodulatory activities of statins. Autoimmunity Rev 2003; 2: 332–8.

73. Abe K, Shimokaya H, Morikawa K, et al. Long-term treatment with a rho-kinase inhibitor improves monocrotaline-induced fatal pulmonary hypertension in rats. Circ Res 2004; 94:385–93.

74. McMurtry IF, Bauer NR, Fagan KA, Nagoaka T, Gebb SA, Oka M. Hypoxia and Rho/Rho-kinase signaling. Lung development versus hypoxic pulmonary hypertension Adv Exp Med Biol 2003; 543:127–37.

75. Liu Y, Suzuki YJ, Day RM, Fanburg BL. Rho kinase-induced nuclear translocation of ERK1/ERK2 in smooth muscle cell mitogenesis caused by serotonin. Circ Res 2004; 95(6):579–86.

76. Shimokawa H, Hiramori K, Iinuma H, et al. Anti-anginal effect of fasudil, a Rho-kinase inhibitor, in patients with stable effort angina: A multicenter study. J Cardiovasc Pharmacol 2002; 40(5):751–61.

77. Tachibana E, Harada T, Shibuya M, et al. Intra-arterial infusion of fasudil hydrochloride for treating vasospasm following subarachnoid haemorrhage Acta Neurochir (Wien) 1999; 141(1):13–9.

78. Scott PH, Paul A, Belham CM, Peacock AJ, Wadsworth RM, Gould GW, Welsh D, Plevin R. Hypoxic stimulation of the stress-activated protein kinases in pulmonary artery fibroblasts. Am J Respir Crit Care Med 1998; 158:958–62.

79. Welsh D, Peacock AJ, MacLean M, Harnett M. Chronic hypoxia induces constitutive p38 mitogen activated protein kinase activity that correlates with enhanced cellular proliferation in fibroblasts from rat pulmonary but not systemic arteries. Am J Respir Crit Care Med 2001; 164:282–9.

80. Lee JC, Kumar S, Griswold DE, Underwood DC, Votta BJ, Adams JL. Inhibition of p38 MAP kinase as a therapeutic strategy. Immunopharmacology 2000; 47:185–201.

81. Parasrampuria DA, de Boer P, Desai-Krieger D, Chow AT, Jones CR. Single-dose pharmacokinetics and pharmacodynamics of RWJ 67657, a specific p38 mitogen-activated protein kinase inhibitor: A first-in-human study. J Clin Pharmacol 2003; 43(4):406–13.

82. Rabinovitch M. Elastase and the pathobiology of unexplained pulmonary hypertension. Chest 1998; 114:213S–224S.

83. Cowan KN, Jones PL, Rabinovitch M. Elastase and matrix metalloproteinase inhibitors induce regression, and tenascin-C antisense prevents progression, of vascular disease. J Clin Invest 2000; 105:21–34.

84. Cowan KN, Heilbut A, Humpl T, Lam C, Ito S, Rabinovitch M. Complete reversal of fatal pulmonary hypertension in rats by a serine elastase inhibitor. Nat Med 2000; 6:698–702.

85. Vieillard-Baron A, Frisdal E, Eddahibi S, et al. Effect of adenovirus-mediated lung TIMP-1 overexpression and role of MMP in pulmonary vascular remodeling. Circ Res 2000; 87:418–25.

86. Srikala S, Shepherd FA. Targeting angiogenesis: A review of angiogenesis inhibitors in the treatment of lung cancer. Lung Cancer 2003; 42:S81–S91.

87. Griesenbach U, Geddes DM, Alton EW. Update on gene therapy for cystic fibrosis. Curr Opin Mol Ther 2003; 5(5):489–94.

88. Ritchie M, Waggoner A, Davila-Roman VG, et al. Echocardiographic characterization of the improvement in right ventricular failure in patients with severe pulmonary hypertension after single lung transplantation. J Am Coll Cardiol 1993; 22:1170–4.

89. Hopkins WE, Ochoa LL, Richardson GW, et al. Comparison of the haemodynamics and survival of adults with severe primary pulmonary hypertension or Eisenmenger syndrome. J Heart Lung Transplant 1996; 15:100–5.

90. Chiu RC. Adult stem cell therapy for heart failure. Exp Opin Biol Ther 2003; 3(2):215–25.

91. Blyth KG, Martin TN, Mark PB, Dargie HJ, Peacock AJ. Late gadolinium enhancement (LGE), a marker of myocardial damage, can be detected by contrast enhanced-cardiac magnetic resonance imaging within the right ventricle of patients with severe pulmonary hypertension. Eur Respir J 2004; 24(S48):S235.

92. Voswinckel R, Enke B, Kohstall MG, et al. Pharmockinetic differences between inhaled treprostinil and inhaled iloprost in severe pulmonary hypertension. Eur Respir J 2004; 24(S48):S109.

93. Raeside DA, Smith A, Brown A, et al. Pulmonary artery pressure measurement during exercise testing in patients with suspected pulmonary hypertension. Eur Respir J 2000; 16(2):282–7.

94. Grünig E, Janssen B, Mereles D, et al. Abnormal pulmonary artery pressure response in asymptomatic carriers of primary pulmonary hypertension gene. Circulation 2000; 102:1145–50.

95. Grünig E, Mereles D, Hildebrandt W, et al. Stress Doppler echocardiography for identification of susceptibility to high altitude pulmonary edema. J Am Coll Cardiol 2000; 35:980–7.

96. Nagaya N, Nishikimi T, Okano Y, et al. Plasma brain natriuretic peptide levels increase in proportion to the extent of right ventricular dysfunction in pulmonary hypertension. J Am Coll Cardiol 1998; 31:202–8.

97. Nagaya N, Nishikimi T, Uematsu M, et al. Plasma brain natriuretic peptide as a prognostic indicator in patients with primary pulmonary hypertension. Circulation 2000; 102:865–70.

98. Torbicki A, Kurzyna M, Kuca P, et al. Detectable serum cardiac troponin T as a marker of poor prognosis among patients with chronic precapillary pulmonary hypertension. Circulation 2003; 108:844–8.

99. Hoeper MM, Hohlfeld JM, Fabel H. Hyperuricemia in patients with right or left heart failure. Eur Respir J 1999; 13:682–5.

100. Nagaya N, Uematsu M, Satoh T, et al. Serum uric acid levels correlate with the severity and the mortality of primary pulmonary hypertension. Am J Respir Crit Care Med 1999; 160:487–92.

101. Voelkel MA, Wynne KM, Badesch DB, Groves BM, Voelkel NF. Hyperuricemia in severe pulmonary hypertension. Chest 2000; 117:19–24.

Index

Acute cor pulmonale, 363–378
  in ARDS, 364, 366, 368–370,
    373–375, 378
  defined, 365–369
  diagnosis, 366–368, 372
  echocardiography, 365–378
  management principles, 374–378
    fluid administration, 375–376
    mechanical ventilation, 375
    vasoactive agents, 376
    vasodilators, 376–377
  pathophysiology, 365–369
  in pulmonary embolism, 370–372
  see also Right ventricular (RV) dysfunction
Acute pulmonary embolism, 201
Acute pulmonary hypertension, 308
  see also Chronic pulmonary hypertension
Acute rejection, 394–395
  see also Chronic rejection; Lung
    transplantation
Acute respiratory distress syndrome
    (ARDS), 364
  acute cor pulmonale in, 364, 368–370
  management principles
    fluid administration, 375–376
    mechanical ventilation, 375
  see also Pulmonary embolism
Acute right ventricular dysfunction, 363
  see also Acute cor pulmonale; Pulmonary
    embolism
Adaptive hypertrophy, 101–103
Adrenomedullin
  imbalance, 53
  see also Vasoactive mediators
AECA, see Antiendothelial cell antibodies
    (AECA)
Aldactone, 235
ALK1 (activin-receptor-like-kinase 1) gene,
    10, 20
  FPAH genetics and, 81
  IPAH genetics and, 81
  mutations and PAH, 66
  PH genetics and, 83–84

Ambrisentan, 296
  ARIES-1 trial, 296
  ARIES-2 trial, 296
  ET receptors antagonists in PAH and,
    297–298
Ambulatory hemodynamic monitoring, 43–44
  see also Invasive testing
Aminorex, 2, 7
Angiography
  CT, 209
  CTEPH, 200, 209–213
  magnetic resonance, 209
  pulmonary, 200, 210–213
Angioscopy
  CTEPH, 200, 210–213
  pulmonary, 210–213
Angiotensin-II, 99
Anorexigens, 57
ANP (atrial natriuretic peptide), 102–103,
    112, 115
  combination with PDE inhibitors,
    354–357
  see also BNP (brain natriuretic peptide);
    CNP (c-type natriuretic peptide)
Anti-centromere antibody (ACA), 151
Antibodies, 151–152
Anticoagulation therapy
  for IPAH, 240
  PAH future directions and, 411–412
  for PAH, 241
  for pulmonary embolism, 239–241
  SSc-PH therapy and, 156
Antiendothelial cell antibodies (AECA),
    151–152
Antihypertensives, oral, 158
Antiphospholipid antibody syndrome,
    203, 205
Antiplatelets, 411–412
APAH (associated pulmonary arterial
    hypertension)
  congenital heart disease (CHD), 20–22
  connective tissue disease (CTD), 20
  drugs and toxins, 23

HIV infection, 23
portopulmonary hypertension (PPHTN),
    22–23
rare condition diseases, 23
see also FPAH (familial pulmonary arterial
    hypertension); IPAH (idiopathic
    pulmonary arterial hypertension);
    PAH (pulmonary arterial
    hypertension)
Apoptosis-promoting genes, 418–419
Appetite suppressants, 2, 57
Arachidonic acid metabolites, 53
ARDS, *see* Acute respiratory distress
    syndrome
ARIES-1/2 (ambrisentan trials), 296
Arterial hypoxemia, 235
Asplenia, 62
Associated pulmonary arterial hypertension,
    see APAH (associated pulmonary
    arterial hypertension)
Atrial septostomy, 383–384
    indications and patient selection, 396–397
    outcomes, 398–399
    PAH and, 396–399
    techniques
        blade balloon, 397
        graded balloon dilation, 397
    see also Lung transplantation
Autoantibodies
    ACA, 151
    CTD-PH and, 151–124
Autoimmunity, 179–180
    see also HIV-PH
"Ayerza's disease", 2–3

Beraprost, 277
    combination with sildenafil, 349–353
    for CTEPH, 222
    see also Prostacyclins
Beta blockers, 187
Biomarkers, 111–113
Biopsy, lung, 44
Blade balloon atrial septostomy, 397
BMPR1A, 64
BMPR2 (bone morphogenetic protein
    receptor gene, 2), 10, 27
    biology, 79–80
    CTD-PH mediators and, 150
    in FPAH, 85
    in IPAH, 78
    mutations, 10
    in PAH, 56, 85

PH genetics and, 73–75
in portal hypertension, 79
in PVOD, 79
screening/counseling, 87–88
statins synergism with, 322–323
targeted therapy, 406–409
see also TGF-β
BNP (brain natriuretic peptide), 102,
    111–113, 115, 235
    combination with PDE inhibitors, 357
    CTD-PH and, 156–157
    for fluid overload, 235
    lung transplantation timing and, 386
    see also ANP (atrial natriuretic peptide);
        CNP (c-type natriuretic peptide)
Bone morphogenic (BMP) ligands, 80
Bosentan, 187
    combination with
        epoprostenol, 355
        iloprost, 355
        inhaled treprostinil, 356
        sildenafil, 357–358
    for CTEPH, 222
    Eisenmenger physiology and, 136
    ET receptors antagonists
    for HIV-PH treatment, 183
    intravenous or subcutaneous prostacyclins
        to oral therapy, transition from,
        343–344
    in PAH and, 287–288
    for PAH, 316
    for PPHTN, 187
    selection aspects, 297
    sildenafil and
        combination therapy, 357
        drug interactions, 314–315
    trials, 287–291
        BREATHE-1, 288–290, 297
        BREATHE-2, 290
        BREATHE-3, 290–291
        BREATHE-4, 291
    see also Endothelin receptor antagonists
        (ERA)
BREATHE-2 trial, 290, 355
BREATHE-3 trial, 290–291
BREATHE-4 trial, 183, 291
BREATHE-5 trial, 130, 138
BREATHE trial-1
    bosentan trials, 288–290
    ET receptors antagonists selection
        aspects, 297
Breathing, sleep-disordered, 242–244

Bronchiolitis obliterans syndrome (BOS),
    395–396
    see also Lung transplantation
Bumetanide, 233

Calcium channel blockers, 246–250
    see also Potassium channel blockers
CAMP pathways
    prostacyclins-cAMP pathway and
        endothelin pathway, combining,
        354–357
    prostacyclins-cAMP pathway and
        NO-cGMP pathway, combining,
        345–349
    see also Combination therapies
Cardiac catheterization, 5
    invasive testing (PAH) and, 42–44
    pulmonary hemodynamics and, 3
    see also Right heart catheterization (RHC)
Cardiac hypertrophy, *see* Hypertrophy
Cardiopulmonary exercise testing
    (CPET), 39
    see also Noninvasive testing
Catheterization, *see* Cardiac catheterization
CGMP pathway
    combination therapy
        nitric oxide-cGMP pathway and
            endothelin pathway, 354
        PDE inhibitors with endothelin-receptor
            antagonists, 354–357
        prostacyclins-cAMP pathway and
            NO-cGMP pathway, 345–350
    PDE5 inhibition and, 306–308
        acute PDE5 inhibition effects on PAH,
            310–313
        acute pulmonary hypertension
            reduction, 308
        chronic PDE5 inhibition effects on PAH,
            310–315
        chronic pulmonary hypertension
            reduction, 309
        CTEPH, 315
        drug interactions, 314–315
        effects on clinical PAH, 309–313
        experimental PAH reduction and, 308
        side effects and tolerance, 313–314
    pulmonary vasculature and, 306–315
CHD-PAH, 20–22, 127–130
    dynamic PAH, 129–130
    Eisenmenger physiology, 134–136
    immediate-postoperative reactive PH,
        131–133

late-postoperative PH, 133
    normal to mildly abnormal PVR states,
        133–134
    see also CTD-PH; HIV-PH
Chest radiography (CXR)
    chronic thromboembolic pulmonary
        hypertension (CTEPH), 204
    noninvasive testing and, 37
    right ventricle (RV) monitoring, 111
    see also Angiography; Angioscopy
Chronic pulmonary hypertension, 309
    see also Acute pulmonary hypertension
Chronic rejection, 395–396
    see also Acute rejection; Lung
        transplantation
Chronic thromboembolic pulmonary
    hypertension, *see* CTEPH (chronic
    thromboembolic pulmonary
    hypertension)
Circulation, *see* Pulmonary circulation
CNP (c-type natriuretic peptides),
    102, 353
    see also ANP (atrial natriuretic peptides);
        BNP (brain natriuretic peptides)
Cocaine, 57–58
Combination therapies, 316
    nitric oxide-cGMP pathway and endothelin
        pathway, 354
    PDE inhibitors with endothelin-receptor
        antagonists, 357–358
    prostacyclins-cAMP pathway and
        endothelin pathway, 354–357
    prostacyclins-cAMP pathway with
        NO-cGMP pathway
        natriuretic peptides with PDE
            inhibitors, 353
        nitric oxide with PDE inhibitors,
            351–352
        prostacyclins with NO, 350–351
        prostacyclins with phosphodiesterase
            inhibitors, 345–349
    rationale behind, 344–345
    see also Targeted therapies
Congenital heart disease PAH,
    see CHD-PAH
Connective tissue disease (CTD),
    see CTD-PH
Continuous positive airway pressure
    (CPAP), 244
Cor pulmonale, acute, *see* Acute cor
    pulmonale
Counseling, PAH genetics and, 87–88
CREST, 146

CTD-PH, 150–151
  clinical presentation and diagnosis
    brain natriuretic peptide (BNP), 155
    Doppler echocardiography, 154–155
    general approach, 155–156
    pulmonary function testing, 153–153
    symptoms and signs, 152
  epidemiology
    dermatomyositis/polymyositis, 150
    mixed connective tissue disease
        (MCTD), 148–149
    rheumatoid arthritis, 149
    Sjogren's syndrome, 150
    systemic lupus erythematosus (SLE),
        148–149
    systemic sclerosis (SSc), 146–148
  pathophysiology, 59
    autoantibodies, 151–152
    CTD-PH mediators, 150
  surgical treatments, 162
  see also CHD-PAH; HIV-PH; SSc-PH
CTEPH (chronic thromboembolic pulmonary
    hypertension), 26, 41
  clinical presentation and history, 205–206
  diagnostic evaluation
    chest radiography, 206–207
    CT angiography, 209
    echocardiography, 205
    laboratory studies, 204–205
    magnetic resonance angiography, 209
    pulmonary angiography, 210–211
    pulmonary angioscopy, 211–213
    pulmonary function testing, 205
    RHC, 210–213
    thromboendarterectomy, 213, 215
    V/Q scanning, 207–209
  ET_B-receptor expression, 287
  long-term outcome, 221
  lung transplantation, 223
  medical therapy, 221–223
  pathogenesis
    pathophysiology, 201–202
    risk factors, 203
  PDE5 inhibition effects, 315
  physical examination, 204
  postoperative management, 217–220
  surgery aspects
    approach, 215–217
    outcome, 220
    selection, 213–215
Cytokines
  growth factors and, 99–100
  statins effect on, 324

Deep venous thrombosis (DVT), 204
Dermatomyositis, 150
Digoxin, 242
Diltiazem, 249
Dipyridimole, 352
Diuretics, 114–115
  for fluid overload, 232–235
  PAH future directions and, 410
  RV dysfunction and, 113
  SSc-PH therapy and, 155
DLCO, 153–154
Dobutamine, 235
Drugs, PAH associated with, 20
Dynamic PAH, 129–130

Ebstein's anomaly, 134
Echocardiography, 185–186
  acute cor pulmonale, 365–369
  CTEPH, 209
  Doppler, 154–155
  noninvasive PAH testing, 37
  PPHTN, 185–187
  RV monitoring, 108–110
  sickle cell disease (SCD), 188
  see also Electrocardiography (ECG)
Eisenmenger's syndrome, 21
  bosentan and, 138
  CHD-PAH and, 138–139
  diagnosis, 135–136
  lung transplantation, 386, 388–389
  noninterventional diagnosis approach, 136
  potentially preventable or reversible
        factors, 136
Electrocardiography (ECG)
  noninvasive testing (PAH), 37–42
  right ventricle (RV) monitoring, 111
  see also Echocardiography
Embolism, see Pulmonary embolism
Endothelial cell function enhancement,
    statins and, 323
Endothelin-1 (ET-1)
  bosentan trials, 287–288
  CTD-PH mediators and, 150
  HIV-associated PH and, 177–178
  imbalance, 53
  PAH and, 285–287
  SSc-PH therapy and, 161
  statins opposition to, 323
  vasoconstrictor, 178–179
Endothelin pathways
  combination therapy

nitric oxide-cGMP pathway and
        endothelin pathway, 354
    PDE inhibitors with endothelin-receptor
        antagonists, 357–358
    prostacyclins-cAMP pathway and
        endothelin pathway, 354–357
    hypertrophic signaling pathway, 103
Endothelin-receptor
    blockade, 287–288
    ET_A receptors, 284–287
    ET_B receptors, 284–287
    nonselective, 287
    PAH and, 284
    selective, 287
Endothelin receptor antagonists (ERA)
    ambrisentan trials, 296
    bosentan trials, 287–288
    combination therapy
        PDE inhibitors with ERA, 357–358
        prostacyclins with ERA, 354–357
    future scope of, 299
    in PAH, 285–287, 316
    selection aspects, 297–299
    sitaxsentan trials, 291–295
    SSc-PH therapy, 161–162
Epidemic, idiopathic pulmonary
        hypertension
    aminorex, 7
    second, 8–9
Epoprostenol, 181–182, 187, 258
    administration and dosage, 265–267
    combination of bosentan, 355
    for CTEPH, 221–222
    early case report, 258
    for HIV-PH, 181–183
    for IPAH, 384
    long-term studies
        functional and hemodynamic effects,
            260–262
        survival aspects, 262–265
    monitoring aspects, 267–268
    patient selection aspects, 265
    for PPHTN, 187
    randomized, controlled trials, 258–260
    for sarcoidosis, 188
    for sickle cell disease (SCD), 190
    side effects and complications,
        268–269
    sildenafil combination with, 353
    subcutaneous treprostinil to intravenous
        epoprostenol, transition
        from, 342
    transition aspects

epoprostenol to inhaled iloprost, 343
    intravenous epoprostenol to
        subcutaneous or intravenous
        treprostinil, 343–344
    see also Prostacyclins
Exercise Doppler-echocardiography, 88
Exercise-induced hypoxemia, 236, 237

Familial pulmonary arterial hypertension,
    see FPAH
Fick principle, 4
    see also Pulmonary hemodynamics
Fluid administration, acute cor pulmonale
    management and, 375–376
Fluid overload, 232–235
    diuretics for, 233–235
    intravenous diuretics for, 233–234
    potassium replacement aspects, 235
Fontan procedures, 134
Forced vital capacity (FVC), 40
FPAH (familial pulmonary arterial
        hypertension), 9–10, 19–20
    see also APAH (associated pulmonary
        arterial hypertension); IPAH
        (idiopathic pulmonary arterial
        hypertension); PAH (pulmonary
        arterial hypertension)
    ALK1 mutations, 81, 87
    BMPR2 mutations in, 79
    screening/counseling aspects, 87
Function testing, see Pulmonary function
    testing
Furosemide, 233–235

G protein-coupled receptors, 98, 100
    see also Hypertrophy
Glenn procedures, 134
Graded balloon dilation atrial
    septostomy, 397
Graft dysfunction, primary, 394
    see also Lung transplantation

HAART therapy, 181
    see also HIV-PH
Heart function, right, 110–111
    see also Right ventricular (RV)
        dysfunction
Hematocrit, 238–239
    see also Polycythemia
Hemodynamics, see Pulmonary
    hemodynamics
Hemoglobinopathies, 59, 62

Hereditary hemorrhagic telangiectasia (HHT)
ALK1 mutations, 81, 87
PAH pathophysiology and, 65
Hereditary spherocytosis, 63
High-dose therapy, 235
HIV-PH, 23, 37, 60, 176–178
pathogenesis
autoimmunity, 179–180
ET-1 vasoconstrictors, 178–180
histopathology, 175
HIV virus effects, 176–178
HLA expression, 179–180
NO vasodilators, 178
prostacyclin vasodilators, 179
toxic substances, 180
treatment, 181–183
vasoconstrictors and vasodilators, 178
treatment
HAART therapy, 181
vasodilators, 181–183
see also CHD-PAH; CTD-PH; SSc-PH
HLA expression, 179–180
Hydrochlorothiazide, 233
Hypertrophy
adaptive, 101–103
maladaptive, 97
right ventricle (RV), 103–105
signaling pathways, 101–101
angiotensin-II, 99
endothelin (ET-I), 99
G protein-coupled receptors, 98, 100
mechanical stretch, 100–101
TGF-β, 99–100
TNF-α, 99
Hypoxemia
arterial, 235
exercise-induced, 236
oxygen therapy for, 236–237
Hypoxia
associated PH, 23
PAH pathophysiology and, 57
RV dysfunction and, 113

Idiopathic pulmonary hypertension, 1
aminorex epidemic, 7
hemodynamics, 3–6
NIH Registry, 8
pulmonary circulation, 5–6
second epidemic, 8
WHO
Evian meet (1998), 9
Geneva meet (1973), 7

see also IPAH (idiopathic pulmonary
arterial hypertension)
Iloprost
acute effects of PDE5 inhibition
on PH, 309
combination with
bosentan, 354
sildenafil, 350
tolafentrine, 347
for CTEPH, 315
epoprostenol to inhaled iloprost, transition
from, 343
inhaled, 276, 343
for PAH therapy, 420
Immunosuppressives, 156
In situ thrombosis, 239–241
Inhaled iloprost, 276, 343
Inhaled NO (iNO), 188
for acute cor pulmonale, 377
acute effects of PDE5 inhibition on PH,
308–309
combination therapy with
dipyridimole, 352
milrinone, 352
PDE3 inhibitors, 308
PDE5 inhibitors, 351
prostacyclin, 354
sildenafil, 352
for CTEPH, 315
for HIV-PH, 183
PDE5 inhibition and, 310
for PPHTN, 187
for pulmonary vasoconstriction, 244–246
for sarcoidosis, 188
see also Nitric oxide (NO)
Inhaled prostacyclin, 377
Inhaled treprostinil, 356
Intravenous diuretics for fluid overload, 233
Intravenous epoprostenol
intravenous epoprostenol to subcutaneous
or intravenous treprostinil, transition
from, 339, 42–343
subcutaneous treprostinil to intravenous
epoprostenol, transition from, 342
Intravenous or subcutaneous prostacyclins to
oral therapy, transition from, 343–344
Intravenous treprostinil
intravenous treprostinil to subcutaneous
treprostinil, transition from, 342
subcutaneous treprostinil to intravenous
treprostinil, transition from, 342
Invasive testing
ambulatory hemodynamic monitoring, 43

cardiac catheterization, 42
lung biopsy, 44
vasodilator testing, 43
see also Noninvasive testing
IPAH (idiopathic pulmonary arterial
    hypertension), 10, 18–19
ALK1 mutations, 81
anticoagulation therapy for, 240
BMPR2 mutations in, 78–79
calcium channel blocker therapy for,
    246–250
epoprostenol treatment for, 384
lung transplantation for, 389–391
SERT pathway and, 82
vasodilators for, 245
see also APAH (associated pulmonary
    arterial hypertension); FPAH (familial
    pulmonary arterial hypertension);
    PAH (pulmonary arterial
    hypertension)
Isoproterenol, 240

L-tryptophan, 59
Laboratory testing, 44
additional testing, 45
CTEPH, 206
essential testing, 45
future diagnostic modalities, 45
optional/investigational testing, 45
see also Invasive testing; Noninvasive
    testing
Large vessel obstruction, 202
see also CTEPH (chronic thromboembolic
    pulmonary hypertension)
Left ventricular (LV) interactions, 104
see also Right ventricle (RV) dysfunction
Left ventricular end-diastolic pressure
    (LVEDP), 42
Loop diuretics, 233
Loprost
administration and dosing, 276
clinical studies, 274
inhaled, 276
patient selection aspects, 276
see also Prostacyclins
Lung biopsy, 44
see also Invasive testing
Lung scanning, CTEPH, 207–209
Lung transplantation, 385
outcomes
    acute rejection, 394–395
    bronchiolitis obliterans syndrome (BOS),
        392, 395

chronic rejection, 395–396
complications, 392–396
cost and cost-effectiveness, 391
physiological function, 390
primary graft dysfunction, 394
quality of life, 390–391
survival, 389–390
pretransplantation assessment, 385
transplant activity, 388–389
transplant operation, choice of, 385
transplantation timing, 386–388
see also Atrial septostomy; CTEPH
    (chronic thromboembolic pulmonary
    hypertension)

Magnesium, 233
Magnetic resonance angiography, 209
Magnetic resonance imaging (MRI),
    110, 209
Maladaptive hypertrophy, 103
see also Adaptive hypertrophy
Matrix metalloproteinases (MMPs), 418
Matrix proteins, 418
Maximum voluntary ventilation (MVV), 40
Mechanical stretch, 99–100
see also Hypertrophy
Mechanical ventilation
acute cor pulmonale management and,
    374–375
RV dysfunction and, 375
Mechanics, RV supporting, 419
see also Targeted therapies
Methamphetamine, 57–58
Metolazone, 235
Milrinone
for fluid overload, 235
iNO combination with, 350–351
Mixed connective tissue disease (MCTD),
    148–149
see also CTD-PH
Monocrotaline, 58

Natriuretic peptides
for acute pulmonary hypertension, 308
ANP, 102, 112, 115
BNP, 102, 112–113, 115, 155
cGMP production and, 308
CNP, 102
CTD-PH and, 160
hypertrophy and, 101–103
SSc-PH and, 160
with PDE inhibitors, combining, 357–358

Neurohormonal agents, 410–411
Nifedipine
  for pulmonary embolism, 240
  for pulmonary vasoconstriction, 246
NIH Registry, 2
Nitrates, 187
Nitric oxide (NO)
  for acute pulmonary hypertension, 308
  cGMP production and, 308
  combination therapy
    nitric oxide-cGMP pathway and
      endothelin pathway, 354–358
    nitric oxide with PDE inhibitors,
      351–352
    prostacyclins-cAMP pathway and
      NO-cGMP pathway, 345–353
    prostacyclins with NO, 350–351
  CTD-PH mediators, 150–151
  HIV-PH and, 182
  imbalance, 54
  PAH genetics and, 85
  PPHTN and, 187
  for sickle cell disease (SCD), 188–189
  statins effect on, 324
  targeted therapy aspects and, 420
  vasodilators, 181–183
  see also Inhaled NO (iNO)
Nocturnal hypoxemia, 114
Noninvasive testing, 37–41
  cardiopulmonary exercise testing (CPET),
    39–40
  chest radiography, 40
  electrocardiography (ECG), 40–41
  pulmonary function testing, 40
  six-minute walk (6MW), 39
  sleep studies, 41
  standard echocardiography, 38
  ventilation–perfusion (V/Q) lung
    scanning, 41
  see also Invasive testing
Nonischemic arteritic optic neuropathy
  (NIAON), 314
Nonselective ET receptors, 287
Nonselective ET_A-receptor blockers, 299
Nonselective ET_B-receptor blockers, 299

Obstructive sleep apnea (OSA), 114, 242–243
  see also Sleep disordered breathing
Oral therapy
  antihypertensives, 158
  bosentan, 343–344

intravenous or subcutaneous prostacyclins
  to oral therapy, transition from,
  343–344
  potassium, 233, 235
Orthotopic liver transplantation (OLT), 184
  see also Portopulmonary hypertension
    (PPHTN)
Overlap syndrome, 243
Oxygen therapy
  HIV-PH treatment, 179
  hypoxemia, 235–238
  PAH future directions and, 409–412
  SSc-PH therapy and, 155–162

P38-MAPK signaling, 417
PAH (pulmonary arterial hypertension),
  8, 9, 20
  associated PAH (APAH), 20
  beraprost for, 277–278
  BMPR2 mutations in, 78
  cGMP pathway in, 306
  CHD-PAH, 20, 128–130, 138
  CTD associated, 20
  diagnostic approach, 33–46
    ambulatory hemodynamic monitoring,
      43–44
    cardiac catheterization, 42–43
    cardiopulmonary exercise testing
      (CPET), 39–40
    chest radiography, 40
    electrocardiography (ECG), 40–41
    invasive testing, 42–44
    laboratory testing, 44–46
    lung biopsy, 44
    noninvasive testing, 37–41
    physical examination, 36
    pulmonary function testing, 40
    six-minute walk (6MW), 39
    sleep studies, 41
    standard echocardiography, 38
    vasodilator testing, 43
    ventilation–perfusion (V/Q) lung
      scanning, 41
  drugs and toxins associated, 23
  endothelin-1 (ET-1) and, 284–287
  endothelin receptors and, 287–296
    antagonists, 287–296
    future scope, 299
  epoprostenol for, 258–269
  familial PAH (FPAH), 74
  future directions, 299
    anticoagulants, 411–412

antiplatelets, 411–412
apoptosis-promoting genes, 418
clinical trials and endpoints, 421–422
diuretics, 410
growth factors, 416–417
matrix proteins, 418
neurohormonal agents, 410–411
oxygen therapy, 409
p38-MAPK signaling, 420
pulmonary vascular remodeling, 412
Rho/Rho-kinase signaling, 417
RV supporting mechanics, 419–420
serotonin (5HT), 415
TGF-beta surperfamily, 413–415
vasodilators, 415–416
HIV-associated, 23
idiopathic PAH (IPAH), 9–10, 18–19
iloprost, 420
iloprost for, 276–277
lung transplantation and, 385–396
modifiers and triggers of
nitric oxide (NO), 84–85
potassium channels, 86–87
serotonin pathway, 82–84
pathophysiology
adrenomedullin, 55
anorexigens, 57
asplenia, 62
cocaine, 57–58
conditions associated with PAH, 59–63
connective tissue diseases (CTD), 59–60
endothelin-1 (ET-1), 54
environmental associations, 56–59
genetic abnormalities, 63–65
hemoglobinopathies, 62–63
hereditary hemorrhagic telangiectasia
(HHT), 63
hereditary spherocytosis, 63
HIV-infection, 60
hypoxia, 57
L-tryptophan, 59
methamphetamine, 57–58
monocrotaline, 58
nitric oxide (NO), 54
portal hypertension, 60–61
prostacyclin/thromboxane A_2 mediators,
53–54
rapeseed oil, 58
serotonin (5-hydroxytryptamine), 54–55
serotoninergic genetic abnormalities,
64–65
TGF-beta genetic abnormalities, 27
thrombocytosis, 61

vascular endothelial cell growth factor
(VEGF), 55–56
vasoactive intestinal peptide (VIP), 55
vasoactive mediators imbalance, 53–56
PCH (pulmonary capillary
hemangiomatosis), 23–24
PDE5 inhibition effects, 308–309
acute effects, 309–310
chronic effects, 310–313
drug interactions, 314–315
side effects and tolerance, 313–314
pericardial effusion in, 105–106
PPHN (persistent pulmonary hypertension
of newborn), 24
PPHTN-associated, 22
prostacyclin for, 257–258
prostanoid, 420
PVOD (pulmonary veno-occlusive
disease), 23–24
rare condition diseases associated, 23
screening techniques, 421
suspicion/historical aspects, 34–36
treprostinil for, 270–274, 420
see also PH (pulmonary hypertension);
Pulmonary venous hypertension;
Right ventricle (RV) dysfunction
PAH therapies
anticoagulation therapy for, 240, 411–412
antiplatelets therapy for, 411–412
atrial septostomy and, 384, 396–399
bosentan, 316
calcium channel blocker therapy for,
246–250
cAMP-prostacyclin pathway, 316
combination therapy, 316, 344–358
diuretics for, 410
endothelin-receptor antagonist, 316
neurohormonal agents, 410–411
nitric oxide, 420
oxygen therapy, 409
PDE5 inhibitor (sildenafil), 316
targeted therapy, 406–409
transitions aspects, 338–344
see also Lung transplantation
PAP, 95–96
PDE inhibitors
combination therapies with
endothelin-receptor antagonists, 357–358
inhaled NO, 351–352
natriuretic peptides, 353
nitric oxide, 350–352
with prostacyclins, 345–353

PDE5 inhibition
  acute effects, 308
  acute pulmonary hypertension
    reduction, 308
  cGMP modulation and, 306–315
  chronic effects
  chronic pulmonary hypertension
    reduction, 309
  CTEPH and, 315
  drug interactions, 314–315
  inhaled NO combination with, 351
  PAH reduction, experimental, 308–309
  PAH therapies and, 316
  in PAH, 308
  side effects and tolerance, 313–314
  SSc-PH therapy, 161–162
  tadalafil, 313
  see also Sildenafil
Pericardial effusion, 105–106
  see also Right ventricle (RV) dysfunction
Persistent pulmonary hypertension of
  newborn (PPHN), 24
PH (pulmonary hypertension), 1, 16
  classification, 15, 53, 152–155
    controversies, 27
    functional, 26–27, 153
    Venice classification, 17, 153
  CTD-PH, 150–163
  CTPH, 25–26
  genetics
    ALK1 and HHT, 81, 87
    BMPR2, 73–81
    modifiers and triggers of, 81–87
    pedigree analysis, 74–75
    screening/counseling, 87–88
  HIV-associated, 174–183
  hypoxia-associated, 25
  miscellaneous, 26
  PPHTN, 183–187
  pulmonary venous hypertension, 24–25
  reversible factors
    fluid overload, 232–235, 251
    hypoxemia, 235–238, 244
    polycythemia, 242, 255
    pulmonary vascular remodeling, 250
    pulmonary vasoconstriction,
      244–250, 351
    right ventricular dysfunction, 241–242
    in situ thrombosis, 240, 251
    sleep-disordered breathing, 242–244
    venous thromboembolism, 239–241
  right ventricle (RV), 96–116
  sarcoidosis, 188

sickle cell disease (SCD), 188–190
therapy
  simvastatin for, 325–327
  statins for, 322–332
  see also APAH (associated pulmonary
    arterial hypertension); CHD-PAH;
    FPAH (familial pulmonary arterial
    hypertension); IPAH (idiopathic
    pulmonary arterial hypertension);
    PAH (pulmonary arterial
    hypertension)
Phlebotomy, 239
Polycythemia, 238, 251
Polymyositis, 150
Portal hypertension
  BMPR2 mutations in, 79
  PAH pathophysiology and, 60–61
Portopulmonary hypertension (PPHTN),
  183–187
  diagnosis and treatment, 185–187, 190
  PAH associated with, 22–24
  pathogenesis, 100, 184
  see also HIV-PH
Potassium
  oral, 233, 235
  replacement, 235
Potassium channel blockers, 415–416
  see also Calcium channel blockers
Potassium channels (Kv), 86–87
PPH1 gene, 19
PPHTN, see Portopulmonary hypertension
Primary graft dysfunction, 394
  see also Lung transplantation
Primary pulmonary hypertension, see
  Idiopathic pulmonary hypertension
Prostacyclins
  for acute cor pulmonale, 364
  beraprost, 277
  combination therapy with
    endothelin-receptor antagonists, 354–358
    natriuretic peptides with PDE
      inhibitors, 353
    nitric oxide (NO), 350–352
    nitric oxide with PDE inhibitors,
      351–352
    phosphodiesterase inhibitors, 345–350
    prostacyclins-cAMP pathway and
      endothelin pathway, 354–358
    prostacyclins-cAMP pathway and
      NO-cGMP pathway, 345–353
  for CTEPH, 218–219
  epoprostenol, 258–269
  for HIV-PH and, 179, 183

iNO combination with, 350
intravenous or subcutaneous prostacyclins
to oral therapy, transition from,
343–344
iloprost, 274–277
for PAH, 259–281
pharmacological actions, 257–258
SSc-PH therapy, 155–162
treprostinil, 270–274
as vasoactive mediators, 53–56
vasodilators, 178
Pulmonary arterial hypertension, *see* PAH
(pulmonary arterial hypertension)
Pulmonary artery smooth muscle cell
(PASMC), 82
Pulmonary capillary hemangiomatosis (PCH),
23–24
Pulmonary capillary wedge pressure
(PCWP), 42
Pulmonary circulation
control, 5–6
normal RV and, 94–96
Pulmonary embolism, 25
acute cor pulmonale in, 370–372
acute, 201
anticoagulation therapy for, 240
management principles
fluid administration, 375–376
mechanical ventilation, 375
see also CTEPH (chronic thromboembolic
pulmonary hypertension)
Pulmonary function testing
CTD-PH and, 153–154
CTEPH, 205
noninvasive testing, 37–42
Pulmonary hemodynamics, 3–5
epoprostenol, 258–269
in idiopathic pulmonary hypertension, 6–7
monitoring, ambulatory, 43–44
septostomy, 406
study, 3–5
Pulmonary hypertension, *see* PH (pulmonary
hypertension)
Pulmonary vascular remodeling
PAH future directions and, 411
for pulmonary vasoconstriction, 250
Pulmonary vascular resistance (PVR), 34, 134
Pulmonary veno-occlusive disease (PVOD),
23–24, 79
Pulmonary venous hypertension, 24–25
see also PAH (pulmonary arterial
hypertension)

Quality of life, lung transplantation and,
390–391

Radiography, *see* Chest radiography (CXR)
Rapeseed oil, PAH pathophysiology and, 58
Remodeling, *see* Pulmonary vascular
remodeling
Rescue therapy, 325–327
see also Statins
Rheumatoid arthritis, 149
Rho/Rho-kinase signaling, 417–418
Right heart catheterization (RHC), 152–155
for CTEPH, 208
for OSA, 242–244
for portopulmonary hypertension
(PPHTN), 186
for sickle cell disease (SCD), 190
Right ventricle (RV) dysfunction
normal RV and pulmonary circulation,
94–96
physiology and pathophysiology, 364–365
Right ventricle (RV) in PH
adaptive hypertrophy, 101–103
clinical approach, 113–116
future scope, 116
hypertrophic responses, 97, 111
LV interactions and, 104–105
pericardial effusion and, 105–106
response, 96–97
right heart function effect on PH outcome,
106–107
right heart function monitoring
chest radiograph, 107–108
echocardiography, 108–110
electrocardiography, 118
MRI, 110, 111
RV failure biomarkers, 111–113
RV failure, 115–116
supporting mechanics, 419–420
Right ventricular (RV) dysfunction
acute, 365–369
mechanical ventilation and, 375
as PH reversible factor, 232–251
see also Acute cor pulmonale

Sarcoidosis
pathogenesis, 188
treatment, 188
see also Portopulmonary hypertension
(PPHTN)
Screening
PAH genetics and, 87–88

portopulmonary hypertension
  (PPHTN), 186
  for sickle cell disease (SCD), 190
  techniques, 421
Selective ET receptors, 287
Selective ET_A antagonist, 297–299
Selective ET_A-receptor antagonist, 291
Selective ET_A-receptor blockers, 299
Selective ET_B-receptor blockers, 299
Septostomy, *see* Atrial septostomy
Serotonin
  imbalance (vasoactive mediators), 53–56
  PAH genetics and, 64–65, 82–84
Serotonin transporter (SERT), 82–84
Sickle cell disease (SCD), 188–190
  diagnosis and treatment, 190
  pathogenesis, 189
  see also Sarcoidosis
Sildenafil, 187
  acute effects of, inhibition on PH,
      309–310
  for acute pulmonary hypertension, 308
  bosentan
      combination with, 355–356
      drug interactions, 314–315
  chronic effects of PDE5 inhibition on PH,
      310–315
  combination with
      beraprost, 348
      bosentan, 357
      epoprostenol, 349–350
      iloprost, 355
      inhaled NO, 351
  for CTEPH, 222, 315
  for HIV-PH treatment, 183
  for PAH, 316
  for PPHTN, 187
  for sickle cell disease (SCD), 190
  side effects and tolerance, 313–314
Simvastatin
  open-label clinical trial, 328–332
  rescue study of, 325–327
  toxicity profile and, 328
  see also Statins
Sitaxsentan, 291–295
  ET receptors antagonists selection
      aspects, 291
  trials
      ET receptors antagonists in PAH and,
          287–298
      STRIDE-1 trial, 291–292
      STRIDE-2 trial, 293–295
      STRIDE-2X trial, 293–295

STRIDE-3 trial, 295
STRIDE-4 trial, 295
STRIDE-6 trial, 295
Six-minute walk (6MW), 39, 421
Sjogren's syndrome, 150
Sleep disordered breathing
  CPAP for, 244
  as PH reversible factor, 242–244
Sleep studies, noninvasive testing
  aspects of, 41
SMADS, 79
Small vessel obliteration, 202
Spherocytosis, hereditary, 63
SSc-PH
  autoantibodies and, 151–152
  brain natriuretic peptide (BNP) and, 155
  CTD-PH and, 146–148
  Doppler echocardiography and, 154–155
  pulmonary function testing, 153–154
  surgical treatments for, 162
  therapy
      anticoagulation, 156
      diuretics, 156
      endothelin-receptor antagonists, 161
      general approach, 152–153
      immunosuppressives, 156–158
      oral antihypertensives, 158
      oxygen, 156
      phosphodiesterase-5 (PDE5) inhibitors,
          161–162
      prostacyclins, 158–160
  see also CHD-PAH; CTD-PH; HIV-PH
SSRI, 422
Statins
  benefits, rationale for
      BMPR2, synergism with, 322–323
      endothelial cell function
          ehnacement, 323
      ET-1 actions, opposition to, 323
      hypothesis, 327
      nitric oxide and cytokine pathways,
          effects on, 324
  clinical applications
      favorable toxicity profile, 328
      open-label clinical trial, 328
  experimental evidence
      proliferative pulmonary vascular changes
          attenuation aspects, 324–325
      rescue therapy, 325–327
  side effects, 332
  see also Simvastatin
Stretching, mechanical, 100
STRIDE trials, *see under* Sitaxsentan

Subcutaneous prostacyclins to oral therapy,
    transition from, 343–344
Subcutaneous treprostinil
    intravenous treprostinil to subcutaneous
        treprostinil, transition from, 342
    subcutaneous treprostinil to intravenous
        treprostinil, transition from, 342
SUPER-1 trial, 314
Surgical treatments
    CTD-PH, 162
    CTEPH, 213–215
Systemic lupus erythematosus (SLE),
    149–150
Systemic sclerosis (SSc), *see* SSc-PH

Tadalafil
    acute effects of PDE5 inhibition on PH,
        309–310
    chronic effects of PDE5 inhibition on PH,
        310–313
Targeted therapies
    apoptosis-promoting genes, 418
    BMPR2, 414–415
    growth factors, 416–417
        EGF, 416
        PDGF, 416
    matrix proteins, 418
    p38 MAPK signaling, 417–418
    Rho/Rho-kinase signaling, 417–418
    RV supporting mechanics, 419–420
    serotonin (5HT), 415
    TGF-beta superfamily, 413–415
    vasodilators
        potassium channel blockers, 415–416
        vasoactive intestinal peptide (VIP),
            415–416
    see also Combination therapies
Tetralogy of Fallot, 134
TGF-ß, 10
    genetic abnormalities and PAH, 63–65
    hypertrophic signaling pathway, 100, 103
    PAH future directions and targeted therapy,
        412–413
    see also BMPR2 (bone morphogenetic
        protein receptor gene 2)
Thrombocytosis, 61
Thromboembolism, 204
    venous, 239–241
    see also CTEPH (chronic thromboembolic
        pulmonary hypertension)
Thromboendarterectomy
    chronic thromboembolic pulmonary
        hypertension (CTEPH), 202, 211, 215

long-term outcome, 221
    surgical approach aspects, 215–217
Thrombosis, *in situ*, 239–241
Thromboxane A$_2$ imbalance, 53–54
TIE2, 64
TNF-alpha, 100
Tolafentrine, 347
Torsemide, 234
Toxic oil syndrome, 58
Toxic substances, HIV-PH and, 180–181
Toxicity profile, statins for, 328
Toxins, PAH associated with, 23
Transitions (PAH therapies), 338–344
    from epoprostenol to inhaled iloprost, 343
    from intravenous or subcutaneous
        prostacyclins to oral therapy, 343–344
    from intravenous treprostinil to
        subcutaneous treprostinil, 342
    from subcutaneous treprostinil to
        intravenous epoprostenol, 342
    from subcutaneous treprostinil to
        intravenous treprostinil, 342
    intravenous epoprostenol to subcutaneous
        or intravenous treprostinil, transition
        from, 339–342
    rationale behind, 338–339
    see also Combination therapies
Transthoracic echocardiography (TTE),
    108, 185
Treprostinil
    administration and dosage, 272
    bosentan combination with, 356
    for HIV-PH treatment, 183
    inhaled administration, 274
    intravenous administration, 273–274
    oral administration, 274
    for PAH therapy, 420
    patient selection aspects, 271–272
    randomized, controlled trials, 270–271
    side effects and complications, 272–273
    subcutaneous administration, 270
    targeted therapy, 420
    transition aspects
        intravenous epoprostenol to
            subcutaneous or intravenous
            treprostinil, 339–342
        intravenous treprostinil to subcutaneous
            treprostinil, 342
        subcutaneous treprostinil to intravenous
            epoprostenol, 342
        subcutaneous treprostinil to intravenous
            treprostinil, 342
    see also Prostacyclins

Triamterene, 235
Troponin, 111, 113

Vardenafil, 310, 313
Vascular endothelial cell growth factor
    (VEGF), 55–56, 416–417
Vascular remodeling, *see* Pulmonary vascular
    remodeling
Vasoactive agents, 376
Vasoactive intestinal peptide (VIP)
    imbalance, 55–56
    targeted therapy aspects, 412–420
Vasoactive mediators
    imbalance, 53–56
        adrenomedullin, 55
        endothelin-1 (ET-1), 54
        nitric oxide (NO), 54
        prostacyclin/thromboxane A_2, 53–54
        serotonin (5-hydroxytryptamine),
            54–55
        VEGF, 55–56
        VIP, 55
    PAH pathophysiology and, 53–56
Vasoconstriction
    ACCP recommendation, 248–250
    calcium channel blocker therapy for,
        246–250
    as PH reversible factor, 232–251
    pulmonary vascular remodeling for, 250
    vasodilator therapy for, 244–246
Vasoconstrictors
    endothelin-1, 178–179
    imbalance, 184–185

Vasodilators, 178
    acute cor pulmonale management and,
        374–377
    for HIV-PH treatment, 178–183
    imbalance, 184–185
    nitric oxide (NO), 179
    portopulmonary hypertension (PPHTN)
        and, 184
    prostacyclin, 179
    for pulmonary embolism, 240
    for pulmonary vasoconstriction, 244–250
    for sickle cell disease (SCD), 188–190
    targeted therapy, 409–412
        potassium channel blockers, 415–416
        vasoactive intestinal peptide (VIP),
            415–416
    testing, 43
Venous thromboembolism, 239–241
Ventilation–perfusion lung scanning
    CTEPH, 207–209
    noninvasive testing, 37–41
Ventricular interdependence, defined,
    104–105
Ventricular mass index (VMI), 111
Volume overload, 235

Warfarin therapy, 244
WHO
    idiopathic pulmonary hypertension and
        Evian meet (1988), 9
        Geneva meet (1973), 7
    WHO/NYHA class
        for CTEPH, 221
        for HIVPH treatment, 181–183